THE INVISIBLE EPIDEMIC

THE STORY
OF WOMEN
AND AIDS

GENA COREA

HarperCollins*P*

HarperCollins books may be purchased for educational, business, or sales promotional use. For information, please write: Special Markets Department, HarperCollins Publishers, Inc., 10 East 53rd Street, New York, NY 10022.

FIRST EDITION

Designed by Laura Hough

Library of Congress Cataloging-in-Publication Data

Corea, Gena.
 The invisible epidemic : the story of women and AIDS / Gena Corea.—1st ed.
  p. cm.
 Includes bibliographical references and index.
 ISBN 0-06-016648-7
 1. AIDS (Disease) 2. AIDS (Disease)—United States. 3. Women—Diseases. I. Title.
RA644.A25C665 1992
362.1'969792'0082—dc20   91-58369

92 93 94 95 96 ❖/HC 10 9 8 7 6 5 4 3 2 1

For Nuria Cadenas i Alabernia of Barcelona
and
for Chester S. Weinerman,
my first editor, at the Massachusetts *Collegian*. My friend from the time we were both nineteen years old until his death of AIDS at forty-four in November 1990. Who spoke of my beauty when I didn't know I had any. Who understood that women were the next group to be hit hard by the pandemic, knew the suffering they would endure, and urged me to do something—what each of us always did: write. Who helped me with the book proposal before he got too sick to edit any more. Who remains a strong presence in my life, especially in the autumn.

CONTENTS

1981–1982

....

Until 1978, there had never been a female Catholic chaplain assigned to a jail or prison in the United States. Eileen Hogan, a nun who had previously taught elementary school in Connecticut, became the first when she entered Riker's Island jail in New York City that year. Now, three years later, she felt she was in on something that nobody else knew. Even people in authority. Something strange was happening to women.

She stopped an inmate in the hall at Riker's, the largest jail in the world.

"How's Judy?" Hogan asked about a woman who had been released some time earlier.

"She died."

Hogan was stunned. Judy had been a young woman.

"What did she die of?"

"I don't know. She got sick and died."

"Well, what did they say it was?"

"Pneumonia."

Hogan was disturbed as she turned away. This wasn't the first time.

She observed the women as they came in to jail, especially those she had known from their previous stays. They were changing from incarceration to incarceration. Drug-using women would come in looking undernourished. Many did not fill out after the first six to eight weeks as they should have. Many were returning to the jail very sick. There was that young woman Eileen had sat up with in the infirmary through high fevers. She'd been transferred to Bedford Hills Correctional Facility, New York State's only maximum-security prison for women, and there she died.

None of the sick women knew what she really had.

Hogan lived in the same area many of the women came from—the Bronx—and would sometimes see women she knew from jail in her neighborhood near Fordham University. She had moved to the Bronx in 1981 when the convent in East Harlem she had been living in closed. She was given permission to live outside a convent, but she still wanted to be part of a community. She also felt that to be effective, she needed to experience on a daily basis what the people she served were experiencing. So she moved into a Bronx building abandoned by the landlord and formed a cooperative with other tenants. They eventually bought the building from the city. And she had a new community.

The five-story brick tenements on her block kept the sun out till afternoon and made Hogan feel she was living in a cavern. At least three thousand people were housed in the packed apartments of that one block. So the neighborhood was crowded, noisy with shouts, curses, music blaring, children at play imitating the violence they saw around them. Gunshots were a staple sound of the night.

On the sidewalks and around the buildings, broken glass, empty bottles, and garbage were strewn. There was no gentleness on these streets. Unless you counted Sister Eileen herself, on her way to and from the subway, saying "Good morning" and "Good evening" to the drug dealers who were openly selling on the corners. On such walks, plainclothes cops occasionally ran past her, guns drawn.

It was shocking to Hogan to descend into a subway to the smell of urine and hot stale air, and minutes later, emerge from the underground into another world: midtown Manhattan. Clean sidewalks. Elegant stores with luxurious window displays. Chauffeurs in limousines delivering executives to their meetings. A sea of white professionals exiting taxicabs to enter gleaming office buildings housing banks and ad agencies and *The New York Times*.

It's like no one knows this other world exists, Hogan would think in astonishment. She felt no condemnation of the people in this gleaming city. People in the Bronx had taken her into their world and allowed her to know their life there. It was a gift, this admittance, this knowledge. You had to pray for the people in the gleaming buildings—pray that they, too, would be given the gift, that they, too, would know of the other world that existed, invisibly, alongside their own.

Hogan had grown close to the first group of inmates she had worked with at Riker's in 1978. Eight women in their twenties and thirties, they were like her first class at school. Most used illegal drugs. When they left jail, she gave them her home telephone number and kept in close contact with them, as close as the dire circumstances of their lives allowed.

What Eileen Hogan had no way of knowing was that by 1987, every one of them would be dead.

When it was crucial for the medical community to recognize, treat, and halt a fatal sexually transmitted disease that appeared first in a series of "others"—gay men, African-American and Latino drug addicts, women of color—there was a problem: the medical system itself was filled with contempt for "the other." It was sex-segregated (with 84 percent of physicians men and 97 percent of nurses women) and two-tiered, providing vastly inferior medical care to the poor, racial minorities, and women of all classes. In its well-funded lobbying efforts, the American Medical Association (AMA) has never advocated guaranteed access to medical care for all. As is oft-noted and ignored, the United States is the only industrialized nation besides South Africa that provides no national health plan for its people.

To the medical community, women are so firmly fixed as "the other" that, in 1991, not a single woman served as dean of a single U.S. medical school. Of the department chairs, 98 percent were men. At all levels in medical school faculties, women had disproportionately low status and pay. There were 144 years in which the AMA, founded in 1848, might have chosen a woman to lead it. But it never had.

Men fought hard to keep the female "other" out of medicine entirely. With the aid of the nineteenth- and twentieth-century feminist movements, some women did make it into the profession, but to this day male colleagues and professors harass them verbally and sexually. When a fifty-year-old female brain surgeon on the Stanford Medical School faculty in California resigned in 1991, charging that she'd endured twenty-five years of harassment, the dean readily acknowledged the routine abuse of female medical students and professors. This abuse included a steady stream of insults (such as labeling women who disagree with them at departmental meetings "premenstrual"), smirks, innuendos, fondling, the refusal to inform women of key meetings, the hogging of medical school resources.

As patients, women are "other" than the standard male human being. Therefore, women's pelvic organs—uterus, fallopian tubes, ovaries—are omitted from the standard physical examination.

Male physicians in this medical system have designed studies on heart disease and other ailments that left women out entirely. For example, one heart study begun in 1981 followed 22,000 physicians—all male. The study showed that taking an aspirin every other day could prevent some heart attacks. Because of women's exclusion from the study, it's unknown whether aspirin has the same effect on women.[1] Explaining why women had not been included in the study, the researchers said too few women were doctors to include them as a group. They had chosen doctors because they believed doctors would be more likely than others to follow the study regimen. Various medical boards reviewing the design of this and other studies that excluded women noticed nothing amiss.

Medical textbooks have presented a view of women as neurotic complainers, fostering the assumption in physicians that the symptoms a woman describes may be "all in her head" and handled, not with diagnostic testing, but with tranquilizers. This was to become deadly to women in the AIDS epidemic.

The U.S. medical system has brought to "the other" a host of risky drugs for normal female functions—DES and Depo-Provera among them—and operations performed unnecessarily. (The United States is the hysterectomy capital of the world, and its high cesarean rate would be a scandal in any land where women were valued.)[2]

The AIDS virus thrives on precisely what permeates the U.S. medical system: the notion of "otherness." This is also called "sexism," "racism," and "homophobia"—words too puny and mild-mannered to convey the savagery they represent.[3]

Otherness: We don't need to care for the worthless "others" afflicted with AIDS. They have only themselves to blame. Nor need we take decisive, effective action to prevent the further spread of AIDS among them. Certainly we don't have to worry about catching AIDS ourselves if it is something "others" get.

So a disease, fanned by the winds of "otherness," was moving through the United States.

The epidemic began, in this country, with gay men. In 1981 they were falling ill of the then-mysterious disease. Physicians in New York City and San Francisco saw a handful of such patients with Kaposi's sarcoma (KS), a rare cancer resulting in lesions of the skin, mucuous membranes, and internal organs, and usually found only in elderly Italian and Jewish men and in Africans. Five men in Los Angeles were also reported to the federal Centers for Disease Control (CDC) with pneumocystis carinii pneumonia (PCP). A parasitic infection of the lungs that results in persistent fevers and bronchial infection, PCP was an extremely rare illness.

Both KS and PCP are "opportunistic" infections, so-called because they are caused by organisms that, while harmless in people with healthy immune systems, opportunistically take advantage of a suppressed immune system to move in. When the immune system is weakened, opportunistic infections cause illness or even death.

With evidence coming in from both coasts, the CDC in Atlanta formed a task force, headed by Dr. James Curran, to study the disease.

In June 1981, the PCP cases were written up in the CDC's *Morbidity and Mortality Weekly Report (MMWR)*, a report sent out to forty thousand physicians and public health officials. Though the CDC's report is also sent weekly to 835 reporters, only three found the news of enough importance to write up.

By December, two hundred cases in men of either Kaposi's sarcoma, PCP, or a combination of both had been reported to the CDC. The new disease had no name, though it was so related to homosexual men that some called it gay-related infectious disease, or GRID.

In this same year that AIDS, as it subsequently would be called, was first identified as a distinct disease entity and recognized as an epidemic, the first case of an infected woman in the United States—in the Bronx, New York—was reported to the CDC.

Only one woman was *reported* as an AIDS case. But in fact, an unusual number of young women, particularly drug addicts, died that year. Few noticed. Eileen Hogan was one. Lynne MacArthur of the New York State Division of Alcoholism and Alcohol Abuse was another. She was having worrisome conversations with a colleague who noted the skyrocketing number of death reports coming in from methadone clinics. Addicts were dying. But why?

Deaths of young women from a variety of respiratory infectious diseases thought to be AIDS-related began dramatically increasing in 1981 in those areas with heavy concentrations of AIDS, journalist Chris Norwood would later uncover. But the fatalities have never been counted as AIDS deaths.[4]

In 1981 many more women were on their way to being infected. Katrina Haslip was one of them.

Katrina Haslip, twenty-one, left her duties as a kindergarten teacher in the Islamic community in Brooklyn where she lived with her strict Moslem husband, and took the Amtrak to Niagara Falls, her family's home. Her face veiled, head and body covered, she boarded the train in full Muslim garb. She entered the restroom and, as the train lurched forward, she changed her clothes. In Niagara Falls, she disembarked dressed in a mini-skirt and tight blouse, her face bright with lipstick. She was Lady T ("Trina") now. No matter what she was doing in the street life she would now resume—prostitution, pick-pocketing, shooting drugs—she would behave like a lady. With tact. Decorum.

Katrina had known the red section of Niagara Falls since she was nine. She had grown up in a white suburb—hers was one of the neighborhood's three black families—but when her father, a construction worker, was injured at work and went on disability, he could no longer support his wife and eleven children in a suburban house. The family moved into a city neighborhood Katrina, until then, had been forbidden to enter.

For the first time, she saw poverty.

Two blocks from her new home in one direction, and three blocks in another, the red zone. Walking home from school, she would see johns picking up women, sometimes beating them, and she'd feel afraid and powerless. She saw people lying out in the street.

She heard shouts, curses: the men beating up the women in the neighborhood and the women calling the police and the police dragging out a man who would later return.

Katrina's older brother Troy did not do well in the new neighborhood with his new comrades. He was arrested and imprisoned for a serious crime no one ever explained to Katrina.

She heard gunshots. Screams. Always the sirens—ambulances, police. Sirens at the neighborhood bar, two blocks away, where someone was always being stabbed or shot or was ODing in the bathroom. Johns hung around in front of the bar. Police cars cruised by. The neighbors began to call it the Death Bar and people were afraid to go there.

When she was eleven, Troy escaped from jail outside Buffalo and began working under an assumed name in Detroit. When a neighbor, another black man, beat his wife, Troy intervened. The neighbor shot and killed him. Charges were dropped against the murderer because, Katrina was told, police considered Troy a fleeing felon, armed and dangerous. If the police had caught Troy, they would have shot to kill, they explained. Apparently his life wasn't worth a trial. In that moment, Katrina's resentment of white authorities and "the system" took hold.

By the time Katrina was fourteen, she was angry. She hurt. She didn't feel people should have to live the way people in her neighborhood did. "We're living in poverty because whites put us here," she heard her friends and her brothers say. It sounded right to her. At fourteen, she began drinking beer. Later, she smoked marijuana. Moved to pills. On to cocaine. Then IV drugs.

She hung out with rebels. Drank with them. When she was sixteen, they were all arrested for smoking pot in a hotel. At home, Katrina was well mannered, well spoken. She never brought drugs into the house. She was a good student. Her parents dismissed the arrest as a brief oat-sowing.

That same year, she met a thirty-year-old Moslem, an architect, half African-American, half Palestinian. During their courtship, he made sure they were chaperoned. At eighteen, she married him and moved to Brooklyn. She taught children. No drinking. No drugging. But still lots of pain. She'd get on the train. A visit to her family, she'd tell her husband.

Back home, the neighborhood was as she remembered it. One

summer day, the companion of her twenty-five-year-old sister Kathy arrived and fetched Katrina off the street.

"Kathy fell out," he told her nervously.

He drove her to their home. Kathy was lying on the floor, face-down, unconscious.

"Call an ambulance!" Katrina shouted, dropping to her knees to give Kathy CPR.

He left the room. No ambulance came.

"Drive us to the hospital," she ordered him.

In the backseat, she kept blowing breath into her sister's mouth. Ten minutes after they delivered Kathy to the emergency room, nurses came out and told Katrina her sister was dead. She had 5.8 milligrams of morphine in her system—pure dope, the coroner later reported.

Something was wrong here. Kathy was off hard drugs. She'd told Katrina she'd stopped shooting them because she wanted to make something of her life. They'd talked about it at length. The boyfriend, a drug dealer, had something to do with her sister's death, Katrina suspected. Maybe he never called an ambulance—that's why it didn't come. But the police never investigated the death thoroughly, Katrina thought, as they had never bothered themselves about Troy's death. "Overdose," they pronounced and closed the books.

The boyfriend was real nice to Katrina—gave her drugs to sell, and gifts. She accepted them. Now she dove headlong into drugs. She was trying to kill herself. She didn't deserve to live, she felt. She stood by silently while Kathy's death was covered up.

Six months later, Katrina woke up one morning in her Brooklyn home and told her husband she didn't want to be married anymore. He was stunned. She felt too confined within the Islamic community, within her home, within the veil, she told him.

She could no longer stand the double life. She had to enter one world or the other.

She returned to the red zone of Niagara Falls.

1982

It was immediately obvious to Dr. Joyce Wallace that this new disease was sexually transmitted. Homosexuals were getting it and they weren't all eating at the same restaurant. If the disease was sexually transmitted, women would get it because women had sex. There was no known sexually transmitted disease that only affected one sex.

Wallace, with her private practice in gay-dominated Greenwich Village in New York City, had seen her first AIDS case two years earlier, though she had not known at the time that that was what it was.

Working with other physicians and researchers, she had found a relationship between promiscuity and immune suppression in their male homosexual patients. Promiscuous men (more than fifty partners a year) had more impaired immune functions than did homosexuals in monogamous relationships, they'd reported in a letter to the medical journal *Lancet*. At the city Department of Health meetings, where physicians seeing the new disease in their patients would meet with health officials to talk about it, Wallace kept saying: If people who are promiscuous are more likely to get this new sexually transmitted disease, what about women who are having sex with a lot of partners? How about doing research on women in prostitution? Nobody took her up on it.

Now she had a new patient. A smart woman, Wallace thought. She was a college student studying for a degree in electrical engineering. She paid her tuition and expenses by working in prostitution three months of the year. She was infected with the new disease. She had suffered several opportunistic infections including PCP and thrush. (Thrush is a yeast organism, *Candida*, that normally lives in the intestines but can flourish in other parts of the body during immunosuppression. It is only called "thrush" when it appears in the mouth.)

The college student was worried about the health of her friends. She sent six of them to Wallace for checkups. A colleague referred a seventh woman. Three of the eight women, all working in prostitution, had abnormal immune function.

Wallace wrote up her finding.[5]

Within five months of her first visit to Wallace, the college student was dead.

Wallace brought her study to the Department of Health. It was testing women in brothels for a strain of gonococcus resistant to penicillin. The Health Department let Wallace test the women's blood, with their consent, for immune function. In this very limited and skewed group of twenty-five women, two were immune-deficient.

She and her collaborators wrote in a letter published in the *Lancet* that although the randomly selected sample of prostitutes did not have depressed immune function, ". . . prostitutes in New York City do develop the acquired immunodeficiency syndrome, and a prospective study should be done to determine the risk."

Joe Sonnabend was worried. He telephoned Zena Stein and her husband, Mervyn Susser, an epidemiologist who had consulted on a project to develop an immunization technique for hepatitis. Many blood donors for the vaccine were gay men. Now that this new epidemic had broken out in the gay community, would the public fear the vaccination?

That wasn't the only worry AIDS gave Sonnabend. A primary care internist, he had many gay patients he was trying to advise and treat as they faced the frightening epidemic.

Zena Stein, now in her sixties, had known Joe Sonnabend and his family in their native South Africa. Soon after qualifying as physicians, she and her husband had worked four years in a health clinic in the black township of Alexandra outside Johannesburg. By 1956, their antiapartheid activities had put them on the wrong side of the white supremacist government. In the apartheid climate of the times, the couple were effectively barred from their clinic work.

Now all three South Africans—Stein, Susser, and Sonnabend—were physicians in New York City.

Joe tried to get Zena and Mervyn interested in his theories on AIDS. He believed that multiple sexual encounters and sexually transmitted diseases (STDs) overloaded the immune system, opening the way for various infections.

Susser, then director of the Sergievsky Center for study of the epidemiology of neurological disorders, and Stein invited Sonnabend and a couple of his friends to give a seminar at the Center and discuss with them their theories on AIDS. Robin Flam, a twenty-five-year-old graduate student working with Stein, listened in fascination to Sonnabend's presentation. She had never heard of AIDS. During the discussion, she and Stein asked Sonnabend:

"Can women get this disease?"

"No."

"How do you know?" they pressed.

"No one has looked," he replied.

Neither Stein nor Flam could understand why the disease should appear only in men.

After the discussion, Flam's mind could not leave the disease alone. She couldn't stop thinking how little was known about its *nature*.

In the middle of the night, she woke with a start: "If having a lot of sexual partners is an issue, then for sure this disease is going to affect women, too, because there are many, many women in this world who have a lot of sexual partners."

She knew some of them. The most obvious and well-defined group in that category were women in prostitution. For several years, Flam had worked in a center that had a clinic providing health care to such women.

The next day, Flam approached Stein:

"Why don't we look and see if women *do* get it?"

They began a long series of dialogues:

Was a single agent necessary and sufficient to cause AIDS? Was the disease the result of certain specific sexual behaviors and certain effects those behaviors had, like re-exposure to common STDs? Was a single, newly active agent necessary but not, in itself, sufficient to cause AIDS, the disease only appearing given specific behaviors and biochemical changes associated with those behaviors?

If women got it, what kind of women would get it? Under what circumstances? If Sonnabend's theory were correct and the disease were the result of immunological overload following multiple sexual encounters and multiple STDs, then maybe women in prostitution *could* get it. Or if some men with the disease were bisexual, the prostitutes they used could be at risk.

Stein agreed with Flam that this was a logical next step in the epidemic. If it wasn't the next step, then that fact could be important in ruling out certain causal factors.

They telephoned Sonnabend often and discussed their ideas with him. He agreed that it was worthwhile to start looking at women in prostitution. Flam knew prostitutes were intelligent and probably would be willing to talk.

Stein and Flam worked up their theory carefully and applied to the National Institutes of Health (NIH) for funding. They were turned down immediately.

Flam was shocked. This was cutting-edge work. It was obscene that nobody was paying attention to it.

The "pink sheets," the NIH critique of the proposal, cited research design flaws as the rationale for rejecting the study. Neither Stein nor Flam was convinced that the flaws the reviewers pointed out were good-enough rationales to reject the study. The hypotheses they were posing were so crucial to furthering an understanding of what this new disease was that no reason was good enough to turn it down.

Flam was sure they had a decent study design. While she herself was still wet behind the ears, Stein certainly was not. Stein, a professor of epidemiology at the Columbia School of Public Health and the Sergievsky Center and research chief at the New York State Psychiatric Institute, had been an epidemiologist for decades. She was internationally respected in her field. Stein certainly knew what was good and what wasn't, and if she were willing to put her name on that study, then for Flam that testified to the study design's validity.

But the message from the "pink sheet" was clear: AIDS was a man's disease.

There was, Stein thought, perusing the "pink sheet," an absolute lack of interest in the fact that women might get this disease.

It was a tiny glass room. Guards in the control room at the old Woman's House at Riker's Island jail could observe the four crowded women sitting at the table.

Joanna, a beautiful black woman in her early thirties, dressed in jeans and a blouse, sat nervously beside chaplain Eileen Hogan. She had asked Hogan to accompany her as two officials from the New York City Health Department questioned her on her baby—born prematurely in April and now sick with pneumonia.

Joanna was an alcoholic. She was friendly, gentle, and laughed a hardy, easy laugh. Everyone in the jail liked to see her coming. "How would a nice girl like you be in a place like this?" they would ask her.

They needed to pinpoint why her baby was sick, the health officials told Joanna. They wanted to know whether she or the baby's father used drugs, whom she had contact with at home, whom she ate with, who her husband's friends were. When they began asking her about her sexual activities and partners—who exactly were the fathers of her five children—Joanna was bewildered. She had been with only one man—her common-law husband. What did they do sexually? the officials wanted to know.

Joanna was embarrassed and flustered. She often answered the questions with a confused, "I don't know."

They wanted details on her husband's sex life. Was he gay? Bisexual? Did he sometimes sleep with men?

Joanna bristled. "No. Of course not. No! He'd be so angry if he knew you had even asked such a question about him!"

The officials pressed her, as gently as they could. "Can you say for sure whether or not he ever did?"

"No," she said softly. "No. I can't be sure about anything."

At the end of the hour-long interview, Joanna was devastated. Alone with Hogan before returning to her cell, she cried, "Sister, I was so embarrassed that they were asking me those questions in front of you. But I could never have answered them without your being there, on my side."

It was clear to the women that Hogan *was* on their side. It wasn't her job to judge a woman for taking what few solaces—alcohol, maybe, or drugs—she found in a life steeped in hardships and abuse, but to recognize and treasure the soul in another human being. Dressed, not in a nun's habit, but in a simple skirt and blouse, listening attentively to a woman, speaking, sometimes, in a soft stutter, she called forth trust.

For Hogan, this Department of Health visit confirmed her suspicions.

Several months later, Joanna's baby was dead.

Dr. Wendy Chavkin, working at the New York City Health Department, was examining the women's health service at Riker's Island when a jail doctor, a friend of hers, said, "I'm seeing a lot of women who have sort of diffused lymphadenopathy [chronically swollen lymph nodes], thrush, and malaise."

"Gee," Chavkin said, "that sounds like this thing that the men with Kaposi's sarcoma have. Or very similar."

She thought the CDC should know.

Established in 1942, the Centers for Disease Control is a part of the Public Health Service, which is designed somewhat like a branch of the armed forces. Many doctors and researchers are commissioned, hold rank, and occasionally wear uniforms. The CDC's mandate is to track the incidence and trends of communicable diseases and certain noninfectious diseases.

Chavkin talked with people from CDC about the women's symptoms. Many women at Riker's were jailed for prostitution, Chavkin knew. Since researchers thought the new disease in gay men was related to multiple sexual partners (the first group of gay men afflicted with the disease had had astronomical numbers of them), Chavkin suggested to the CDC that women in prostitution might be vulnerable to the disease.

CDC sent some people to Riker's but nothing much came of that. Chavkin found them focusing on prostitutes as potential sources, rather than sufferers, of infection.

Lady T woke up at six in the evening, showered, ate breakfast, dressed, and went to work picking pockets. She'd hit the busy avenues or the airport or high-class bars or clubs. She drank a little, smoked marijuana.

Her refined language was much admired in the fast life. Her mother had never allowed her to use slang. Whites were "Caucasians" to her. Street life was "uncouth."

On the avenue, a john would pull up to her in his car and she'd talk to him through the driver's window.

"Are you going out?"

"Well," she'd ask him, "what do you want?"

They'd discuss price while she placed a hand in his pants. She was actually in his wallet. When she got the money, she'd say, "No, honey, I don't think you're spending enough," and walk away, discreetly counting his money.

She was taking advantage of men, she felt. She liked that.

Sometimes the john would catch her, chase her, beat her. To avoid the beatings, she got more skilled at pickpocketing. She knew the streets were wild, that prostitutes were raped and killed all the time—strangled, stabbed. She kept high and she went on.

··· ···

"Edith, you've got to help us with this disease," Luis Palacio Jimenez, a gay social worker, told his friend Edith Springer, a social worker assisting drug addicts.

She'd love to help, a harried Springer told him, but she couldn't take on any more work. She just couldn't split herself into too many pieces.

Springer, a slim, energetic woman with long black hair attractively graying, dangling earrings, and large brown eyes, was devoted to her drug users. For years, she had been one of them. Addicted to heroin, she remained a nice Jewish girl, going to work every day. She was a secretary, not a criminal. Determined to detox or die in 1973, she succeeded, suffering a full year of withdrawal symptoms.

She graduated from Hunter College and later got a master's degree in social work. She knew she wanted to help drug addicts, and she never forgot the severity of the pain she had tried to numb with drugs, the contempt that had been heaped on her as an addict, or the paucity of help available to her when she wanted to get clean. She knew that, despite conventional wisdom, her spirituality had been alive and well throughout her addiction. Now, she treated her clients with great respect.

A short time after her conversation with Palacio, a client told her that her husband had this new gay disease. Then another client herself came down with the strange illness that had no name.

Edith telephoned Luis Palacio. "Luis, you gotta help me."

When cyanide was discovered in Tylenol capsules in the Chicago area on October 1, 1982, network evening news programs devoted the entire first segments of their newscasts to it; many major metropolitan dailies placed the story on their front pages. *The New York Times* ran a Tylenol-poisoning story every day for the rest of the month, as journalist James Kinsella reported in a study of media coverage of AIDS.[6]

In contrast, it would be another seven months before the *Times* ran its first front-page story on the epidemic the CDC named this same year: acquired immune deficiency syndrome (AIDS). United Press International (UPI) and Associated Press (AP), the sole sources of science and medicine stories for most small and medium-sized newspapers, ran, respectively, ten and nineteen stories on the AIDS epidemic in all of 1982.

While the Tylenol poisonings had claimed seven lives by the end of 1982, nearly eight hundred cases of AIDS had been reported since the beginning of the epidemic. But the Tylenol poisoning was a major news story and the AIDS epidemic a minor one. Why? Tylenol threatened "us"—normal, white, heterosexual people in "the general population," while AIDS only affected "them"—abnormal, black and Latino, homosexual, drug-addicted people.

The federal government showed as little interest in combating the epidemic affecting homosexuals and drug addicts as the media did in reporting it. In April the Reagan administration allotted no money in its budget proposals to fight AIDS. Although CDC funding remained stable in these budget proposals, funding for the National Institutes of Health, the major bodies within the Public Health Service responsible for financing AIDS research, was reduced.

But the line between "us" and "them" kept shifting. By July, the CDC reported the first case of the disease among hemophiliacs, supporting the theory that AIDS might be transmitted through infected blood or through the exchange of bodily fluids in sexual activity. Then in December, the CDC published a report on a small number of infants afflicted with AIDS. This drew more media coverage than any previous revelation about the epidemic. In a belated act of concern and fear, Congress appropriated $2.6 million for the CDC's AIDS research. Two categories of "innocent victims"—babies and blood recipients—had now joined the stigmatized "guilty victims."

In 1982 the CDC issued the first of what would be several surveillance definitions of AIDS—definitions used for reporting the extent of the disease throughout the United States.[7]

AIDS is not one fixed disease but a set of conditions and diseases that can change. Which particular conditions particular infected people get may vary depending on such factors as their general state of health, endocrine differences, age, and sex. Women—who have vaginas, uteruses, fallopian tubes, and ovaries—may get conditions or diseases in those organs that men will never experience.

So AIDS is an illness characterized by one or more of a list of "indicator" diseases. The surveillance definition, used for reporting

the extent of disease throughout the United States, included no gynecological symptoms. This first definition was based on what was
observed in a minuscule number of mostly white gay men. The conditions considered to constitute an AIDS case for national reporting
were PCP, Kaposi's sarcoma, cryptococcal meningitis, and certain lymphomas. As the epidemic evolved, gynecological symptoms of the disease were found in women but were never added to the AIDS surveillance definition. This was to have serious consequences for women
dying from the disease who could not qualify for the governmental
assistance available to men.

Of the first eight hundred reported AIDS cases, fewer than one
hundred were in women. Twelve percent of those cases in women were
believed to have been acquired through heterosexual contact. Yet the
CDC classification system for AIDS had no category for heterosexual
transmission.

In the public silence where danger warnings to women might have
sounded, women could hear the message: this is not our epidemic.

"I have to stop this," Katrina Haslip would say to herself, reeling from
the sirens, stabbings, beatings, drugs. "I have to get out of this. This is
crazy."

She read books and hungered to learn more. She wanted to do
something constructive, she told herself. She registered for business
school and, later, a community college. To get away from the street
madness, Katrina would sometimes stay with her new white, middle-
class college friends out in the suburbs—the suburbs she, too, had
inhabited before her father lost his job.

"I don't want to live like this anymore," she repeatedly told herself. But she didn't know how not to. Again and again, she'd drop out
of the street life, saying "I'm not going back," only to be drawn in
again. It was crazy. The more she prostituted herself, the more she felt
herself fill up with "disgustingness." Marijuana and a drink or two
were no longer enough. She would get high on anything now:
cocaine, Valium, whatever numbed.

She had dropped the demure, obedient-wife mask when she left
her husband, as she had earlier dropped the good-student, well-
behaved-daughter mask. Now, under a junkie mask, she drank,

injected, carried a knife, and looked out at the world with dulled eyes through which, somehow and sometimes, the gleam of sharp intelligence still broke through. She heard faintly, saw dimly, felt nothing—no anger, no love, not even, on the violent streets, fear. The world was dulled, dimmed, muffled, and thus bearable.

Sometimes she'd be on the street all night—picking johns' pockets, prostituting, drugging—and then get on the bus and go to college in the morning. Sometimes she'd pick a professor's pocket.

She hadn't wanted to become like the other street people—*she* was a lady, Lady T—but now she could see that she was one of them.

1983–1984

Sandra Elkin could talk easily with anyone. Leaning back in her swivel chair, telephone against her ear, she could effortlessly switch from joking with a Mafia hit man in prison who was a key source for a writer she represented as a literary agent, to helping a Vermont housewife she'd gone to high school with figure out what was going on in her marriage. With another switch of a telephone button, she'd negotiate a contract with an editor, firmly warning him not to mess with her author's payment provisions.

Slim, dark, small, and feisty, Elkin loved problem-solving, whether in a computer video game, a three-thousand-piece jigsaw puzzle she'd complete in a lazy August on Nantucket Island, or number-crunching on a spread sheet.

Planning a feminist guerrilla action, she would pad around her Manhattan loft in jeans and bare feet, silent. She was thinking. If you looked in her eyes, you could see the rapid clicks and sudden flashes going off in her mind.

Elkin lived and worked in one of the shiny buildings of Manhattan, the kind Sister Eileen Hogan saw when she traveled from the invisible Bronx into Manhattan.

Elkin always called Fred when she needed a haircut. An old friend, he'd been the hairdresser for the PBS show "Woman" she had produced and hosted in the 1970s out of Buffalo, New York. Now both lived in New York City. Fred would come over to her apartment and cut her thick black hair in the bathroom while they caught up on each other.

This time, they were talking about the mysterious new gay disease caused by what would eventually be named the human immunodeficiency virus (HIV).[1] They had both read in the newspapers the new theory that the "poppers" some gay men used were helping it to spread.

To Fred, who was gay, the theory was ridiculous. But Sandra pressed him. Did he ever use poppers? What about his friends?

Fred talked about a gay friend of his who was clearly ill. He'd been sick on and off for the last year; in fact he'd been seeing a woman for a while but . . .

The information stunned Sandra. Her mind clicked through a sequence of pictures.

"Oh, my God!" she exclaimed to Fred. "This new disease is going to hit women, too!"

The realization took her breath away. Of course! How foolish— how incredibly foolish—to think that anything could be a "gay" disease or a "heterosexual" disease! The whole concept was outrageously misguided.

A few days later, she was talking with another friend from her Buffalo days, Dr. Anke Ehrhardt, professor of clinical psychology at Columbia University.

Well, of course, Ehrhardt said. Human sexual behavior is a continuum, with exclusive heterosexuality at one end and exclusive homosexuality at the other. There's lots of behavior in between. Call it "bisexuality" or whatever you like—sexual relations with members of the opposite sex are a common phenomenon among "homosexuals" as are sexual relations with the same sex among "heterosexuals." Though it's rarely discussed, it isn't necessarily true that a person is exclusively homosexual or exclusively heterosexual over the course of a lifetime. The majority of even strongly gay-identified men have had sexual intercourse with women, Ehrhardt said.

(In fact, as Ehrhardt later learned in a study in the New York City gay male community, 72 percent of 205 respondents had had female sexual partners at some time in their lives, the median number of partners between three and four per man.[2]) Ehrhardt felt sure that if you took a detailed history of heterosexual men, many of them would have had homosexual encounters at some point in their lives.

Bisexuality was such a taboo behavior that there just weren't any good estimates of its prevalence around, Ehrhardt told her. There hadn't been a sex survey in the United States since the Kinsey Report, based on data collected in the 1940s, was published in 1952. But there was clearly a common misconception: When people say there aren't many bisexual men, what they mean is that there are very few men who *identify themselves* as bisexual. Men who sometimes have sex with men may identify themselves as heterosexual as long as they are always the "inserter" in sexual activity.

So the realization slowly sunk in. In the AIDS epidemic, women were not just caretakers of sick and dying men. Women were going to be hit, too.

At forty, with an already grown son, Marie Tulman of Brooklyn, New York, married again in 1983. Her new husband, Lamont, had used drugs in the 1970s but when she met him in the spring of 1982, he'd been drug-free for two years.

She herself had long been in recovery from alcoholism. After hundreds of Alcoholic Anonymous meetings and supportive conversations with women in AA, she was a strong and serene woman.

Marie Tulman had read about AIDS in the newspaper. As far as she knew, it was something gay men got.

Years later, after Lamont had died, she would tell a group of women training to be AIDS educators that if she had known in 1983 that women were at risk, she wouldn't be in the fix she was then in. She would introduce herself to the group this way: "I am a forty-eight-year-old HIV-positive grandmother. I married into the virus."

No matter how often Katrina Haslip vowed to lead a straight life, she could not get off the street. She knew what easy targets for male violence she and other streetwalkers were. But she was as fearless as she was hopeless. With a shot, a sniff, or a swig, Katrina placed every emotion that arose in her under general anesthesia.

She knew what had happened to Sally, her friend from the age of five. One day a john got rough with Sally in his car. She tried to get out. He pulled her back in, whipped her with his gun, shot her in the back, and kicked her out of the car.

Sally was in the hospital for months, paralyzed from the waist down. Katrina and other women from the streets often went to see her.

"You guys gotta stop doing this," Sally told them on each visit. But they didn't. Katrina would get high and hit the streets again.

Even when Carol was found nude, strangled to death, Katrina did not stop. The night after her funeral, she went out looking for johns. Each high eliminated the immediate past nightmare.

In 1983, two years after Sister Eileen Hogan recognized that something was happening to women, Dr. Judith Cohen, an epidemiologist teaching at the School of Public Health in Berkeley, California, met Elizabeth Prophet. She looked down the corridor at San Francisco General, the county hospital where the poor came, and saw a tiny woman chained hand and foot walking between two burly guards. Wearing the orange jumpsuit of a prisoner, Prophet was grinning and wisecracking.

She looked awful. Still a young woman, she could be taken for fifty. Her nails appeared to be rotting off. A fungus had infected them. Her skin was blotched. She was losing weight. Jail authorities were sending her to be assessed at the hospital AIDS clinic—the first such in the country—that had recently opened.

Prophet was the first woman with AIDS Cohen met. Her elder child, who died in 1978, was the first AIDS baby reported in the medical literature. In 1980, Prophet, a prostitute and an addict, gave birth again. That child also died. There must have been women other than Elizabeth Prophet then infected and dying, Cohen later realized—women with "pneumonia" who were never counted in the AIDS statistics. But Prophet she could document. A bona fide case of AIDS in a woman.

News coverage of the epidemic was still generally sparse, though early in the year, when the number of AIDS cases passed the one-thousand mark, there had been a rash of news articles. Even *The New York Times,* a late bloomer on the AIDS issue, ran its first-ever front-page story on AIDS.

The conservative Reagan government was in no rush to provide public education on an epidemic affecting a population so distastefully "other" as gays, and what coverage the media provided hardly filled the information gap. One story in particular intensified the public's fear of coming into contact with HIV-infected people. In May the *Journal of the American Medical Association* published a study by Dr. James Oleske that suggested AIDS could be transmitted by "routine household contact." In an editorial in the same issue, Dr. Anthony Fauci, director of the National Institutes of Health, seemed to give credence to the casual-contact claim. Most major media outlets, including the television networks, United Press International, and Associated Press, ran the story. Fauci's follow-up, in which he refuted the casual-contact theory, was not well reported.[3]

Soon after Prophet appeared, Cohen and two other women began talking about AIDS and women in conversations at the coffee pot at the end of the hall at San Francisco General. Dr. Constance Wofsy, head of the Infectious Disease service and one of the first to see and treat PCP in young gay men, and Lori Hauer, a research nurse with a long history of community activism, felt, as Cohen did, that something wasn't adding up. Hadn't they seen their first clear case of AIDS in a woman? Hadn't the CDC in January documented AIDS cases among female partners of men with the disease? Yet AIDS was being studied only in men. That violated common sense. Of course this new disease was going to hit women, too! It was becoming clear that the disease was infectious and sexually transmitted and none of them had ever encountered a sexually transmitted disease that confined itself to one sex. At some point, many more women would follow Elizabeth Prophet through their doors.

And more confusing yet, letters were appearing in the medical journals stating that women did not get AIDS and that it could only be transmitted homosexually. To the women around the coffee pot, this made no sense even on a physiological level. If the risk behavior for the disease were anal sex, was it to be argued that women never had anal sex with men? Or that bisexual men never slept with women?

Cases of the disease were beginning to be reported among intravenous (IV) drug users in New York, although most of these cases were among men. Again, if the risk factor were IV drug use, was it to be argued that women didn't use IV drugs?

But when the women brought up the issue of women's risk with male epidemiologists, the response was always one of dismissal. Studying AIDS in women was a waste of time, Cohen's department chairman told her. If she spent any of the time he paid for on such work, she had better find another job, he added. Which is just what Cohen later did.

Seeing women's health issues trivialized and underfunded was not a new experience for Cohen. Growing up in a Jewish family where men were expected to pursue a career in the professions and women were not, she had been discouraged from going to medical school. She went to graduate school at her own expense, finally managing to get a doctorate at forty.

She had been hired by the University of California at Berkeley in 1974 during the great wave of affirmative action for women. Each fall, at student orientation in the School of Public Health where she was the only female faculty member, the professors would tell the students, "This is Dr. Smith and Dr. Jones and Dr. Brown and Judy." None of the women got tenure.

"They had to hire us but, by God, they didn't have to keep us," Cohen later summed up the women's collective experience.

One explanation for her tenure denial was the supposed triviality of her research. It was trivial because it concerned women's health. Cohen was looking at gender differences in coronary disease. The apparent lower coronary rate in women was then attributed to women's hormones. But that explanation did not fit the data, Cohen concluded. The difference in coronary rates between men and women in various countries varied widely. Cohen didn't believe that women in France had different hormones than women in Italy. But attempting to bring clarity to the question of coronaries in women was judged unimportant.

Now the three women decided to design a modest inquiry to see if there were women at risk of AIDS. They would ask people in the medical community and those conducting research studies whether they were encountering infected women—such as companions, wives, and widows.

There was no interest in the research project at all. They could find no funding. None from the city or county of San Francisco. None from the state of California. None from the university itself. Their colleagues told them they were wasting their time.

The women—Cohen, Wofsy, and Hauer—were not convinced. They decided to find out on their own, without funding, whether women in San Francisco thought AIDS was a woman's problem. In the autumn they rented the Women's Building auditorium and put out photocopied flyers: "Are you concerned about AIDS and women? Do you provide care to AIDS patients? Are you a woman who thinks you yourself might be at risk for this disease? We're sponsoring a day to come together and talk about our concerns."

Since there was no publicity other than the flyers and word of mouth, they expected they might get a hundred women. About five hundred showed up, overflowing the auditorium of the ramshackle, colorfully painted Women's Building. There were a range of women from the community, including some representing political and women's health advocacy groups. Many health-care providers who worked in prenatal and drug treatment clinics and in facilities for adolescents also came to the meeting in the working-class Mission District of the city. The organizers spoke and then the women broke up into groups to discuss risks to adolescents, drug users, partners of bisexual men, and women in prostitution.

The women talked together all day. While they didn't know too many women who had AIDS, they believed many were at risk. Before the day was out, the following questions were asked and organizing efforts planned to get them answered: Could they develop programs or networks or some ways of anticipating the spread of the epidemic and starting prevention? What *were* preventive measures for women? Gay organizations were distributing safe-sex guidelines for their community. But what would safe sex be for women?

That Christmas season, Dr. Cohen looked down the corridor at San Francisco General to again see Elizabeth Prophet—this time accompanied by police officers and a reporter and photographer from the *San Francisco Chronicle*. The newspaper had apparently found out about Prophet, notified the police, and gone out on the streets to find her. The police were bringing her into the hospital so the doctors could tell them if she had AIDS—a request the physicians refused.

Front-page headlines the next day trumpeted the threat of AIDS to the male heterosexual community. It wasn't Prophet's health that was a concern. It was the health of the men who used her.

The next day, the mayor's task force on AIDS called a special meeting. Cohen and other women made quick phone calls and tried to get female staffers to attend, providing themselves with a meeting more receptive to their message. When the task force members wrung their hands, crossed their legs, and said, "What can we do?" the women replied, "We need research." Cohen and Wofsy, as co-investigators, got $40,000 to launch a study, and a suggestion that they go to the jails and test the prostitutes. Finally, a hunk of money had become available for an inquiry into AIDS in women.

Maybe they would have a better chance at getting an NIH-funded study if they first did a little pilot study, Dr. Zena Stein and epidemiology graduate student Robin Flam thought. Their idea was to set up a woman's cohort within the Multi-Center AIDS Cooperative Study (MACS), a study that, in 1983, began enrollment of five thousand subjects, almost all of whom were white gay men. Through a pilot study, Stein and Flam would determine if including women in the MACS were realistic. Stein's friend, Joe Sonnabend, advised them to apply to the American Foundation for AIDS Research (AMFAR). They did so and got a very small grant.

Flam met and interviewed twenty-three women in prostitution. Could she get their cooperation for a long-term study? she asked them. Would they be willing to go on seeing the researchers regularly over a period of years and have their blood drawn for testing? Did they think other women in prostitution would be recruitable for this study?

Yes on all counts, the women replied.

Returning to her Bronx apartment after a long, hot summer day, Riker's jail chaplain Eileen Hogan dropped her grocery bag and headed for a cooling shower. She turned the faucet on full force but only a trickle of water responded. The neighborhood children had opened the fire hydrants to cool themselves and the water was flowing in the streets, not in her pipes. Disappointed, she gave up on her shower. As loud music entered the open windows on air that never cooled, she tried to sleep.

Hogan finally had a name for the "something" that was happening to women: AIDS. There had been no one shocking moment of revelation, but simply a gradual process of connecting the conditions she was seeing in the women at Riker's with what she was reading and hearing of AIDS in the media.

One Riker's Island inmate with AIDS was a woman in her mid-twenties, thin and weak. She did not respond to any medications. Estranged from her mother, she made a few feeble attempts to telephone her. Hogan took the mother's number and reached her in Boston. She was excited that Hogan had called to let her know where her daughter was. Hogan arranged for the two to talk. When the fever-racked daughter was transferred to Elmhurst Hospital from Riker's, Eileen called the mother. She came to New York and spent the last week of her daughter's life with her.

Katy Taylor, a lesbian attorney in New York City, figured she'd better get herself into a position where she could fight back because for sure a battle was coming.

An antigay backlash stimulated by the AIDS epidemic was certain to come and she knew lesbians would be included. But other attacks were coming as well. Taylor, through her activism on behalf of women in prostitution, was familiar with the history of venereal disease; women were always blamed for it. AIDS would be their fault, too; the old view of women as spreaders, not sufferers, of disease would again surface, she was sure.

AIDS was a disease transmitted in the blood and through sex. That, Taylor knew, meant some women would be infected through drug use.

Plus, she knew that the burden of taking care of those afflicted would fall to women, too. She remembered reading about "the daughter track" phenomenon: the average U.S. woman spends seventeen years raising kids and eighteen years caring for elderly relatives. It was the "daughters" who had been giving long-term health care to the elderly, and now the unpaid, unseen, unrecognized, taken-for-granted, massive labor of the "daughters" would be mobilized for family members with AIDS.

Taylor had better be in a position to wage the coming war. When the new AIDS Discrimination Unit of the New York City Commission on Human Rights opened, she went after a job on it and got it.

One of the first cases she dealt with at the Commission was that of a Bronx woman whose young adult daughter had just died of AIDS. The woman could not find a funeral home to bury her daughter. As soon as a funeral director learned it was an AIDS death, he refused to handle the body. The woman was bereft. She didn't want to press any charges; she just wanted her daughter to have "a decent burial." Taylor gave her referrals.

Though this was the only problem the woman volunteered, Taylor discovered in talking with her that she actually faced a whole web of problems. Her daughter had left behind three children, two of whom were infected with the AIDS virus. The grandmother was old, blind, and living in a one-room apartment. She could not care for the children herself, find foster care, or even find an agency that would help her locate foster care.

It was about 1:30 A.M. on a Saturday. Katrina decided to turn in for the night. She'd already been in a few pockets. Back home, she discovered she was out of cigarettes. She went out to buy a pack. Two of her girlfriends were talking to a john in a car. As she walked by the car, he shouted out that he wanted to talk to her. Katrina said she was in for the night.

"No, please. I like the little one," he said to one of the women. "Call her over here."

"No," Katrina told her friend, "I don't want to go out with him."

"He said he'll give you fifty dollars just to come over to the car and talk to him."

She went to the car. He gave her a crisp fifty-dollar bill.

"I just want to talk to you," he told her. "If you get in, I'll spend whatever you want to spend. I just want to go out with you. I think you're cute."

"Why don't you go out with one of the other girls? I'm finished for the night."

They went back and forth. She began to feel uncomfortable with him. As she raised her hands to say "I'm sorry" and got ready to walk away, she saw the knife coming, saw the glare of it under the lamp. She couldn't move fast enough. He stuck her and drove off.

"Son of a bitch!" She held her stomach, lifted up her shirt. A little puncture. At the hospital they stitched her up. Then she spit blood. When she woke up, two surgeons were standing over her telling her that she'd needed abdominal surgery, that she had had a hole the size of a silver dollar in the lining of her stomach.

She was in the hospital twenty-one days. Eight pints of blood were transfused into her veins.

When she got out, she went back to the street.

Gladys Thompson, the thin woman sitting opposite Dr. Kathy Anastos at Montefiore Hospital in New York City, had AIDS.[4]

She was not the young physician's first female AIDS patient. In 1982 a woman who had never used drugs had been Montefiore's first documented case of heterosexually acquired AIDS. Her husband had had AIDS and had died of PCP before she was admitted to the hospital in July. Still in her twenties, she had died completely demented, curled up in a ball in bed at the hospital. In fact, in the same year in which Anastos first saw AIDS cases at all, she had seen this case in a woman. And there had been others in recent months.

Now, here sat Gladys Thompson, mother of three young children. Thompson had never used drugs. She had been with only one man, her husband, for the past fifteen years. And here she was: living with AIDS.

As Gladys Thompson sat there talking about her infection and the issues it raised in her life, Anastos wept. It could have been her. Anastos also had three young children. It could have been her sitting in that chair knowing her children would soon be left without her, knowing she herself would die young. In these early days of the epidemic, Anastos couldn't sit in the same room with an AIDS-infected woman, a mother of young children, without crying.

At home, reading medical journal articles on AIDS, she felt disgusted. None of the physicians or scientists talked about the women with AIDS as being sick themselves. They all saw women simply as vectors of disease to men and fetuses, as organisms, like insects, that transmit a pathogen. Women were discussed in perinatal and prostitute studies: Those innocent babies getting it from those irresponsible moms. Those bad women in prostitution giving it not only to innocent men—the johns—but to "good" women, the johns' wives. As if this guy in the middle had nothing to do with it. And the reason it mattered that the "good" women were getting AIDS, according to the physician-experts, was not that they would suffer from the disease but that they would give it to the innocent man's innocent babies.

As one of five children raised by her divorced mother in suburban Boston, Anastos grew up with middle-class privilege ("you can be anything you want") without middle-class money. She dropped out of college in 1970 because she couldn't figure out what she was doing there. She worked on a Virginia vegetable farm and later, in Washington, D.C., as a bicycle messenger. On the farm, she discovered her own physical and mechanical skills. Repairing a tractor one day, she thought, "This is what men think is such a big deal? This is nothing. This is obvious." She also saw female farmworkers, despite their competence, assigned the less-prestigious chores. Anastos became a feminist.

She returned to college in 1973, and later entered medical school, a culture of such privilege it astonished her. Many of her classmates did not have Social Security numbers because they had never worked. This was the first time Anastos had met adults who had never held a job.

She hated medical school. Its rote learning stifled her mind, and as an unmonied woman and a feminist she felt out of place. It was when she entered a social medicine residency at Montefiore Hospital explicity aimed at improving the health status of the urban poor that she finally felt at home in medicine.

She had become a doctor both to earn her living and to work for social change. Caring for Gladys Thompson and the many women who would sit in her seat in the years to come, Anastos would learn just how deadly the forces were that needed changing.

Women in the audience seethed. As attorney Katy Taylor and two other feminist activists spoke on AIDS at the first National Organization for Women (NOW) Lesbian Conference in Milwaukee in January 1984, years of pent-up resentment in the women found expression.

How could they be urging women to support men in their

health crisis, when gay men had never supported women in their own massive, long-standing crises?

The previous spring, the Gay Men's Health Crisis (GMHC) had held a fund-raiser—a sold-out performance of the Ringling Bros. and Barnum & Bailey Circus at Madison Square Garden and raised something on the order of a million dollars.

"In our entire fifteen years of activism in the women's health movement, we were never able to raise what men raised in one night," one woman angrily exclaimed.

Now, asked to put their time and energy into something that appeared to be affecting men, the women balked: Women were always doing the giving. When had men ever formed a Gentleman's Auxiliary to help deal with battered, raped, or unnecessarily hysterectomized women? Were women now to turn their attention away from their own crises in order to help men?

Taylor argued that the backlash against homosexuals, spurred by the AIDS epidemic, would affect lesbians, too; that since many lesbians had gay male friends, it was a matter of time before some of their close friends would be dying; that some women *were* getting sick with AIDS, though people were hardly aware of this; that women, as prostitutes, were being scapegoated in the epidemic; and that women were the primary caregivers of people with AIDS.

This was news to the conference-goers.

Donna (a pseudonym) was making a stab at staying straight. One of the women in chaplain Eileen Hogan's first group at Riker's Island in 1978, she had been in and out of jail for years. Home again in 1984, she was sick. Something was wrong with her blood. She had high fevers and they couldn't get them down. Hogan knew it was AIDS. Donna probably did, too, but she never called it that. Hogan visited her when she was hospitalized with endocarditis, an infection of the heart valves. Donna knew her troubled blood could kill her. But, she told Hogan, the nurses had explained to her she could live a normal life for years if she took care of herself.

Once released from the hospital, she did that. She managed to stay off illegal drugs, though it was a struggle to hold onto her abstinence.

She took vitamins and ate the right foods. She had a job. She cared for her baby—a baby with AIDS. Donna lived in the same Bronx neighborhood Eileen did. Eileen, who saw her at least once a week, had been present at the baby's birth. The two women became close.

While Donna was struggling with her addiction and thinking of trying to get into a long-term drug treatment program, Hogan, knowing such programs offered women no child care, volunteered to care for her baby if she did that.

Donna's daughter was about two years old when Donna's boyfriend stole the money she had long been saving up for a washing machine. That threw her. She began using drugs again, stole to pay for them, and ended up back at Riker's for two weeks.

She was devastated that she was back in jail. She was weak. Jail authorities discharged her with full-blown AIDS and no support services. From home, she called Hogan immediately: "I am very sick. Can you come over? Please!"

Hogan came. She took a look at her friend and called the ambulance. Two days after her release from jail, Donna went into a coma. Four weeks later, she was dead.

After her death, Hogan often stayed with the baby Donna's boyfriend now cared for. The child took three steps once but never walked again. She didn't survive long after her mother's death. Hogan watched her, held her, as she got sicker and sicker and finally died, an experience so painful she could never find words to communicate it.

As women from the jail continued to die, Hogan felt bewildered, then angry at how disposable the women were, how little it mattered that these women suffered and died.

"Something is hurting poor women badly, something is killing them, and it doesn't matter."

"I can't even walk to a car because I'm afraid they'll blow my head off," a newly notorious young woman in prostitution told a *New Haven Register* reporter. Street people were now treating her like she had the plague, she told him. She was afraid of the men who came in cars to the women who stood in streets. They wanted to hurt her to get her off the street, she feared. She emphasized that she had not been diagnosed with AIDS.

Her public trouble had begun in January 1984 when a Yale University student publication and later the *New Haven Register* reported that a young woman in prostitution was suspected of having AIDS. State and local officials and legislators, newspapers, the Yale University chaplain, a physician at Yale–New Haven Hospital—that is, much of the local power structure—all saw her as a Problem. News coverage of the case generated a debate on whether people with AIDS should be quarantined.

While the debate raged, a few weeks after the news articles appeared New Haven police arrested the twenty-nine-year-old woman for disorderly conduct. The police had been told by "street sources" that the woman might be an AIDS carrier, the *Register* reported. During the arrest, police claimed they found drug paraphernalia in the squad car in which they transported her. She asserted it was a plant.

After the arrest, police scrubbed out the vehicle in which they conveyed her. The young woman was placed in an isolation jail cell. Jail matrons were equipped with plastic gloves, and a guard wearing protective gloves escorted her to court. The newspaper failed to report the uselessness of such procedures since it was known that AIDS could not be transmitted by casual contact.

At the arraignment, the judge set a trial date of March 15 and ordered the woman into a drug rehabilitation program in Middletown. She was not to leave the hospital until she returned to court.

The newspaper reported: "State and local officials are worried that if [the woman] does have AIDS, she might infect her prostitution customers."

Sent to the hospital February 11, she left a few days later, setting off a six-day police manhunt that ended when she turned herself in at Superior Court in New Haven on February 27.[5]

Two weeks later, the *New Haven Register* headlined an article on the woman "AIDS Hooker Is Back in Jail," though the first line reported that the woman was only "*suspected* of carrying the deadly disease." The woman was back in jail after getting medical tests for pneumonia at Yale–New Haven Hospital, the article reported. A hospital spokesman confirmed for the newspaper that a guard had been posted outside her door and that rubber restraints were sometimes used to keep her in her hospital bed. Her lawyer told the newspaper that the restraint, which he described as made of heavy rubber-coated metal, was "absolutely barbaric. It boggles the mind that in 1984, a person would be treated this way."

New quarantine legislation was quickly introduced into the Connecticut General Assembly. At this point, AIDS Project New Haven (APNH) called attorney Katy Taylor at the AIDS Discrimination Unit of the New York City Commission on Human Rights for help in lobbying against the statute.

Richard Tulisano, Democratic cochairman of the Assembly's Judiciary Committee, said his statute didn't specifically mention AIDS but would cover "individuals unable or unwilling to conduct themselves in such a manner so as not to expose other persons to the danger of infection." He acknowledged that the statute was drafted in response to the New Haven case.

The statute would have allowed a quarantine to be evoked on the signature of appointed county health representatives who did not need to be physicians.

AIDS was mostly seen as a matter concerning gays, Taylor knew. There were plenty of calls for quarantine but there were always vociferous objections to it each time it was brought up.

Except this time.

When it involved women.

In this instance, she noticed, everyone's objections "kind of disappeared."

Throughout the epidemic, Taylor later reflected, there were many efforts to deal with AIDS through control and repression: quarantine; automatic testing of women in prenatal clinics; mandatory testing of prostitutes; tattooing of the HIV-positive; installing electronic devices on people suspected of having AIDS such that if they strayed more than two hundred yards from their home, the police were notified. Such efforts suceeded on those occasions when women, and sexist stereotypes of women, were used to facilitate and justify them, Taylor observed.

In sharp contrast, they generally did not succeed when the focus was on *men* as carriers. In most places where inroads had been made in increasing control and intrusion, women—as prostitutes threatening to pass the disease to heterosexual men or as mothers threatening to give it to babies—had been used as the rationale.

A national television news program did a story on the New Haven prostitute, interviewing Assemblyman Tulisano and others. Katy Taylor recalls the segment as one in which white men interviewed each other: male journalists asking the opinions of lots of other men— police officials, divinity professors, health officials, legislators—all saying basically the same thing: We have to get this woman off the streets. We have to lock her up. We have to call for a quarantine.

It was obvious to Taylor that the woman had become totally dehumanized to the men. She was a "prostitute." If a gay man's confidentiality and dignity had been violated as the woman's had, Taylor thought, everyone would have been up in arms. But because she was a whore, no one was thinking twice. It was as if she had it coming, she was a loaded gun, and while *she* was a scumbag who deserved to die, she was also a vector of deadly disease to people they did *not* think were scumbags worthy of death—namely her customers, men of their own middle class, "innocent victims," dignified "constituents."

The train from New York City passes north through sunlight-dappled green woods and arrives at Bedford Hills, one of the most affluent suburbs in the United States. A few miles from the tiny town center stands Bedford Hills Correctional Facility, New York State's only maximum-security prison for women. High wire fences enclose eight buildings housing 850 inmates. On land dominated by a hill stand four dormitories, a mess hall, a gym, the infirmary called IPC (In-Patient Care). Two recreation yards are swamped with geese. The smaller is the "elite" yard where women gather for quiet conversation, chess games, or folk songs sung around a guitar-playing inmate. In the more boisterous yard, women walk around in state greens—pants or skirts—and their own blouses.

The buildings are always noisy: Jangling keys of guards locking and unlocking doors. Gang locks snapping shut. Voices of women.

Elaine Lord, a quiet woman who, while in a pre-med program at the University of New Hampshire in the 1960s, had become intrigued with criminology, had come to Bedford two years earlier as deputy superintendent of programs. Now she was superintendent.

Influenced by the feminism and critical thinking of the 1960s, she tried to make Bedford as humane as possible until better solutions than prisons were found for crime. She never wanted to put an angry woman out angrier.

There had been no feminist books in the prison library when she arrived. Now the library had a women's studies section and Bedford had the only National Organization for Women (NOW) chapter in the nation's prison system.

Lord did not believe people changed because outside powers forced them to. People changed themselves through an inner process. By bolstering the women's self-esteem, she tried to create an atmosphere that supported their efforts to change.

In her attempts to provide esteem-building programing for the women, she had the support of Linda Lofredo, a dynamic feminist and a program associate in the Division for Women at the New York State governor's office. The two women had met a year earlier. The Division for Women had helped get funding for programing and Lord had maintained close ties with it. She appreciated not only Lofredo's support for her work, but her ability to pose the right questions. "Superintendent," Lofredo would often ask in discussing an inmate proposal, "why not?"

The year before there had always been one or two women in IPC with serious illnesses. Carmen had a baby in the prison's kibbutzlike nursery who became very ill in 1984, needing oxygen and respirators. Carmen's mother took baby Jesse home to live with her. Finally, Jesse died. Lord did not recall the child's illness ever being referred to as AIDS. Then Carmen got sick.

At the same time, Rachael, a tiny young woman living in the prison unit for the mentally ill, became increasingly sick. When Lord made her rounds on the unit, Rachael would take Lord's hand and walk the rounds with her. It was like having a little kid, Lord felt. Rachael was hospitalized several times. Then she died. No one called it AIDS.

By 1984, confusion and panic about AIDS reigned in the prison. Not only was the prison population at high risk for the disease since many had injected drugs intraveneously, but there was also near-hysteria stemming from the erroneous reports the year before that AIDS could be spread through casual contact.

Could the women get AIDS by drinking at the water fountain?

By sleeping on a mattress that had been used by a person with AIDS or PWA, as she was called? By washing the blouse of a PWA in the laundry? What if water splashed off a showering PWA and touched the skin of an inmate in the adjoining stall?

Not a week went by that Superintendent Elaine Lord did not receive a letter from a panicked inmate: "I just got here and you've got AIDS here and now I'm afraid I'm going to get it. I don't want to go to the mess hall. Can't I just stay in my cell all the time?"

Women became suspicious of one another. Who was infected? Rumors erupted over women who went to nurse's screening for a doctor's appointment. A woman had only to lose five pounds or run an overnight fever for it to be rumored that she had AIDS. Once a woman who had been seen coughing often and had been to nurse's screening argued with another inmate over use of the public telephone. "Oh, go ahead, you AIDS bitch," the other woman finally shouted at her. "Use the phone. You can't be waiting for it too long. You're going to die soon."

Whispers at mess hall, in the gym, in the yards ("Marilyn went to an outside hospital twice and she's losing weight." "Stay away from Sheri. She has a cough and she signed up for nurse's screening twice this week." "They should put these people somewhere else.") poisoned the prison community. In that atmosphere, knowing they would be shunned, women alone in their locked cells at night panicked: "What if it's in me? How many times did I share needles?"

More and more women were getting sick. HIV-infected women were isolated in what the inmates considered the dark and dirty IPC where paint peeled off the walls.

The confusion, fear, and ignorance of correctional officers was at least as high as that of inmates. Taking women to outside hospitals, they would assume the inmates had AIDS and drive into New York City, masked, gowned, and gloved. Simply transporting an inmate with pneumonia from her cell to IPC, the terrified guards dressed as though on a moon walk. The sight of guards insulated in space-age protective gear fueled the panic and suspicion rampant in the prison.[6]

In Manhattan, far from the snapping gang locks of Bedford Hills prison, the Gay Men's Health Crisis (GMHC) had been running an

AIDS crisis telephone line for a year. Katy Taylor attended an inter-agency task force meeting on AIDS with three men: the head of the crisis line, another worker, and GMHC's director, Rodger McFarland.

They were discussing solutions to the problems in running the hotline. Taylor had acquired a vast knowledge of crisis intervention. She had both worked on and run a rape, incest, and battery crisis hotline for years. But no matter how relevant her points, the other participants—all men—ignored her input, almost indignant that she presumed to have any information or expertise. They were thinking, she felt, "But she only dealt with rape and this is about something important. This is about people *dying*."

Angered, Taylor began talking about sexism, addressing her remarks largely to McFarland, whom she felt had more respect for women than the other two men.

Women were serving as buddies, as care partners, to men with AIDS, Taylor pointed out. They were demonstrating, fund-raising, and typing. Most of these women were lesbians and they were involved because AIDS was affecting people they cared about.

Taylor leaned forward.

"Rodger," she asked, "do you think that if the situation were reversed and it was lesbians being hit by an epidemic, that gay men would be coming forward to work on AIDS?"

"No way," he replied.

Katrina Haslip took a john to a hotel room and picked his pocket. He caught her. To get away from the angered man, she pulled a knife and ran. He went to the police and picked her out from mug shots. She was arrested. While out on bail, she robbed another man. He picked her out of a lineup. She was sent up to Albion prison, sentenced to five and a half to eleven years.

With the completion of the pilot study of women in prostitution in New York City demonstrating that a larger study of women was feasible, Zena Stein and Robin Flam applied to NIH again, this time for funds to do a follow-up study of the women. In their proposal, they pointed out that since 1982, AIDS had been appearing in women in Africa, a fact Stein knew through her African contacts.

But NIH again turned them down. There would be no study of women. NIH enclosed the customary "pink sheet." The proposal critique revealed no understanding of the problem of AIDS for women, Stein felt. There was just a complete disinterest in the fact that women were getting this disease in Africa and might be in line to get it in the United States as well.

It was shattering. That even after their pilot study NIH flatly turned down their proposal appalled Stein and Flam. The research they were proposing was important in understanding the epidemic; they were convinced of this. It baffled them why, then, it wasn't being funded.

Well, they'd have another go at AMFAR—the American Foundation for AIDS Research—for the funding. AMFAR, too, turned them down on scientific grounds.

But for *what* scientific reasons Stein didn't know because there were no scientific reasons for doing *any* of the studies except to look. So little was known about the new disease that *all* studies were speculative.

She and Flam had to abandon their research on women. They wrote up their work for a book, *The Social Dimensions of AIDS: Methods and Theory.*[7] Flam got a job and left Columbia School of Public Health. Stein turned her attention to other research.

1985

In July 1985, the media trumpeted the news: Rock Hudson, the film star whose roles had romanticized and glorified heterosexuality, was gay and had AIDS. In October he was dead. In those three months, the media focused unprecedented attention on the disease and heightened public awareness of it. National media swelled with additional coverage when Ryan White, an Indiana teenage hemophiliac with AIDS, was refused entry to school. That month, President Ronald Reagan, in his first public utterance on AIDS, announced at a press conference that he could understand why parents didn't want their children "in school with these kids" who have AIDS.[1] The president of the United States, endorsing "the politics of otherness," provided no positive leadership in shaping public attitudes toward AIDS. Succeeding Reagan, George Bush would also fail to lead.

Early this same year, NIAID (National Institute for Allergy and Infectious Diseases) released a test it had developed to detect HIV in blood. New York City confined the test largely to research purposes in 1985. It was only available from a small number of designated physicians.[2]

Despite the attention belatedly drawn to AIDS, women remained invisible in the epidemic. But attorney Katy Taylor, from her vantage point on the New York City Human Rights Commission, could see some of them. Ludicrously suspected of harboring the virus, some women were pressured to prove they were not, even though the HIV test was generally unavailable.

For example, a woman from Staten Island called the Human Rights Commission, not to report a violation of her civil rights but only to learn where she could get the HIV test. Her boss knew she had an unmarried son in his forties living in Greenwich Village. He concluded that her son must be gay and must have AIDS and that therefore his mother must be an "AIDS carrier." Unless she could prove she did not have AIDS, her boss told her, she would be fired. She was trying to comply. "Where am I going to get another job at my age?" she asked when she called.

A Brooklyn woman whose boyfriend had died of AIDS also called to find out where she could get the test. She had confided to a coworker the cause of her grief. Soon after, no one in the office would speak to her. She called because she had just been told by the personnel director that she was being placed on "indefinite leave without pay" until she could "prove" that she didn't have AIDS.

Disturbing calls to the commission revealed other hardships imposed on women as the epidemic picked up speed. A Red Cross home attendant called to report the poor treatment one of her clients was receiving in a Brooklyn hospital during a bout of AIDS-related pneumonia. When the home attendant visited her client, she found that she and her roommate, who also had AIDS, had not been cleaned in three days. Nor had their beds and clothing been changed. Their food trays were left in the hall. The Red Cross worker was so upset that she cleaned both women herself, made their beds, and took their soiled clothes home to wash. The hospital staff treated the women like lepers, she told the commission.

A woman in Queens called the commission anonymously. Her husband was dying. Terrified that her friends and neighbors would discover he had AIDS, she was trying to quietly arrange for his burial. She feared that she and her two children would be subjected to the hysteria and discrimination she had seen reported on television. But she could not find a funeral home that would bury her husband. The only one willing to do it wanted several thousand dollars above its usual fee and she didn't have the money.

A church worker who dealt with prostitutes told Katy Taylor she was worried about the AIDS backlash she saw affecting women on the streets. There had been increased arrests and harassment of the women and attacks on them from johns. But these were invisible women being invisibly attacked, dark shapes falling in dark shadows.

Women were only dimly more visible in government health statistics. In 1985 CDC changed the AIDS surveillance definition, distinguishing between "with laboratory evidence of HIV" and "without," and adding several cancers to the list of indicator diseases. This revision of the AIDS definition still included no gynecological conditions. It hardly could when women with the disease often were not recognized or counted at all and the pelvic organs of those who were usually went unexamined. So who knew what was going on in vaginas, uteri, and ovaries?

By 1985, AIDS cases reported to the CDC in men numbered 8,062, in women 569.[3] Women were twice as likely to die the same month of their AIDS diagnosis as men. To Dr. Ruth Berkelman, chief of the CDC's Surveillance Branch in the Division of HIV/AIDS, looking at that fact five years later, physicians weren't recognizing AIDS in women.[4] Therefore, women must be being diagnosed and treated later than men.

While still in 1985 almost nothing was appearing in the media about women with AIDS, Chaplain Eileen Hogan continued to see these women before her eyes. She could look at a woman and tell whether she had it. Some women were coming to jail in advanced stages of the disease though they would never be given the official AIDS diagnosis until the CDC gave its blessing on it. And, although most AIDS-associated diseases like PCP apply equally to women, the CDC definitions of AIDS ignored the additional conditions specific to women. A woman had to be very, very sick to be declared a bona fide person with AIDS, Eileen knew. (If tested, she would be diagnosed as having HIV, but that was not AIDS. AIDS was the end-stage of HIV disease.) Hogan estimated that more than half the women in the prison then had the disease.[5]

The official total number of women with AIDS at Riker's Island was three.

Several inmates assigned to clean IPC, the infirmary at Bedford Hills prison, told Superintendent Lord that the two HIV-positive women living in IPC were lonely.

"You know," they said, "we gotta do something here. You need four or five people to have a card game and there are only two of them."

Lord met with the two PWAs. They said they wanted companionship, something to do. An inmate volunteered to teach them how to knit. A few others came to play cards with them.

For Sonia Perez, a petite, long-haired Latina in her early thirties, card games were not enough. She was ready to jump out of her skin. She felt healthy and wanted to be doing something with people. But here she was, cooped up in IPC. Before her diagnosis, she'd worked on the yard crew. She wanted to be back out there.

After Elaine Lord and her deputies talked over how the staff and women might react if Sonia went out into the general prison area, they decided she could go back to mowing the lawn. But they'd ease her back slowly.

They asked the yard crew to leave a lawnmower for her near IPC. She mowed her section, waving at the yard crew as she worked. The women, talking among themselves, were wary of her. But after a few days, they began waving back. After two weeks, when the yard crew gathered round the officer to get their assignments, Sonia was there chatting with them. Then she took her lawnmower and went to mow her section. They had accepted her back.

Would others accept her at a Family Day picnic, when the inmates' children and spouses visited all day? A picnic was coming up and Sonia wanted to participate.

Lord agreed. She met with Sonia and the five women who visited the inmates confined to IPC. Together, they worked out a plan.

On Family Day morning, Lord met with the group at a picnic table and asked one woman to bring Sonia out of IPC. Sonia sat at the table. They all talked.

Inmates looked at them in astonishment: There was the superintendent sitting and chatting with "AIDS-ridden" Sonia.

Food was served buffet-style. Since inmates might be worried about eating the food if Sonia had been anywhere near it, Sonia suggested that this first time, to reduce anxieties, she not go to the buffet table. Instead, she would take a plate of food another inmate brought her.

Sonia had been a popular inmate before her diagnosis. Now, after some time passed, women came to sit at the picnic table with her, bringing their babies and older children with them.

That was a step in breaking down the isolation and stigmatization of women with AIDS.

The Prostitute Study.

That's how some male colleagues of Dr. Judith Cohen, Dr. Connie Wofsy, and Lori Hauer referred to the study of HIV in women they launched in San Francisco. This, despite the fact that the majority of women in the study were not prostitutes and prostitution had never been a criterion for inclusion.

The researchers had worked with potential subjects to design the study in which participants would be tested and counseled every six months. "What do you need to make it possible for you to participate?" they asked.

The women wanted people like themselves, some of them former drug users, to interview and counsel them so they did not have to be talked down to by authority figures. They wanted the option to remain anonymous. They wanted the meetings to be held, not in the AIDS clinic, but in places in their own neighborhoods where they felt comfortable. Finally, they wanted researchers to share with them what they learned from them, and give them medical and social service referrals.

So that's the way it was.

Cohen and Wofsy presented data on the 180 women in their study at the International AIDS conference in Paris the following year. Their data was interpreted as fascinating information on prostitutes, Cohen found, though less than a third of the women they described were prostitutes. At conferences that followed, they were asked to give presentations on their "prostitute study."

A black minister in Los Angeles, launching a project to help parishioners affected by AIDS, called Dr. Vickie Mays at UCLA and asked her for help. People in distress were telephoning him. Some were suicidal. He needed a skilled counselor to help.

An African-American clinical psychologist, Mays was just back from a research stint at the University of Michigan where she'd become keenly aware of the AIDS epidemic. She volunteered to do telephone crisis intervention.

Born and raised on the South Side of Chicago in a tightly knit black neighborhood, Mays had been involved in community activity since high school when she first volunteered in a local prison. After getting her Ph. D. in clinical psychology, she had joined UCLA's faculty in 1979.

As Mays worked with the community-based AIDS project in Los Angeles, Juan Ramos, director of the Office of Prevention and Special Populations at the National Institute of Mental Health (NIMH), was identifying key ethnic minority researchers concerned with AIDS who he thought could eventually come up with ways to deal with the epidemic in minority communities. Mays was one of these key researchers. He called meetings in various locations around the country, giving the researchers a national perspective on the epidemic.

In visits to places like Belglade, Florida, and in her community work, Mays could see the disease affecting a group of people who were not like white gay men. Some were married men worried about being infected because they might have had sex with a man at some point.

Mays knew that men who identify themselves as heterosexual may still have sex with men under certain situations, in prison, say, or in the armed forces. These men, not identifying as gay or bisexual, were not people who would show up for a risk-reduction workshop at Gay Men's Health Crisis. Handing them a brochure was no way to educate these men.

They were worried about their health and they didn't know where to go to get information on AIDS.

Studies and reports on women and AIDS and then on babies and AIDS poured into the South End office of Dr. Hortensia Amaro at Boston University School of Public Health, where she was an associate professor. The "baby" pile dwarfed the "woman" pile. In the stacked piles, she could see it before her eyes: the federal focus was on pediatric AIDS, even though there were many more women infected than children and even though pediatric AIDS was in fact a reflection of AIDS in women.

This neglect of women was par for the course in medicine and public health, Amaro knew. Though most women spent a small portion of their lives bearing babies, women's health was almost exclusively seen as "maternal and child health"—those aspects of their health related to reproduction.

You could see it at the Massachusetts Department of Public Health. The Women's Health Unit was a subdivision of Maternal and Child Health, though logically, Amaro thought, it should be the other way around. The reality was that, even within Maternal and Child Health programs, women's health was not really studied or dealt with. Instead, Amaro saw, health professionals in those programs studied *how a mother's health adversely affects her child's health.*[6]

What had drawn Amaro into research on HIV prevention and, eventually, to accumulate these two stacks of documents was the HIV infection, illness, and death of her younger brother, Armando. After her family immigrated to the United States from Cuba in 1960, her parents worked several jobs and attended English classes while Hortensia cared for Armando, eight years her junior. The two became very close.

Her research on drug use among women and adolescent girls also brought her painfully in touch with the effects of the epidemic on women she knew and valued.

The more deeply she delved into HIV research, the more clearly she saw that in preventing, studying, and treating AIDS in women, the questions chosen by scientists, by physicians, and by the federal agencies that fund the science were defined through the lens of women's reproductive function. The central question was always "How does this impact the children?" Any women's experience of AIDS that didn't relate to their reproductive function was ignored.

Viniece Walker, an inmate at Bedford Hills who became active in AIDS counseling and education, comments that the federal government "seems to view women-and-children as a package deal. You buy one, get one free. When you take the children away, we don't count anymore. Once we are not able to bear these children or say, 'No, we're not bearing no more,' then it's out to pasture. And we just graze for the rest of our lives 'cause we don't matter. We served our purpose."

From the beginning of the epidemic, the issue around pregnancy and HIV that would be highlighted in public discussions was the possibility of women harming fetuses by passing HIV on to them. Since women in and of themselves were not important, the possibly injurious effects of a pregnancy on the health of an HIV-infected woman never became a significant topic of public discussion.

The primacy of the fetus and the unimportance of the woman in governmental and scientific thinking on AIDS led to a series of concerns for those, like Amaro, who *did* consider women valuable. Basically they were that HIV-infected women would not be making their own decisions about their reproduction and health but would be coerced into doing what fetal-centered policymakers wanted them to do. The issues were: coercive testing of pregnant women to prevent HIV transmission to fetuses; hostile counseling; potential criminalization of childbirth for HIV-infected women; medical treatment of the pregnant woman that neglected her needs, withholding treatment *known* to be beneficial to her but *suspected* of being harmful to her fetus; the exclusion of women of childbearing potential from clinical drug trials; the coercion of women into abortions and sterilizations; conversely, the denial of abortions to those women who wanted them.

1. *Testing:* Many national groups have advocated offering testing to all pregnant women or to all pregnant women in "high risk" groups and some organizations have called for counseling that directs women away from becoming pregnant or bearing children.

Confidential rather than anonymous testing means that test results will go into the women's medical records and will be available to people who have access to that medical record, perhaps placing women at risk for stigmatization in the community and loss of job.

"The full extent of the potential misuse of results from confidential testing is yet really to be seen," Amaro warned.

In December 1985, the CDC published guidelines purportedly to help prevent HIV transmission to fetuses. It recommended that pregnant women in risk groups for AIDS take the newly developed HIV test and that infected women "be advised to consider delaying pregnancy until more is known about perinatal transmission of the virus."

Many state and city health departments followed the CDC lead and recommended that pregnancy in HIV-infected women be postponed. Women at this time were often advised that the chance of their having an infected baby was high—70 or 80 percent. Only a few years later, however, the chances were actually found to be 30 percent, and even lower in some European studies.

Since there was little likelihood of a cure for the virus in the next few years, HIV-infected women in fact were being urged never to bear children.

AIDS was appearing most in poor minority communities. So talk of not bearing children became a political issue. Some critics, knowing the history of forced sterilization of poor minority women, and the promotion of risky contraceptives like Depo-Provera for them, suspected that such advice was motivated by a willingness to let the black race die off.

2. *Hostile posttest counseling:* Counseling is not reimbursed appropriately, Amaro notes, and in busy inner-city clinics, not much time is devoted to it. In a project she runs, Amaro has encountered women counseled elsewhere who, on being given the devastating news that they were HIV-positive, had been told such things as "Well, what do you expect, with your background?" She and her colleagues had to do a lot of cleaning up to help women deal with the consequences of judgmental, unkind counseling. She knows of no studies that examine the attitudes of medical professionals toward women with HIV, especially women who are pregnant or drug-using, and how those attitudes may affect counseling.

3. *Criminalization of childbirth:* If women chose to bear babies, would they be prosecuted for willful transmission of HIV? By 1990 twenty-two states had made it a felony or misdemeanor to knowingly expose or transmit HIV infection. Only one—Texas—exempted HIV-positive mothers of infected infants from criminal penalties. Women in Idaho with AIDS or HIV who knowingly breast-feed their infants could be found guilty of a felony.

"While no state has prosecuted a woman for knowingly transmitting the virus perinatally," *Intergovernmental AIDS Reports* observed, "the omission of specific exemptions for HIV-infected women makes the potential for criminal action possible."[7]

Considering such laws, along with recent court cases charging women who used drugs during pregnancy with child abuse and neglect,[8] Amaro could foresee a time when HIV-infected women who knowingly become pregnant could be charged by the state with intentional homicide or child abuse.

While that might seem farfetched to some, it did not to Amaro, director of a project to aid drug-using pregnant women in Boston. Concern with "fetal rights," she knew, had already been used successfully to compel women, under court order and police escort, to submit to cesarean sections they rejected on religious grounds or out of disagreement with the physician's assessment of the need for surgery.

In fact, a national survey published in May in the *New England Journal of Medicine* found that physicians had obtained court orders for cesarean sections in eleven states, for the detention of pregnant women in hospitals in two states, and for intrauterine blood transfusions into the fetus in one state. Among twenty-one cases in which court orders were sought, the orders were obtained in 86 percent. Eighty-one percent of the women involved were black, Asian, or Hispanic. Almost half the heads of fellowship programs in "maternal-fetal medicine" (what used to be "obstetrics" until physicians raised the fetus to "patient" status) thought that women who refused medical advice and thereby endangered the life of the fetus should be detained.[9]

4. *Medical treatment concerned less with the woman's health than with that of the fetus:* Providers, knowing that women with a severely lowered immune response would benefit from the drug AZT, have often withheld it until after the twelfth week of pregnancy out of concern over the unknown effects of AZT on the fetus.[10]

As late as 1990, there were still federal documents stating that physicians attempting to prevent a predictable bout of PCP in a woman should not prescribe pentamidine for her until her pregnancy is completed. What that suggested was that if a physician were treating a woman with a severely compromised immune system, in whom it could be predicted both that the woman would progress to an opportunistic infection during the pregnancy and that pentamidine would help prevent that, the physician should withhold that information from the woman and withhold that treatment.

5. *Exclusion of women from clinical drug trials:* The primacy of fetal health—even the health of a nonexistent but *imaginable* fetus—

and the unimportance of women's well-being were also reflected in the criteria for inclusion in an AIDS Clinical Trials Group (ACTG). Created in 1987, funded and managed by the National Institute of Allergy and Infectious Disease (NIAID), ACTG is the system of cooperative medical institutions conducting federal clinical AIDS drug trials. Through this system, forty-seven institutions are funded to do clinical trials. As late as 1989, the criteria for an ACTG read: "Pregnant and lactating women and *women of childbearing potential* are excluded."[11] So women were largely left out of studies. After activist protests, the complete exclusion of women of childbearing potential was dropped, but women were now required to provide proof they were using an "adequate" means of contraception. Still only 5 percent of clinical trial participants are women. Such exclusionary criteria is one reason there is now so little information on what HIV disease does in women's bodies.

The Ob/Gyn Subcommittee is where NIAID officials direct inquiries regarding enrollment of HIV-infected women into an ACTG. All members of the ob/gyn subcommittee are either pediatricians or obstetricians. Again demonstrating the primacy of the fetus and the subordination of women, *Ob/Gyn is a subcommittee of the Pediatric Committee.* Pediatrics is a core committee within the ACTG structure; ob/gyn is not.[12]

Nineteen ACTGs assess various substances for efficacy and safety in treating children with AIDS. Not one trial is designed to evaluate treatments for AIDS and AIDS-related opportunistic infections in women.

6. *Pressuring of women into abortions and sterilizations:* As the New York City Task Force on Women and AIDS points out in its 1992 "Policy Document," the CDC guidelines stating that women should be encouraged to "postpone" childbirth set the stage for efforts to pressure women into abortion and/or sterilization.

7. *Denial of abortion services:* Though women who don't want abortions may be pressured into them, women who do choose to end the pregnancy often have difficulty doing so. A majority of states deny HIV-infected women Medicaid funding of abortions. Another barrier was revealed in 1989 when a survey in New York City found that 64

percent of abortion clinics refused HIV-infected women an appointment for an abortion.[13]

The issue around pregnancy and HIV that has never been publicly highlighted is the degree of physical debilitation a pregnancy imposes on a woman infected with HIV. Little is known about it since few studies exist. There's some reason to suppose that pregnancy may accelerate disease progression. Concerns about this are based on evidence of a deteriorated immune status in pregnancy.[14] But the "preliminary and inconclusive nature of the data," as one ob/gyn who treats HIV-infected women notes, makes it difficult to counsel women and difficult for the women to make their decisions.

What little information is available indicates this:

- that HIV disease does not seem to worsen in women in an asymptomatic stage of the disease, at least in the short-term (long-term effects are unknown)
- that women with AIDS (the end-stage of HIV disease) are likely to get sicker more quickly if they carry a pregnancy to term

But even this hypothesis—that the effect of pregnancy on HIV infection may vary according to the severity of the illness—has little information available to support it.

"Information about disease progression during pregnancy is not available from a prospective study of symptomatic HIV-infected women," two epidemiologists wrote in 1990.[15]

Francesca was not at chapel that Saturday on Riker's Island. But she always came. Where was she? a friend asked. She had just been taken to the hospital with a high fever, she was told.

Eileen Hogan went to the hospital to see Francesca, another woman in her original group of eight.

"They think there is something wrong with my blood," the fever-racked Francesca told Eileen.

She recovered and was sent to Bedford Hills for just under a year. She was released, feeling pretty good. The next week she went into a coma and died.

1986

The two-year-old child had been referred to Dr. Helen Rodriquez-Trias, who ran a pediatric clinic at Newark's Beth Israel Medical Center in New Jersey. "Failure to thrive" was the diagnosis. A clinic nurse who had often nursed children with cancer took one glance at him and said, "He looks immuno-compromised."

So there it was. They did the workup. He was HIV-infected.

Rodriquez had seen her first children with AIDS in 1984 when she was directing the primary care division of the Department of Pediatrics at St. Luke's–Roosevelt Hospital in Manhattan. Most medical professionals she worked with were not alarmed by the infected children. "Well, they are the children of drug addicts, and drug addicts are a minority and not an important one." That attitude was in the air Rodriquez breathed in the hospital corridors and examination rooms. "This is happening in people who are marginal, who are not like our real clientele, not like us."

At fifty-six, Rodriquez, slight of build, has the face she deserves: kind, smiling, with eyes radiating intelligence, warmth. Never a distanced professional, her manner is natural, easy.

By the time Rodriquez started work at Beth Israel in 1985, it was obvious that physicians were dealing with a major epidemic and one that was affecting women and children. They began to pick up children who had been undiagnosed at the general pediatric clinic at the Newark hospital because physicians were unaware that maybe the children who were losing weight were actually HIV-infected.

The mother of the two-year-old boy Rodriquez was treating had no idea that her child and she herself were both infected with the AIDS virus. Now Rodriquez was faced with giving her the news. The woman, in her mid-thirties, had used intravenous drugs years ago, had been clean for some time, and was now devoting herself to her family. This early in the epidemic, before the development of various preventive treatments, an HIV diagnosis was a death sentence. Sitting in Rodriquez's office, hearing that sentence, the woman was devastated.

In the horror of telling the woman, Rodriquez felt, too, the horror lying in the background: that there must be many, many more women out there who were infected, and physicians knew nothing of them. The only ones coming to their attention were the ones who happened to have had children who had become symptomatic.

Rodriquez had the distinct impression that at Beth Israel Hospital, medical professionals did not want to be identified as people treating HIV and did not want the hospital to become known as an HIV center. They referred most pediatric in-patients to an infectious disease specialist at University Children's Hospital in Newark rather than care for them themselves. They were concerned about whether they'd be able to recruit residents and nurses, and whether they'd scare off other patients if they didn't keep a low profile on HIV.

No one ever said, "Look, we don't want to be known as an HIV center." The message was delivered through the referral patterns and by the fact that no thought was given to developing a designated HIV unit.

This was an implicit policy on AIDS, not an explicit one. Rodriquez's nostrils were sensitive to the odor of implicit policies. She had first smelled it in 1959 when she was a fourth-year student at the School of Medicine in San Juan, the only medical school in Puerto Rico. In 1959 she went to Columbia-Presbyterian Hospital in New York as a medical exchange student in the ob-gyn rotation. The oral contraceptive was then being developed; women in Puerto Rico were the experimental subjects. One of her ob-gyn professors in New York talked about it: "Oh, that's the study that's going on in Puerto Rico with the Pill." Rodriquez was embarrassed because she, who had been right at the center of academic medicine in Puerto Rico being taught the latest research findings, knew nothing about the study. Some of her professors in Puerto Rico were actually participating in it. While people at the school customarily talked about their research, Rodriquez never heard the Pill experiment discussed.

This—1959—was before tight guidelines for an institutional review of medical experimentation on human beings had been issued. It was before the unethical Tuskegee study hit the news. (Physicians following poor black men with syphilis in a long-term study that began in Alabama before an effective treatment for the disease existed allowed the men to go untreated for years even after penicillin had become widely available. They wanted to go on following the natural history of syphilis, so they withheld from the ailing men the information that a very effective treatment now existed.) Physicians and scientists were doing all kinds of human research that did not require consent from the people being researched on or an experimental design compatible with human rights.

The study in Puerto Rico involved 132 Puerto Rican women who took the Pill for one year or longer, and 718 other Puerto Rican women who took the drug for less than a year. Five of the young women died during the study, three with symptoms suggesting blood clots. No autopsies were performed. It was on the basis of this study that the Food and Drug Administration approved the Pill for mass use in the United States.[1]

So as a medical student, Rodriquez learned that there was an implicit policy to use Puerto Rican women as research subjects in a major study in which some of her professors were participating. That policy had never been stated and was never discussed.

The second time the odor of implicit policy hit her nostrils was during the campaign to sterilize women in Puerto Rico. The opening up of sterilization as a massive phenomenon on the island began gradually in the early 1950s and soon accelerated. Again, no one made an announcement: "The U.S. government has a policy of restricting population in Puerto Rico that requires that we sterilize." Or: "We have a policy that sterilization be the main method provided Puerto Ricans for ending their fertility."

It was not discussed. Yet, as Rodriquez later learned, there were pamphlets given out to persuade factory owners in Puerto Rico to establish in-factory birth control clinics. The pamphlets talked dollars and cents on the savings to owners if the women didn't get pregnant. Owners wouldn't have to give maternity leave, provide health benefits, etc.

The sterilization campaign was going on all the time that Rodriquez was a young attending physician at San Juan's University Hospital, the central hospital in Puerto Rico. Yet she did not know about it until the late 1960s when she read studies conducted by a demographer showing that an outrageous 38 percent of the women of childbearing age in Puerto Rico had been sterilized.

In late 1975, Rodriquez and other activists in New York City (where she had come in 1970 to direct the Department of Pediatrics at Lincoln Hospital) formed the Committee to End Sterilization Abuse (CESA). CESA developed a slide show it used in public forums, one that included a shot of the pamphlet given factory owners. That same year, she became a charter member of the National Women's Health Network that linked the grass-roots organizations of the women's health movement.

Implicit policy, like body language, communicates powerful messages but because words are never spoken, the policy is hard to combat.[2] Implicit policy has high deniability, Rodriquez knew. If you confronted anyone, saying, "Well, wait a minute. Is there a deliberate policy here that we are not going to beef up our capability to provide services for HIV-positive people?" the response would be: "What do you mean by that? We just don't have the beds."

Marie St. Cyr, a thirty-four-year-old Haitian-born social worker, sat in the tiny office she shared with two other employees of the Haitian Centers Council preparing a quarterly report to a funding foundation. The Centers ran a variety of programs—employment, after-school, family counseling, and the Haitian Coalition on AIDS to which St. Cyr devoted much of her time. St. Cyr felt that the other employees in the suite of four small offices in downtown Brooklyn kept her at a distance. She spoke often, publicly and privately, about AIDS and met with PWAs routinely. Perhaps her colleagues were associating her and her Coalition coworkers with anxiety they felt about their own risk of AIDS. Whatever was going on, it didn't make for a comfortable work environment.

With the report in front of her, looking at the number of AIDS cases the Coalition had had a year ago and those it now had, she saw a startling change. The previous year, less than 10 percent of its clients had been women. Suddenly, in 1986, 22 percent were women.

St. Cyr was stunned. Not because there were women with AIDS: it had been a logical deduction that, of course, they would begin to see ill women. No. What was stunning was that it had happened so fast.

St. Cyr, a large woman whose regal presence commanded attention, had immigrated to the United States with her family in 1966 when she was sixteen. She went to high school on Long Island, and, retaining her lilting Haitian accent, earned two degrees in social work from the University of Pennsylvania. She had first worked with clients with AIDS in 1982 while directing a social services health project for the Lutheran Ministries of Florida in Belglade, where up to seven thousand Haitians and other migrant workers were concentrated.

Now, as she sat at her desk, she saw it: Here, predictably, were the ill women. What she found frightening was that there were no services at all to help the women she was encountering. Nowhere was the issue of women with AIDS being addressed.

Other women working in various health settings such as the Gay Men's Health Crisis or in social, administrative, or research agencies were also suddenly encountering HIV-infected women and finding the same complete lack of services. A group of fourteen, including St. Cyr, began gathering and talking about one thing: Where could the women turn? Even to talk to someone about what they were going through?

A sympathetic minister at the United Methodist Church in Manhattan's Greenwich Village opened the church's day-care center to the group. The women sat in chairs built for four-year-olds. After laughing at the awkwardness of their seats, their somber discussions moved from accounts of infected women they were encountering at work to fearsome thoughts of their own risk.

Sister Eileen Hogan telephoned Linda Lofredo, the program associate in the Division for Women at the New York State Governor's Office. Hogan and Lofredo had met some months earlier at a conference in Queens on women and corrections and had talked occasionally since then.

Lofredo was a passionate advocate for women in prisons, her

ardor fanned by an extraordinary hearing she and Superintendent Elaine Lord had helped arranged the year before at Bedford Hills on the relationship between incarceration and domestic violence.[3] Sitting in the prison gym, listening to the testimony of the women inmates, Lofredo had been stunned by the extremity of the violence the women had been subjected to before they committed a crime—sometimes the crime of murdering a mate who had battered them for years—and by the depth of their suffering. The hearing changed the way she thought about women in prisons. If you took the issue of women in prisons long enough and deep enough, she had seen then, you waded through layers of sexual abuse, incest, violence against women, substance abuse, homelessness, the self-contempt abuse generated in women.

Now Sister Eileen Hogan was on the phone. Lofredo respected her. When she called, Lofredo paid attention.

"Four women I knew from Riker's died of pneumonia over the space of one month," Hogan told her. "Linda, I know it's not pneumonia."

There it was: AIDS in women. Lofredo felt dread. For some time, in moments of quiet reflection, she had thought, "This disease can't be confined to one sex. If it is a virus, it doesn't make sense that only men would get it."

But she had not had the numbers to suggest any state-run AIDS program for women, such as AIDS awareness and prevention. The CDC statistics showed so few women affected by the disease—569 at that point.

Lofredo had felt immobilized in a fog of uncertainty; the numbers demonstrating a problem just weren't there. Hogan's phone call blew the fog away. They needed to get moving on this. AIDS had to be put on the agenda for women. The numbers would not stay low for long.

She called Lynne MacArthur, the forty-year-old feminist employed in New York's Division of Substance Abuse Services, and told her she thought AIDS would be the next big issue for women. The two women had worked together earlier on a project for the homeless. Now they were going to tackle AIDS.

MacArthur's agency, where she had worked since 1972, dealt with drug abuse issues and she had already taken a course in AIDS. The course leader was the indefatigable social worker Luis Palacio

Jiminez, who quickly became a friend. When he disclosed that he had AIDS, the tragedy of the epidemic hit home.

MacArthur and Lofredo decided to bring together a group of women who were dealing with the disease in women and needed a place to talk about the issues.

In September twelve women met in the Governor's Library in the World Trade Center.[4] Over the following months, they brought more women in—Marie St. Cyr and attorney Katy Taylor among them—and founded the Women and AIDS Project.

It couldn't be an advocacy group since it was a part of the Governor's office. But such a group that could speak up for women, as the Gay Men's Health Crisis spoke up for gay men, was clearly needed.

Marie St. Cyr and others decided to form a community-based organization that could respond to the dearth of services for women in the AIDS crisis: the Women and AIDS Resource Network (WARN). After a laborious fund-raising process, they finally got $45,000 from several foundations and began. St. Cyr became director.

On the Lower East Side of Manhattan, on Second Avenue, stands a big solid Renaissance building erected in the 1880s as a clinic for German immigrants. The building maintained its dignity when the neighborhood became, in the 1960s, home of the Fillmore East and the disco-saturated Electric Circus and one of the city's major drug-dealing centers. The mesmerizing vibrations of the Jefferson Airplane's "White Rabbit" have long ceased and hippies are no more, though the drug dealing and a few head shops linger on.

In the 1980s, the neighborhood partially gentrified—there's a Gap on the corner next to the clinic—but Ukrainian and Polish restaurants and delis surround the building, still giving testimony to the Lower East Side's immigrant past. The Electric Circus of the 1960s becomes the Twelve-Step Building of the 1980s, its rooms filled not with flashing psychedelic lights but with one drug-free disco and the programs of Alcoholics Anonymous, Overeaters Anonymous, and Narcotics Anonymous.

Now the building houses the community-based Stuyvesant Polyclinic, owned by the private Cabrini Hospital and the first HIV test site opened in New York City. In the spring of 1986, women, mostly white, in their late twenties and early thirties began flocking to the Polyclinic. Some were recovering or current IV drug users or partners of users. They came in for tests, discovered they were positive or negative or that their partners were infected. Some were sick. Some were dying. Many worried that sickness and death lay directly before them.

Dr. Dooley Worth listened to the women and to the harried nurses to whom they poured out their pent-up feelings. New in the work world, she had started graduate school in her thirties after her marriage ended. Through a combination of student loans, scholarships, and part-time jobs, she'd gotten through the tight student years and now had a doctorate in medical anthropology.

Almost none of the women Worth saw felt that they could tell anyone what they were going through. So they carried it all inside. Then they would come into the clinic and sometimes break down. Some told how, on their few, timid attempts to tell a friend or family member about their overwhelming problems related to HIV, they had watched them recoil in horror. Yet the nurses had no time scheduled in their duties for listening and they were getting upset at what they were hearing.

Some women would come in and say that their husbands were sick. "How are we going to explain to our parents who are on us to have grandchildren that there won't be any grandchildren?" they'd ask. "How can we do that without letting them know that he used drugs?"

So it was never just about AIDS, Worth found. It was also about other secrets that were as stigmatizing and distancing as the disease itself.

The women were more closeted, in a way, than gay men, Worth realized, listening to them. Men had the Gay Men's Health Crisis, a place where supporters would advocate for them and receive them warmly. Although GMHC welcomed women, there were so few of them that the women felt uncomfortable in those groups discussing personal, especially sexual, issues.

In 1986 it seemed that all at once women revealed this need across the board, and no services existed to fill it.

Worth felt she had to do something. Angered by the woman-blaming she was seeing everywhere (women were blamed for the breakdown of the family, for the street crime attributed to family breakdown, for children not doing well in school, for being poor, for being on welfare, for being abused, for using drugs), she had the drive and energy to do it. She called her friends working in settings where they had to be seeing the same need she was: drug treatment programs, social and health services for minority women. But her friends were overwhelmed. Working in understaffed, underfunded institutions, they had no time or energy to take on more work. To learn more about AIDS, she called people at GMHC. When she heard that Dr. Joyce Wallace was seeing women with AIDS in her Greenwich Village practice, she talked with her.

Worth next wrote to a New York State AIDS Institute official describing the acute, unmet need she was seeing in women. The Institute asked her to write a position paper about it. With computer printouts from the city Health Department breaking down AIDS figures by gender, she and an epidemiologist colleague pieced together a picture of AIDS' impact on women from 1981 to 1986. The state did not respond to their report. But two women in the city Health Department—the assistant commissioner for AIDS and the director of the city's HIV hotline—did. They didn't have any funds but they gave what they could: the services of a group counselor for what was soon called "the women's group" and referrals from the HIV hotline. The Stuyvesant Polyclinic donated Worth's time and a meeting room.

The women's group ran with no money except for two private donations amounting to less than $3,000 used to purchase educational materials. There was almost no funding to apply for because there was still little attention given to the heterosexual spread of AIDS or to the impact of the disease on women.

The program drew not just the expected neighborhood women but women from the whole region and even from New Jersey, Rhode Island, and Connecticut. These women had nowhere else to go. Worth and her colleagues had planned to provide AIDS education for women at risk but quickly realized that more than information, the women needed to talk, without being judged, about what they were going through. They needed support as they dealt with their fears for their children, the impact of AIDS on their relationships, their need for medical care and social services that, for women, did not exist. They needed to understand how the disease affected women. This they learned, as best they could, not from any medical articles—those weren't being written—but by sharing information with each other.

("Look, I get vaginal infections and they're bad and they keep coming back.") They needed emotional support and a community where they could break out of their isolation. So in the first month, the program was reformulated to give the women a safe place to talk and share.

In 1986 the antiviral drug AZT (azidothymidine) began slowing the progress of AIDS in some men. Developed by the Burroughs Wellcome Company, the drug, also called zidovudine, continues to be controversial for several reasons, including its high cost. The only way to get AZT in 1986 was to be in an experimental trial. But women in general and drug users, many of whom were female, were excluded by design from the first trial.

This infuriated social worker Edith Springer, who worked with many sick and dying drug-addicted women. Researchers explained that they were excluding drug users because it would be impossible to tell the effects that illicit drugs were having on the experiment. But when a therapeutic community of former drug users volunteered its members for a trial, the researchers turned them down. The truth was, Springer believed, they just didn't want to deal with drug users. They didn't think they had a right to survive.

Former heroin addict Springer saw that hatred expressed in the abusive treatment of her clients in hospitals.

One client, Rosemary Star (a pseudonym), was terminally ill with AIDS. They were unable to diagnose what turned out to be a brain tumor, but it was obvious that the woman would soon die.

The doctor entered Star's room while Springer was there. The woman was racked with pain, cancer eating her up. Parts of her mouth and throat had disappeared. He wanted to do a bone marrow test, the doctor told her.

"Is it going to hurt?" she asked.

"No. You'll feel some pressure, okay?" he replied.

Springer's eyes bulged out of her head. She, a medical social worker, knew a bone marrow test could be extremely painful (although not always; the pain depends on the placement of the anesthetic injection and other aspects of technique). He left the room. Star turned to her and said, "Edith, this doctor is fucking lying. The woman down the hall had it last week and she was in terrible pain."

"Well, it's up to you whether you want this test or not. He's trying to come to a diagnosis about what's going on."

"I don't want the test."

"Do you feel comfortable telling him?"

She said yes. Springer left. When she next visited Star, she was lying in pain from the bone marrow test.

"I thought you weren't going to do it," Springer said.

"He wouldn't leave me alone," Star replied.

Rosemary Star died shortly after that. There had been no need to arrive at a diagnosis.

Another client, June Winkler (pseudonym), lived four months in the hospital. Although the black woman was perfectly well much of the time, she was homeless and the hospital could not legally discharge a person with ARC (AIDS-related complex) into the street. Winkler was unattractive. She had a loud, vulgar mouth. She told people off. The hospital personnel hated her and treated her badly.

Winkler had no teeth. While she was rapidly dropping weight, they gave her food she could not chew.

Although she could not leave her room, Winkler was the only patient on the floor who had no telephone and no television. At seven dollars a day, she couldn't afford the hospital television.

Winkler's telephone, her only means of reaching people, including Springer, broke. Telephone company employees refused to enter the room of an AIDS patient to fix the phone. So Springer asked that her client be moved into another room with a phone. The request was denied. A week later, they decided to paint the room and found a way to move Winkler.

She wanted photographs taken of herself with Springer and with her doctor from the drug program, whom she loved. Springer brought in a camera and the three took pictures of one another. When she opened the door at one point, the head nurse saw a flash and confiscated the camera and pictures.

"Why?" Springer asked her.

"There's a rule. You can't take pictures of a patient in the hospital."

"The patient is taking the pictures. She wants the pictures."

"This is against the rules of confidentiality," the nurse persisted.

"These are her pictures," Springer protested. "You have no right."

"Well, this is to protect her."

"From who? Who are you protecting her from?"

After much wrangling, Springer finally got her camera back, and Winkler her pictures. Winkler kept those photos by her bed. They meant a lot to her.

One day an arrangement was made for Springer to take the woman out to lunch. Everything had been approved. When Springer arrived on the floor, the head nurse said: "You can't take her off the floor because if anything happens to her, I'm responsible."

Winkler, cooped up in one room for months, burst into tears. There was no reason why she could not have been allowed to leave the hospital escorted by a social worker. But she remained inside.

One Sunday Winkler called Springer at home.

"I gotta get out of here," she told her. "They're treating me like shit and I want out."

"Listen," Springer said. "I'll come in tomorrow and we'll discuss this."

"I'm getting out of here tomorrow, one way or the other," the woman replied.

The next morning, Springer got a telephone call in her office. The woman was dead.

There was no medical reason for her death. She was free of illness, kept on in the hospital only because she was homeless. Springer and others in the hospital believed Winkler had bought tranquilizers from other patients and overdosed. Springer ordered an autopsy. The hospital canceled it. Springer was convinced the hospital, attributing Winkler's death to heart failure, was covering up a suicide. There was no reason for a thirty-eight-year-old woman to suddenly die of heart failure.

When Springer championed the needs of the drug addicts she was serving and protested abusive treatment of them in the hospital, her social work department always sided with the hospital rather than her. It was the same old thing, she felt. Social workers don't like drug addicts either.

When people would ask Springer how to treat drug addicts in the hospital, she would answer, "You treat them like your mother or your sister. That's how you treat them. You don't have the right to treat them differently just because you don't like them."

Springer was grateful when her friend Luis Palacio introduced her to Dooley Worth, who was also working with female drug addicts. Both women felt isolated and unsupported. Meeting each other, they immediately became close.

Springer was burned out. She began pulling away from direct work with AIDS patients. It got to her—the emotional devastation of watching people die, particularly the women who died so quickly, with such meager support and sometimes surrounded by hostility as they breathed their last breath.

You just can't watch young people die right and left and not be affected by it, she thought.

In 1986 crack, a cheap, smokable form of cocaine, invaded the inner cities. By 1987, it had become available in forty-six states and the District of Columbia, the Drug Enforcement Agency reported. Many longtime heroin users switched to crack. Crack was cheap (five- and ten-dollar packages were available), gave a brief high, and induced paranoia—a quality that sometimes led to violence.

But crack was only the latest in drug fashions. In the 1960s and 1970s, heroin had prevailed in the inner cities.

Edith Springer had two theories on why inner-city women who'd used heroin for years switched to crack:

1. Women want their anger. Crack lets them keep it. Heroin, blotting out all unpleasant feelings, takes their anger away.
2. Crack makes women feel good. They don't have any other way to feel good.

"They have no hope," Springer said, explaining one of a variety of theories on drug addiction. "At our Harlem AIDS Project, we call it a poverty of spirit. It's not about being poor. There were many poor groups that came to America. But they had hope and they knew they were going to do better if they worked hard and minded their P's and Q's."

One factor that determines whether a person uses a drug recreationally, without harming herself, or compulsively and self-destructively is the cultural setting.[5] Crack is not instantly addictive in all settings. As Springer explains: "A black woman in Harlem who has nothing: no home, no family, no one who cares about her. Who knows this is a racist society. Who knows she ain't going nowhere—the American dream is not for her. She takes crack cocaine and she feels good. She says, 'My God, I'll do anything to have this feeling.'"

In an intact community where women do have some hope, give women crack and they'll say, "This is okay. I could see myself doing this once in a while."

What's the difference? It's not the drug. It's the setting. It's how they feel about themselves. It's how much hope they have.

But the famine of hope stems not only from life in a community marginalized by racist policies and practices, but from an insidious attack on the spirit of individual women. Women who abuse drugs are not social deviants, exhibiting bad personal behavior, as conventional thinking would have it. More likely, they are victimized women blotting out the pain of childhood abuse. Women exist in a society in which widespread sexual abuse of females is overlooked, tolerated, trivialized. In fact, a minimum of 80 percent of female drug addicts have been sexually abused, according to Gloria Weissman, deputy chief of the Community Research Branch of the National Institute on Drug Abuse (NIDA).

Many female heroin addicts have been raped or incested before their addiction. Since long-term heroin use depresses sexuality, some researchers believe that women may adopt intravenous drug use as an escape from sexual trauma into an asexual world.[6]

As former addict Marilyn (T.J.) Rivera of New York City explains it, heroin is an opiate that "sleeps your feelings." Abused, first in the family; told, in words or in blows or through twitching facial muscles or contemptuous glares, that they were ugly, stupid, incompetent, valueless; failing in a school environment that, with its order and predictability, seemed to have come from another planet—certainly not the one they lived on—many women have feelings of hurricane force they want put to sleep.

With heroin, Rivera explains, the world could come tumbling down and you just wouldn't care. Before the arrival of crack, women generally did not cop (get, buy, barter) heroin for themselves. If they tried, the dealers would cheat them. Women waited for men to bring the heroin home to them. For the men there was a sexual ritual, precise and suffused with fantasizing, involved in setting up the drug paraphernalia, tying up the woman's arm, and sticking her with the needle.

Childhood abuse—sexual, physical, emotional—along with poverty and oppression underlies numerous addictions, psychologist Charlotte Davis Kasl explains.

"Childhood abuse is a betrayal of the deepest part of a human being," Kasl, author of *Women, Sex and Addiction,* said in an interview.

A person—small and vulnerable—trusts people who then hurt and use her. So her ability to trust and bond with others is damaged or almost destroyed.

"Abuse is so beyond the capacity of a little person to handle that she reaches for something to distract and comfort her, like food or fantasy," Kasl said. "It's easier to eat too much food and have a stomach ache than to know that the only people you have to protect you are not protecting you and to face that aloneness and the terror that maybe these adults are going to kill you."

Young children might escape into a fantasy world. They might fantasize that they are adopted or are beautiful princesses or are in charge and can order these adults killed.

Eventually, as the children age, they might bump into a different fantasy world—the world drugs open up to them. Drug use is a way of controlling the pain that's so unbearable.

As Davis notes, "It's preferable to be high, stoned, or drunk than to think that nobody loves you."

Which mood-altering substance or activity people use is partly dependent on what's available in their neighborhoods and on the typical ways people hide in that particular culture.

"For privileged white men, it's workaholism and money and status, along with drugs, very often," Kasl said. "That's what they are taught."

In an inner-city neighborhood, people would have easier access to hard drugs. In the suburbs, women might use food or alcohol to alter their moods.

Abuse, particularly sexual abuse, is a setup for drug addiction.

People use drugs compulsively, Springer believes, when they feel a great deal of pain.

"When I was a kid experimenting, I went to the feel-good drugs, psychedelics, marijuana," Springer recalls. "When I was full of pain, I wouldn't touch a psychedelic. I didn't want my consciousness expanded. I wanted to be closed down. I went for the heroin."

When crack hit the inner cities, women could cop it on their own rather than waiting for men to bring it to them. If need be, they could sell themselves for it. Crack gave a mega-hit. For a moment, it made the woman feel powerful, in control, surrounded by a bubble of protection. It was a lie, Rivera says.

After serving in the U.S. Army and working as an apprentice mortician, Rivera had, through a companion, tried heroin, been addicted to it for eight months, then entered a methadone program for another eight months. While detoxing in the fall of 1985, an acquaintance from her methadone group had taken her to a crack house in Queens, one of the first in the country. The crack alleviated the withdrawal symptoms she was experiencing.

Unlike heroin, which was a depressant, crack was a sexual stimulant—at least for men. Women began using crack partly because men, thinking women liked cocaine, would give it to them to make the women more available to them sexually.

Crack dealers, who were almost exclusively male, used crack's sexually stimulating quality as a key selling point to new male customers. Its lure for male teenagers was of a spectacular sexual experience and the ultimate orgasm. For women, Rivera said, sexual pleasure was often the last thing on their minds. They wanted that sensation of power induced by the drug. Sex was a tool they sometimes used to get the drug; the drug was a tool they used to make the sex endurable.

With crack, men developed a new, particularly degrading form of prostitution for women.

"Drug dealers eager to bring in new clients may promise a woman along with the drug," Dr. Mary E. Guinan of the CDC wrote. "Women crack addicts are sometimes kept at crack houses and given the drug in exchange for sex with the dealers or clients. The women become virtual slaves to both the drug and the dealers."[7]

Men would give crack to women in exchange for the performance of sexual stunts. It's called "tossing." The woman who exchanges sex acts for crack is a "toss-up"—an object to be exploited, used up, and "tossed" away. Rivera called the stunts women were called upon to perform a "side show." The men would have a woman perform sex acts with a dog as they all watched. Or they would instruct a woman to perform oral sex on all the men in the room. Or they would gang-bang. The women were there at their disposal, Rivera said. The men could do whatever they liked.

Sometimes women would be in the crack house smoking non-stop for days, Rivera said.

"When your stuff ran out, you had to think really fast how you were going to get your next hit," she said. "So you were enslaved. Once you started selling everything and everything was gone, what's left? Your body."

In the most depressed areas of Oakland, California, young women were going door to door offering sex to pay for their crack, researchers were told.[8]

Psychologist Kasl has worked extensively with women in prostitution.

"The shame in coming out of prostitution is so profound," she comments. "The annihilation of spirit and of self—we should all grieve, as a society, that anybody has to go through that kind of pain. We get righteous about some hostages in Lebanon and whether they were tortured, but women are getting tortured every day."

Crack combined with sex-for-barter led to a rise, particularly and disproportionately in young women, in sexually transmitted diseases—syphilis and gonorrhea. These diseases plowed fertile ground for the planting of HIV. Syphilis had been found to be a cofactor in facilitating the transmission of the AIDS virus during intercourse.

The answer to how some women are getting AIDS is intimately bound up with the sexual abuse of women and with the notion that sexual access to women's bodies is a male birthright, Dr. Janice Raymond, professor of women's studies at the University of Massachusetts, said in an interview. It is always placed in the background of any discussion of AIDS or ignored completely. Until it is pushed to the foreground and addressed, she argued, AIDS cannot be prevented in women. The strategy of preventing AIDS is intrinsically linked with the strategy of preventing sexual abuse and abusive sexual access to women.

One begins to see the outlines of a cycle: A female is sexually assaulted. She uses a drug to numb the pain of that experience. To procure the drug, she submits to further sexual degradation and humiliation. Now an even greater pain requiring anesthesia throbs within her.

The attacks, through abuse, on a woman's spirit, on her self-esteem, on her very capacity for developing an ego, an identity, a self, a sense of "I am," plow the ground for drug addiction. This, in turn, creates an environment ripe for HIV infection.

Helen Cover's mother was a heroin addict from New York City. Her father, also an addict, left for Georgia soon after her birth. When Helen was two months old, her mother could no longer care for her or her three sisters. They were sent to relatives in North Carolina.

Abused and beaten there, the girls were taken in by other, kind relatives.

When Cover was six, her paternal grandmother, who had been looking for the girls for years, finally found them and brought them back to New York. Her father, dying of cancer, came to live with them.

The next year, the grandmother became too ill to care for the four girls. They were sent to a children's home. Two years later, Cover's young mother died a drug-related death.

At sixteen, Cover, pregnant by another teenage resident of the children's home, was thrown out. Her boyfriend abandoned her. She returned to her grandmother. A year later, she and her baby daughter moved to Boston, where one of her sisters lived. Cover thought she was in love again. But the man was a drug dealer who encouraged her to inject cocaine, beat her, and tried to force her into prostitution.

Her grandmother rescued her again, sending her money to come home. Back in New York City, she got off drugs, got a job as an executive secretary, and returned to school.

But she didn't want to raise her daughter in the rough city. Remembering Syracuse from summer visits through the Fresh Air program for inner-city children, she moved there.[9]

She wanted something from life and Syracuse was where she was going to get it. She knew she had to work for it. In the early 1980s, she completed a nurses'-aide program at Sidney Johnson Vocational Center.

Mario Tomasetti, the center administrator, respected her. As he saw it, she was a personable woman who, through nursing, hoped to make a better life for herself and her child. Her dedication was admirable. In training, she would stop in the room of a young man comatose from an automobile accident, hum music, and talk to him. One day Helen Cover noticed the man move a finger and informed her supervisor and the other staff. When the young man came out of the coma, Tomasetti thought Cover's care had a lot to do with it.

Life was good for Helen. She was successful in school and once again she was in love.

In the fall of 1986, she enrolled at Onondaga Community College and had finished one semester when her boyfriend Tim decided to go to school in North Carolina. Pregnant, she didn't want to be left behind.

Love ended her college days. She followed Tim. When they couldn't make it financially in North Carolina, they moved to New Jersey to live with her sister. Her sister's boyfriend was on cocaine. Cover tried it; it hooked her.

She had one bout of drinking and drugging that got her so sick she had to be hospitalized. A doctor, apparently alert to the possibility of AIDS in drug users, tested her blood. One morning he broke the news to her: she had the virus that appeared to cause AIDS.

She felt stripped of everything. She had no future. Her life would be over before she got something out of it.

Marilyn (T.J.) Rivera, smoking crack for two weeks almost nonstop, had exhausted all her assets, burned all her bridges. She had, since getting hooked on the new drug, moved from a house to an apartment, and finally to a room. She had panhandled, turned tricks, and now, her mind scurrying to find other ways to get money, she decided to rob.

She put two sets of clothes on a body withered into thinness. She went out, planning to shed the first set of clothing as she made her getaway from the crime scene. Near Columbia University in Manhattan, she saw an old woman leave a supermarket. One hand held a grocery bag. From the other swung a beige pocketbook.

T.J. walked behind and grabbed the bag. The old woman was strong and held on. T.J. yanked the bag, hurling the woman into a telephone booth on the corner, and ran. A crowd ran after her. As she raced down Riverside Drive, adrenaline surging, her mind played her a video. It showed her her dead body lying on an embalming table and, in the next scene, her corpse under the earth in a grave. She was terrified. She knew that if she did not stop, she would die. She would kill herself or kill someone else.

She stopped running. For a minute, she stood alone on Riverside Drive, waiting for her pursuers. Then the crowd caught up with her. Still terrified, her instincts took over and she tried to persuade the people to let her go. She was on parole; give her a chance, she pleaded. She was so convincing they were on the point of doing so when someone escorted the old woman through the crowd to her side.

The woman's face was bloody. An eight-inch gash ran over her eye. T.J. had not realized how elderly she was.

"I'm sorry," she said to the woman, stricken.

"Honey," the woman said, "if you had just asked me to help, I would have."

T.J. sobbed.

She no longer pleaded to be let go. The police arrested her. The judge gave her three to six years in the maximum-security Bedford Hills Correctional Facility.

There was a lot for T.J. Rivera to get used to in prison: the constant banging of the doors and jiggling of keys, the screaming, the never-ending voices, the lack of privacy. More than that, she was now in the company of big-time criminals: Kathy Boudin and Judy Clark, convicted of the 1981 Brinks robbery in Nyack, New York.

Both Boudin and Clark had been in the leftist Weathermen. Boudin had gone underground in 1970, after an explosion in the basement of a Greenwich Village townhouse that she and other radicals had converted into a bomb factory. Three Weatherpeople were killed in the explosion. Boudin and one other woman escaped with their lives. Beginning in 1974, underground fugitives began surfacing one by one. Before the Brinks robbery in which a guard and two police officers were killed, Kathy Boudin had been the most prominent political fugitive still at large. She had been on the FBI's "Most Wanted" list.[10]

"Wow!" Rivera thought when she heard that Boudin and Clark

were inmates, too. "I'm in here with some real live criminals! They're notorious! You have to be a heavyweight to go through something like that Brinks robbery."

But when she actually met Boudin and found her gentle and soft-spoken, she was astonished.

"She's a pussycat!" Rivera thought.

A small, slight, dark-haired woman with deep-set brown eyes, Kathy Boudin had had more than twenty years' experience as a political activist and organizer. While a sophomore at Bryn Mawr College, she had helped organize African-American janitors and maids on campus. After graduating magna cum laude, she'd worked four years in Cleveland with welfare mothers. Now she was serving twenty years to life for second-degree murder and first-degree robbery.

Judy Clark, also of slight build with short, dark curly hair, was an equally experienced organizer, intelligent and articulate. She had been sentenced to life imprisonment.

Rivera respected Boudin and Clark for their commitment to the liberation of African-American and Hispanic people, but, as she first began talking with them, she was wary, concerned that they would try to influence her into accepting armed struggle.

"Listen," she told Boudin straight off. "I'm not with that shit."

But Boudin never tried to brainwash her, she felt. They just talked. When T.J. told Boudin that her father had been a founder of the Puerto Rican Day Parade in New York City, Boudin made her realize for the first time the importance of his work and the political legacy he had left her. T.J. felt proud of him.

Boudin and another prisoner, Luce, encouraged her to write and paint. Rivera read plays and then wrote one. She taught herself to sketch, drew cartoons, and later experimented with oil painting. (Birds always appeared in her paintings, the same birds that came to her in dreams and, with the wind under their wings, promised her freedom from prison.) Boudin lent T.J. her guitar and taught her three chords. Rivera, who had always sung, began composing songs, all written in those three chords. To her, Boudin had become her "white dove sister."

The women talked for hours. One of the things they talked about was the panic over AIDS rampant in the prison. Despite earlier informal educational efforts, they were now seeing the panic spread and poison relationships among the women. The problem had to be named: they were living in terror and in ignorance of a fatal, communicable disease. They had to do something. They met with a few other women to talk about the problem: Diane Gouch (a woman whose gift for writing would soon become invaluable to them), Mohammed Arleen, and Rosie Barbott.

It was a relief to put their fears into words. There had been mean and frightened whispers in corners. Everyone had felt the terror but no one had talked about it. Now, at least in this small group, it was out in the open.

They wrote a letter to Superintendent Elaine Lord: AIDS is clearly becoming a reality in here. We don't know anything. We need education and we need to know what the prison policy is. We believe that as peers we would be the most effective in AIDS education, counseling, and building a community of support. Our goals are: to save lives through preventing the spread of HIV; to create more humane conditions for those suffering HIV-related problems; to support and educate women with fears, questions, and needs related to AIDS; to build bridges to outside community groups so women reentering the community will have support.

Lord invited the women to meet with her. She accepted their proposal for an organization they would later name ACE (AIDS Counseling and Education Program). They agreed that they didn't want to live in a community where fear reigned and some were stigmatized. They had valued the earlier efforts to challenge the stigmatization—Sonia Perez leaving IPC to rejoin the lawn crew—but now a sustained program was called for. Women needed information on AIDS. They began searching for it. Inmates in the general prison population could visit and befriend women with AIDS in IPC, they also agreed.

Despite their worries, women began visiting their friends in IPC whom they had not visited out of fear that they, too, would be stigmatized. Each woman would "patch herself up" to a particular woman with AIDS, visit regularly to feed her, bathe her, give her massages, read to her, take her out on strolls, talk—about their children, their childhoods, their former lives on the street, their fears.

To make the place look cheerful, some women painted IPC and hung bright curtains.

Women began to listen to one another, began to ask, "How can I help?"

All this, they later understood, was building community. But they did not understand at the time that that was what they were doing.

Boudin was teaching vocabulary and spelling in a basic education program for prison women with no or minimal literacy. She chose AIDS as the key issue and, in her project, the women learned and discussed AIDS-related words like "immunology." Out of that project, the students decided to produce a play in which the women's concerns about AIDS would be played out in scenes in the yard, the mess hall, and the visiting room with the family.

These were inmates who did not read. But they wrote the script and learned to read and memorize it. The play was a hit.

In their organizing efforts, the ACE core group both loved and hated Superintendent Lord. She was their sister in struggle. They knew they would never be able to organize if she did not allow it. They knew that officials in male prisons had transferred out inmates who tried to develop AIDS education for their prison mates, saying, "Docs will handle this."

They knew that if Lord had not supported them, they would have been transferred. They had seen her sitting with Sonia Perez at the picnic table, acting as a role model. They knew that at a conference of prison superintendents, other superintendents had shot darts at her for allowing ACE. They admired her for standing firm under attack. That she was willing to struggle with them made them feel bonded with her. Knowing that she had put her trust in them and was taking risks for them, they felt they had to prove she had not misplaced her trust.

But Lord was also their warden. She was their keeper, their guard. She made or enforced the rules they were compelled to live by. She controlled their lives, their movements, what they wore on their bodies. She was both a sister in struggle and keeper of the prison keys.

One inmate later referred to the intrinsic contradiction in a program that empowered women who were locked inside a prison. She called it "empowerment on a leash."

Penny Abernathey, twenty-four, the daughter of an Episcopal priest and a third-grade teacher in Austin, Texas, attended nursing school for two and a half years, left, and became a secretary. She began dating Mark Knox, a thirty-year-old car mechanic, in 1983.

As the two came to know each other better, he confessed that he had shot drugs a few years back.

"Okay, so you did drugs," Penny said. "Big deal. Let's just go on with our lives."

They married in 1984. On weekends, they camped in the country. Penny bicycled as often as she could. She had traveled to seven states on her bicycle, pedaling up to eighty-five miles a day. Mark raced motorcross. Penny loved watching him: on a dirt track on his springing motorcycle, he'd fly into the air off a big hill, land hard, jump, turn sharp. It was fun.

In 1986, Penny delivered their son, James. When he was hospitalized at seven months old with a minor bone infection, Penny and Mark, spending nineteen days in the hospital, watched a lot of television, an unusual activity for them since they spent most leisure time outdoors. They saw several specials about AIDS, each, at various times, murmuring, "Oh, those poor homosexuals!"

Six weeks later, Mark came down with pneumonia. In the hospital, physicians told him the pneumonia was PCP and he had AIDS. Penny and baby James had better be tested, they said. The baby tested negative, but Penny was infected. Eleven days after Mark's diagnosis, on December 7, he died.

Penny was stunned. It had never, ever entered her head that Mark could have been exposed to AIDS through his drug use. In those television specials, the people with AIDS had been almost all gay men. She had never seen a woman with AIDS on television. Now she, a *woman*, was infected!

Later she thought, "If I had seen a woman on television like me saying, 'My husband died in eleven days because of something he did years before I married him and now I have the virus,' maybe I would have looked at Mark and said, 'Hey, bud, we need to get tested.'"

1987

For the second time since 1982, CDC changed the AIDS surveillance definition used to track the epidemic. Overnight, many more women had AIDS. The proportion of women diagnosed with AIDS shot up 39 percent in 1987. The illnesses HIV-infected women were getting had not changed, only the way CDC classified information about those illnesses.

In 1983, 162 women made it into the official AIDS case count. In 1987 there were 2,569. The proportion of women who were reportedly infected through intercourse with men jumped to 30 percent, up from 12 percent in 1982.

Epidemiologist Dr. Judith Cohen had had problems with the CDC's definition of AIDS early on. It was a politically arbitrary set of definitions, she believed.

In 1982 the conditions included in the AIDS definition were those appearing in predominantly gay white men. In this new 1987 definition, conditions appearing exclusively in HIV-infected children were added. Cohen, director of AWARE (Association of Women's AIDS Research and Education), believed this was because child welfare organizations had lobbied for attention to children with AIDS. Even though pediatric AIDS was becoming a reflection of AIDS in women, conditions appearing exclusively in women were still excluded from the definition.

To determine what conditions to add to the definition in 1987, CDC had followed the same procedure it had used to define AIDS symptoms in gay men. It had gathered together physicians who were treating children with AIDS, along with other experts, and asked them what they were seeing.

With this revision, CDC also added HIV wasting syndrome, HIV dementia, and certain lymphomas (tumors of lymphoid tissue) to the definition. The 1987 definition change now allowed physicians to "presumptively" diagnose AIDS in HIV-infected people who showed symptoms of certain conditions. That meant physicians no longer had to order the expensive laboratory tests that would prove the presence of those conditions.[1]

Adding a few new symptoms and diseases and the presumptive diagnosis resulted in many new AIDS cases among women, blacks, Latinos, and IV drug users, and a significant rise overall in reported AIDS cases. Before the 1987 revision, 67 percent of the AIDS cases meeting the CDC definition were in homosexual or bisexual men and 23 percent in IV drug users. In the first year following the new revision, the percentage of people with AIDS who were IV drug users shot up from 23 to 43 percent; who were blacks, from 24 to 36 percent; Hispanics, from 13 to 16 percent; and women, from 2.6 to 3.6 percent.[2]

"Compared with patients who meet the pre-1987 definition, a higher proportion of patients who meet only the 1987 definition were female, black, or Hispanic or were intravenous drug users," the CDC itself noted in its August 1990 HIV/AIDS surveillance report.

Yet many conditions appearing in drug users and in women were left out of the revised definition. The physicians seeing the disease in drug users were in no position to document their observations. They were overworked residents or emergency room docs in public hospitals. They had no time to write up their observations for medical journals or consult for the CDC. Nor did they have the expertise or staff to collect essential information or write sophisticated grant proposals to fund research on their populations. Unquestionably, some of the people with AIDS they saw were women. These women were never counted.

If a woman staggered into an emergency room with really bad pneumonia, Judith Cohen knew, no one would suspect that woman had AIDS. She would just be a poor woman, in lousy shape, more susceptible to pneumonia than the middle class.

Because women were not expected to have AIDS, similar symptoms in both women and men were interpreted and treated differently. In one study in Los Angeles, researchers looked back at the records of every HIV-infected person who was in the hospital with PCP and in the Intensive Care Unit. What had happened, they found, was that when women came to the emergency room to be treated, they were being told they had upper respiratory tract infections and sent away. Sometimes men were told that, but more of the men were being admitted for pneumonia and PCP. The outcome of this failure to recognize AIDS in women was that many more of the women than the men experienced respiratory failure, ended up in the intensive care unit, and died.[3]

In San Francisco, Connie Wofsy and Judith Cohen were seeing a range of symptoms in women that concerned them. At scientific meetings on AIDS, they talked about them with other physicians and researchers who had similar concerns even before 1987.

Pediatrician friends of Cohen had told her they had treated babies clearly sick with HIV but not classified by CDC as HIV cases because the children had childhood, not adult, illnesses. Adults don't get otitis media, inflammation of the middle ear. Kids do.

It's not the individual disease or diagnosis that's the issue, Cohen thought impatiently. It's the fact that whatever that disease is, it doesn't respond to treatment; it progresses aggressively, and returns the minute you stop treating it. It's a matter of what that condition ordinarily is versus what it is when the person's immune system is compromised. None of those things were part of the CDC list.

When you questioned CDC officials on this, they responded: our classification only includes serious, life-threatening diseases. Well, Cohen thought, it just was not true. Kaposi's sarcoma was on the list. When people (almost exclusively male) were diagnosed with it, they might have a couple of spots. That was hardly life-threatening.

If CDC opened the definition up still more to include AIDS symptoms in women, Cohen was convinced, the number of women with AIDS would shoot up still higher.

The way CDC was tracking AIDS, feminist activists believed, was guaranteed to keep the number of AIDS cases lower. Bar women's

AIDS symptoms from the AIDS definition and you have a manageable epidemic. Include the symptoms of women and drug users, and you've got a disaster.

Authorities at Albion prison transferred Katrina Haslip to Bedford Hills January 3 as a disciplinary action. Segregated in a small cell in the Separate Housing Unit (SHU). Katrina was allowed out only for a shower and a recreation period. In SHU she met political activist Judy Clark and, through her, Kathy Boudin.

On a bitter cold February day, Linda Lofredo from the New York State Division for Women went to visit a pediatric AIDS units at Einstein Hospital in New York City. The social worker who accompanied her introduced her to the women standing by the beds of the sick babies. Most were grandmothers. Their daughters had already died of AIDS.

One grandmother told her with quiet dignity: "It's tragic. It's horrible. I'm sick about losing my child. But the thing I can't cope with as I care for her baby is that I live in a walk-up apartment and there's no heat or hot water."

Helen Cover, twenty-five, returned to Syracuse from New Jersey. Her HIV infection had become full-blown AIDS. She gave up her aspirations and returned to injecting drugs. High one March day, she fought with a woman in her apartment house over a radio. Helen picked up a bottle, smashed it, and cut the woman with the broken glass.

Police arrested her.

Maxine Wolfe saw a man selling "Silence = Death" T-shirts at the Lesbian and Gay Pride March in New York City in March. Just the week before, a friend had told her an AIDS activist group was forming and here was someone from that group.

She approached him: "Are there women in your group?"

"Sure," he said.

The next evening, Maxine Wolfe sat in a meeting of several hundred men and four women at the Lesbian and Gay Community Center.

With thirty years of political activism in leftist, feminist, and lesbian groups, Wolfe had not found a political home for several years. The groups she had worked with earlier had been unwilling to reach outside their known constituencies, she felt. Their rigid politics could not be questioned without making oneself suspect.

Now, in March, a group of largely white, upper-middle-class gay men were forming ACT UP, the AIDS Coalition to Unleash Power, "to hold the government publicly accountable for the genocide it has perpetrated on our community and others," as one of its leaflets explained. "We believe the government failed to act swiftly and effectively against AIDS because it was seen as a disease of expendable minorities: gay men, IV drug users, and people of color." ACT UP would fight against official indifference and ineptitude and "bear witness to the criminal negligence that has devastated our community. We do so through direct action."

Wolfe was impressed with the activists in ACT UP. They focused on ending the AIDS crisis, period, and would listen to anyone with a good idea. As ACT UP developed, Maxine and the handful of other women involved began holding a series of "dyke dinners" to build a support system for themselves within an organization so predominantly male.

The issue of women in AIDS drug trials came up early at these dinners. Federal money had been allocated for AIDS clinical trials and what subsequently became the AIDS Clinical Trials Groups (ACTGs) in 1987. Ten thousand people were supposed to be enrolled in the first year. When only eight hundred were, ACT UP protested. The women began to look at who was actually getting into the trials. As their investigations continued over the years, they became increasingly savvy about the more subtle barriers to women's participation. They found these obstacles:

• The requirement that participants have a private physician excluded the majority of women with HIV/AIDS who, for lack of money, use public health facilities.

• Both the Food and Drug Administration (FDA) and National Institute for Allergy and Infectious Diseases (NIAID) guidelines for clinical trials excluded women of "child-bearing age" from any trial unless they could provide definitive proof of an "adequate" contraceptive, often judged to be the IUD or the Pill. The IUD can set up an infection that may be life-threatening if the women are immunosuppressed, the activists noted, and no one knew how the Pill interacted with HIV. While condoms and diaphragms posed no health risks to women, they were not being promoted.

Why? As Wolfe deduced, they didn't think most women were smart enough to use them routinely.

In certain drug trials, the few women included were tested every month and dropped from the trial if found pregnant, they learned.

• Decisions on where to locate the trials effectively kept women out. The highest caseloads of HIV infection among women were in Newark, New Jersey, and Brooklyn, New York. Federal planners ignored both cities as trial sites.

• Drug trials were set up in ways that were convenient for the researchers but had nothing to do with how women live their lives. No child care or transportation was provided. A participant might have to be in the hospital for a few days, and there were no child care provisions for those days. Testing was scheduled without consideration for school hours and dinner times.

• One criterion for trial participation—the necessary level of liver functioning a participant had to have—could eliminate women. About half the women in New York who had AIDS or HIV had gotten it through intravenous drug use, a practice that often impairs the liver.[4]

When a clinic signs a contract with NIAID to be one of NIAID's clinical sites, it has to state that it will provide certain kinds of professionals on its team and certain kinds of services. NIAID did not require that anyone on the team be a gynecologist. The few women who did make it into the trials were simply examined according to the male model. Pelvic exams were not performed on them. So researchers did not learn such facts as, for example, this: if the woman started out with a pelvic infection, did it get worse or better after AZT was administered?

Since so few women were enrolled in ACTGs, the ACT UP

activists argued after their investigation, no treatments for HIV-related infections were adequately tested for women. Symptoms, dosages, and side effects unique to women remained unstudied and unknown.

The women were angry. It was June, and the Third International Conference on AIDS was being held in Washington, D.C. With its emphasis on women as "vessels of infection [for men] and vectors of perinatal transmission [to fetuses]," the five-day conference left the impression that women are "almost an invisible pass-through," Dr. Constance Wofsy told *Medical World News* reporter Pat Thomas. "Very little addressed women as the human beings they are, what happens in their lives, or how their choices about childbearing are affected. What little attention has been given to women affected by HIV has been inappropriate, offensive, and a perpetuation of negative stereotypes."

A spontaneous committee of women wrote and distributed an open letter to conference planners during the business meeting. Only nineteen of approximately 370 speakers (5 percent) touched on women and AIDS. Eight discussed heterosexual transmission, four speakers spoke of prostitutes as vectors of disease, and seven speakers of women as infectors of infants. There were more scientific papers and panel presentations on blood transmission of AIDS, which represented only 3 percent of AIDS cases, than on women, who accounted for 7 percent. And this, despite the fact that the number of blood cases was dwindling while women were the fastest-growing group of U.S. AIDS patients.[5]

Dr. June Osbourne, dean of the School of Public Health at the University of Michigan, delivering a closing speech at the conference, read the women's statement to the entire conference. For Katy Taylor, sitting in the audience, this was the first time women had been mentioned in the AIDS epidemic in anything other than a vessel/vector role.

Solemn presentations at scientific conferences on AIDS like the one in Washington, D.C., made it appear that prostitutes were spreading HIV to innocent men. So did headlines in some city newspapers ("AIDS Hooker Is Back in Jail").

Was this true? Let's take another look.

In the United States, no federal agency can present research showing large numbers of men whose HIV infection can be traced to prostitution. Many studies, including one conducted by the CDC in seven different sites around the country, suggest that HIV rates in women in prostitution are about the same as in other women not in prostitution in the same geographic area. As the Center for Women Policy Studies points out: Almost all prostitute-john encounters are single episodes, and the likelihood of female-to-male transmission in a single encounter is remote. Most such encounters involve oral, not vaginal, sex. The risk of HIV transmission to the male in oral sex is extremely low.[6]

But are men who use women in systems of prostitution endangering them by infecting them with HIV? This never became a hot question—either at solemn scientific congresses or in bold newspaper headlines.

In the United States, there is no evidence of high rates of HIV among prostitutes. Yet on a worldwide basis, AIDS is certainly a danger to women in prostitution. In Thailand, where sex tours by foreign males are a major source of the country's tourism income and of foreign exchange, the increase in HIV infection among prostitutes rose from 3.5 percent in 1989 to 10 percent in 1990.

The sprouting of an enormous commercial sex industry selling impoverished women to wealthier Westerners, Japanese, and Arabs puts Asian women at risk of AIDS. The sex industry emerged in the mid- to late 1960s when it served American military men on five- to seven-day R&Rs (rest and recreation leaves) from Vietnam. Thai women, considered the property of the father or head of household, were often delivered to the sex industry to relieve the debts of a poorer, typically rural family. The sex industry expanded in the mid-1970s when chartered jets flew European, American, Japanese, and Middle Eastern men into Bangkok for sex tours. Most tours offered the use of Thai women. Far fewer, Thai men. (About 10 percent of prostitutes in Thailand are male.)

As an official from the United Thai Council of North America explains it, some homosexual and bisexual Thai men are sexually used by Western male tourists in a sugar daddy/sugar baby process. Seen by Westerners as gentle and compliant (i.e., submissive), men of such countries as Thailand, Laos, and the Philippines became, in the 1970s, the exotic, the preferred sexual object.

In Thailand these male "sugar babies" often have girlfriends and the girlfriends may be being used by, for example, German business-men traveling on sex tours. Or the male sugar babies are married.[7]

Because of the strong elevation of sons and devaluation of daughters common to many Asian cultures, the male sugar babies—both homosexual and bisexual—are pressured to marry, produce children, and become proper patriarchal heads of household.

Thai women are endangered with HIV infection both directly by Western men (and some Asians and Arabs) on sex tours and through the Thai men who marry them after or while being sexually used by foreign men.[8]

They are also endangered by the Thai tradition of widespread male use of women in prostitution. Dr. Janice Raymond, international coordinator of the Coalition Against Trafficking in Women, reports these facts gathered by the Thai Ministry of Public Health in its efforts to deal with the AIDS epidemic: There are half a million women and children in prostitution in Thailand. Most Thai men—75 percent—have been to brothels. Every young male is expected to be sexually initiated through the use of prostitutes, and by age sixteen, almost half of all Thai boys have been to prostitutes. Under the custom of Ruen-pee at Thai universities, upperclassmen take undergraduates to brothels and buy women for them. With 450,000 Thai men visiting prostitutes every year and most objecting to the use of condoms (59 percent of Thai men say they have never used them), men are spreading sexually transmitted diseases to their wives and lovers.

So the beliefs of Thai men that it is their right to have access to sex at cheap prices, that they themselves bear no responsibility in the prevention of STDs, and that they have the right to forgo condoms in their sexual use of women place women in danger of AIDS.

The danger men subject women to in prostitution is clear in other countries as well. For example, among Central African prostitutes, the HIV-positive rate ranges from 55 to 80 percent; among those of the Ivory Coast, 32.8 percent. Among those in Bombay, India, the rate is up to 70 percent.[9]

Prostitution is dangerous for women—much more so than for male users. Women have a ten-times greater chance of being infected by a man through intercourse than a man has of being infected by a women, as Dr. Helen Rodriquez, medical director of the New York States AIDS Institute from 1988 through 1989, said in a 1991 interview. But male researchers and government and military officials have stood the facts on their head. Dr. June Osbourne, as chair of the U.S. National Commission on AIDS, referred to a time in the epidemic when AIDS and HIV were virtually unrepresented in the Philippines, except for two gay men out of several hundred tested, and forty-nine women. All forty-nine of the women with AIDS in the Philippines were bar girls in the immediate vicinity of the U.S. military base.

"I was still trying to absorb the import of those numbers," Osbourne told an audience in 1991, "and was wondering what kind of outraged response the Philippine government would have to such importation [of AIDS], when I learned that the U.S. military had substituted a good offense as the best defense, accusing those bar girls of putting Americans at risk and demanding that they be incarcerated, or at least moved far away from the bases."[10]

In the face of the savage harm prostitution does women, many defend the institution as a "career choice," unjustly stigmatized, that some women freely make. When radical feminists name prostitution as an institution oppressing women, as a cornerstone of patriarchy, this is often misrepresented as an attack on and defamation of the women themselves, as a repressive, prudish, "antisex" stand.

But these critics of radical feminists themselves do not rail against economic sexism and sexual harassment in the workplace that keep women's income and position on the employment hierarchy low, thereby ensuring a steady stream of women who will "choose" prostitution. (Equal pay for equal work, which we still do not have, is a *radical* demand, as feminist Andrea Dworkin long ago made clear.) Instead, these defenders of prostitution present prostitution as simply a job like any other, the women as "sex workers" in the labor force.

In a powerful refutation of prostitution as "choice," Jane Anthony, now a novelist and formerly a full-time prostitute, writes of "the psychic trauma that grows from having one's most private self routinely entered by one stranger after the next, day after day, week after week," and of the "ghost of prostitution" she still lives with years later in her most vulnerable moments: "the sense of being non-human."[11]

What is the consequence of the upside-down framing of the public discussion on HIV and prostitution? Focusing on women as prostitutes vectoring disease in what Sandra Elkin calls "prurient research" has helped create the dangerous myth that only flagrantly "promiscuous" women are at risk of AIDS.[12] One result of the dangerous myth is that early in the epidemic, U.S. women who were not in prostitution and not using drugs tended to believe that as long as they weren't having intercourse with numerous men a day, they were safe.

But "faithful" women are not safe. As physicians treating women with AIDS point out, many of the women are like Gladys Thompson: homemakers; the working poor; women whose partners' drug injection or sex practices—not their own—have been the source of HIV transmission.

As a Rhode Island study would find in 1990, the median number of lifetime sexual partners of the women infected with HIV heterosexually was only three.

The data from Puerto Rico, where women are hard hit by the epidemic, shows that infected women, by and large and more so with time, do not fall into the category of "women with multiple sex partners."[13] Many of the women had only one partner. But that one partner was infected. That one partner was enough, since numerous sexual encounters with him were involved.

The slogan "faithfulness, abstinence, and celibacy" has been promoted worldwide as an AIDS-prevention strategy for women, implying that the women who get infected have had large numbers of sexual partners. But such admonitions are inapplicable to infection prevention in women, as Australian AIDS expert Elizabeth Reid points out:

"At the current stage of the epidemic [in 1991], it can be estimated that each day now, 1,500 faithful women [worldwide] are infected. That is, every day, just now, there are 1,500 women who have no sexual partners other than their husbands who are becoming infected. This number will increase as the number of infected men increases."

Preliminary data from African studies indicates that 60 to 80 percent of all HIV-infected women have one and only one sexual partner, Reid notes.

That such advice as "faithfulness, abstinence, and celibacy" can actually *be* the AIDS education offered to women in many parts of the world is one of those "Wake up!" slaps on the cheek that force women to face our actual status in the world. Male assaults on females have not become a hot topic at international AIDS conferences or one boldly headlined in newspapers. Yet for the large numbers of women and young girls assaulted in rape and incest, "faithfulness, abstinence, and celibacy" is an irrelevant admonition, Reid notes. When violence is the transmission mode, women have no power to bring about "abstinence."

As the situation in Thailand shows and as the worldwide statistics on sexual subordination of and assaults on females demonstrate, power differentials are critical factors in the spread of HIV. Social justice protects public health. In contrast, male supremacy provides the wings on which the human immunodeficiency virus flies around the world.

The Women and AIDS Resource Network (WARN) had no office. But it did have a telephone number listed in various publications. The number was transferred day by day to the homes of the various WARN organizers who took turns handling the calls that poured in.

One woman called from Washington State to get information to relay to her HIV-infected daughter. The daughter lived close by WARN in New York but because of the HIV stigma, she was afraid to call for the information herself.

One young woman, infected with HIV, traveled to New York from Canada, where all AIDS-related services near her were geared to gay men. She spent six hours with WARN director Marie St. Cyr discussing grief, dying, anger, and whether it was still possible for her to have a sexual life. She had no one else to talk with.

To be so sharply confronted with such great need from women was traumatic for St. Cyr. In her native Haiti, women survived as best they could in a society molded for men. Arriving in the United States as a teenager, she had thought that here, at least, women got a fair shake. Her parents could not send their seven daughters through college, but each struggled and did it herself. So St. Cyr had felt: Women have a chance here. Here, women are not downtrodden.

The onslaught of the AIDS crisis, however, dramatically revealed that no matter what strides they were making, women were considered second-class citizens.

This was the stark reality, St. Cyr realized. As she figured it, we knew that AIDS was transmitted sexually. We knew about bisexuality. We knew about IV drug transmission. So we knew women would be infected. But there was no notion of doing something about it. None. There was no planning for women at all.

When the small group of women started WARN, they thought they would have money to run it, for there was hardly another organization providing services to women. But it was very difficult to get funding. While St. Cyr felt grateful to the van Ameringen Foundation for its support, few others leaped to WARN's aid. WARN would get $30,000 here and $20,000 there, but service was costly and that money did not go far.

Route 26 in rural Maine winds past white picket fences, moss-capped tombstones in cemeteries, lots filled with trailers, antique shops, fairgrounds, a trailer housing Milly's Hair Design, flimsy two-story houses with sagging porches and dying sheds.

Off Route 26, American flags wave from poles in front of one-room white post offices. Gray, Poland Springs, Falmouth, Yarmouth, Cumberland—pretty little towns.

Off Route 26, dirt roads with muddy puddles creep into woods where rusting auto bodies park for eternity next to trailers.

School dances were sinful, her grandmother told Patricia Daugherty (a pseudonym) when she was growing up. Lipstick and nail polish, too. Shameful to dance with boys, to paint your lips, your nails. How to make sense, then, of Uncle Harry's penis rubbed between Patricia's legs when she was four, five, six. That didn't happen, her mother said. Besides, Patricia led him on. Patricia enticed him. Patricia was to blame and the fault was hers and she made it happen and how ashamed she was. But it didn't happen and she was a liar.

In country stores off Route 26, country music from the radio. Walls cluttered with mounted rifles, moose heads, pewter antiques. Grocery shelves of Wonder Bread, two-liter Coca-Cola bottles, and motor oil, twelve, thirteen different kinds, regular, super, outboard. The motor oil covers the length of two shelves.

Men in boots, oil-stained pants, flannel shirts over hard, protruding bellies, red and white visor caps, elastic on each side to stretch for big heads. The men buy lottery tickets, pick up the paper, drink coffee at the lunch counter. One injects sex into every word the scrawny, hard-muscled waitress says. She has back trouble, gets massages for it. From a man or a woman? the man asks, leering. Her face goes blank. He turns to the other men on stools. Goin' to be a big crackdown on welfare, he says. He's all for it. Can't tolerate these women on welfare. Too lazy to work. He never applied for unemployment once in his life and many's the time he's been out of work.

Off Route 26, Uncle Harry taking Patricia's dress off, grandmother walking into the barn, and Patricia, five, nude, and Uncle Harry with his pants down, and grandmother, so angry at Patricia, spanking her hard—nasty girl!—switching her legs as she marched her into the house. Shame on you! Shame!

Strict Irish Catholics. Patricia and her friends coloring their fingernails with red crayons and—quick!—scrape the red off before you got home, and Sunday Mass, Patricia and her two sisters in matching pink dresses and pocketbooks, petticoats, ribbons in hair, gloves, white socks, and black-patent-leather shoes. Patricia laughed in Mass and her aunt and the deacon's wife took her upstairs and questioned her to find out what was wrong with her. She laughed because the man was snoring and it was funny. Shame! Shame on you!

At home, Patricia told her mother, her father. She wanted Uncle Harry to stop. Her mother got mad and called her a liar and afterward Uncle Harry kept taking her to the barn, and at night, touching her in her room. She was afraid of night.

Patricia grew. Uncle Harry took her younger sisters to the barn, leaving her alone.

Happy times playing. Playing in the woods, on those three gray steps of the church. She climbed trees and heard her mother and aunt talking about her, how she moved her body like a boy. They were worried. Patricia, a tomboy.

Daddy had girlfriends and Mom knew. Patricia heard the talk between her aunts and Mom. Sometimes Mom would drive by the girlfriend's house to see if his truck was parked outside it.

When Patricia was fourteen, she telephoned the girlfriend and swore at her, spitting out every dirty swear word she ever heard, yelling she hated her and she hated her father, and her father, sitting right there with his girlfriend when Patricia called, jumped into his pickup truck, sped to the house, and yelled at Patricia's mother, indignant, How dare she?! What kind of a daughter was she raising? To do such a thing?!

Patricia wanted to study French but the guidance counselor at school didn't think it was a good idea. She took home economics as expected. She would get married when she graduated, she knew. Everyone knew. She was reared to be a mother.

It was a pretty good life. A princess life, really, she was so pretty and everyone told her so. She could have been a model, with that long, thick black hair, those high cheekbones, brown eyes. She was some beauty. She had good friends in school, had good times, and all in all, if you took it as a whole, her life was pretty much fine.

Soon as she got out of high school, in 1971, Patricia married her boyfriend John and had the first of her three sons. John took her to see porno flicks so often she got to feeling that's what people did—had supper, went to the porn flicks.

Patricia loved to talk and joke. Always had been high-spirited, popular at school. But once married, John'd damp her down when she was flying high in company.

"How could you act like that?" he'd say in the car driving home. "Stupid—like a silly dumb broad. God, you're so stupid sometimes!"

As the years went on—and there were pleasures in those years, moments with her three sons, though actually, she thought much later, she would not have had children if it had occurred to her that it was possible not to—as the years went on, she wanted to go to college.

"Oh, Patricia, you're so stupid," John said. "No way you could handle it. Besides, we don't have the money. And who'd take care of the kids?"

Fifteen years of marriage and John cutting her down in sarcastic remarks and with contemptuous faces and didn't anyone ever do anything besides watch porn flicks? He was always talking about sex and sex was in his looks at her and she didn't like things he did to her and sometimes he smacked her around and he was always threatening her—he'd kill her and the kids if she didn't—and sometimes thoughts of suicide comforted her but there were good times with friends and with her sons and, if you looked at it as a whole, she had a pretty good life, she thought.

She stopped going to Mass and joined a fundamentalist Christian church her physician introduced her to. Women couldn't speak in the service, only men. Patricia and the physician's daughter, Ida, started drinking martinis together in the afternoon—one day at Patricia's house, the next at Ida's. Then they started partying, going out to bars.

Patricia knew: she had to get out. Get away from John. She was scared. Martinis gave her courage. She was so brave when she was drinking, brave enough to stand up to her husband.

People in church started talking about her. Then they had a meeting and voted to shun her. They wouldn't talk to her anymore. She didn't go back to church. She felt ashamed.

Patricia drank but she didn't eat. She was too fat, too ugly. She had to be slim, had to be pretty. It was hard at first, not eating, but then she got used to it and it was nothing. She was never hungry. Once a day, she ate. Patricia Daugherty's purpose in life was to burn calories. From morning to night everything she did revolved around using up calories. Running, always moving. Her life was one sustained aerobic exercise. She got down to ninety-five pounds.

She stopped running only to drink. For courage. Pouring fire-courage martinis into her belly so she could act up, get out of line, walk out.

Then her niece Katy, her brother's child, five years old, complained that Uncle Harry was rubbing that thing between her legs. Katy's mother believed her, called the cops, brought in investigators and social workers. Patricia, now thirty-two, erupted in pain and anger. How many other little girls had he used in all the years since he'd taken her to the barn? Now she told the whole family what Uncle Harry had done to her. Katy must be telling the truth, she said; he'd done the same to her.

In twos and threes, Patricia's family came to see her in her kitchen. She was a liar, they told her. And Katy set poor Uncle Harry up. She was a sly one, that Katy. They would all go to court and testify for Harry.

Patricia, sinking, retracted, denied. No, Harry hadn't done anything to her. An investigator came and interviewed her. No, she told him. Uncle Harry couldn't have done those things to a child.

She drank more martinis. She watched her three sons begin to act toward her the way John did: she was one of those who cooked, cleaned, and served. Patricia drank, drank some more, felt the warm power of alcohol flow through her body. Then she did the unthinkable: she divorced. Drinking got her out of her marriage.

Somehow, through all the years, she knew: no matter the cost, she had to leave that marriage. Somehow, she knew she was not stupid. She knew she could go to college. She knew she could do something with her life.

She got herself a trailer and moved out with the kids. She got a good job as a dental assistant, got into therapy, started college at night. She looked in amazement at teenagers in college. All they had to do was study. What a piece of cake! Anyway, caring for three kids and studying in various stages of exhaustion, she got nearly all A's. So she *was* smart, after all. She loved being free of the porn flicks and John's daily put-downs.

But still, everyone she knew seemed to want her back where she had been and they let her know it. It was a hard time. She got through it by drinking.

John still scared her. He'd push his way into the trailer without knocking.

"We gotta talk," he said one day. "Get in the truck."

He drove ninety miles an hour down Route 26, shouting he was going to kill her as she screamed in terror. When she came to pick up the kids at his place after a weekend visit, he locked them all in his trailer and drove off. He continually threatened to kill her, the kids, and then himself. She believed him. So did they.

She called Maine's Child Protective Services and the man at the other end lambasted her: She'd divorced that poor man and caused all this. John was doing the best he could. There was nothing at all she could do to protect her children, he told her. She was responsible for it all.

Her parents were outraged that she'd left John. A woman endured anything to stay married.

"You've got three kids! What's the matter with you?"

Patricia had gone back to the Catholic Church after being

shunned by the fundamentalists. But now, divorced, she was too ashamed to go to Mass and face the priest and parishioners.

When she saw her family doctor, he asked her about her sex life. She answered. She was single. When her sons stayed over at their father's, she would go to a dance or a party or a bar, drink, joke, laugh. She had some one-night stands. She told him, felt him judging her, felt ashamed.

Her second son was getting bad grades. She went in to talk with the junior high guidance counselor.

"Well, you know the divorce has to be affecting him," the guidance counselor told her accusingly.

"Think about what you're doing to your kids," her friends urged her reproachfully.

Were her cheeks a perpetual red? She was shamed by her parents, her church, the school, her doctor, her friends. To avoid running into people she knew, she began shopping at night. *Monday* nights, specifically. When the aisles of the grocery store were empty.

With her therapist, Patricia began looking at her life, first to deal with her drinking problem. She saw that she had no self; she was whatever her parents, her school, John, her church wanted her to be. She began experiments to learn what she liked, what she didn't. She set up boundaries around the self she was developing. It exhilarated her to be who she was. She refused to spend time around people who treated her without respect. She stopped denying what Uncle Harry had done to her.

His trial on the child molestation charge was coming up. His lawyer expected Patricia to testify that, a year earlier, she had told the investigator her uncle could not possibly have done it.

"No," she told him. "If you think I'm going to get up there and say he didn't do that, you're out of your mind."

Hearing of her resistance, her uncle came to her trailer. She was working in the yard.

"Don't go in," she told him when she saw his hand on the trailer handle.

"You know," he threatened, turning to face her, "if you don't go to court, they're going to put you in jail."

"You look here," she said, cold and angry. "I'm not the one that sexually abused that little girl. You did. They're going to put *you* in jail."

When she confronted him on what he had done to her, he denied it at first and then, unable to continue, said, "Well, you were living with me." As if that justified it.

"I was a child," she said firmly, looking straight into his wavering eyes. "I lived wherever my parents put me."

She was wrong; they didn't jail Harry. He plea-bargained, was put on probation, and told to stay away from children. Alone of all her family, Patricia did not testify on Harry's behalf. Outraged, some of her family stopped speaking to her.

She was lying, her mother accused her, when Patricia reiterated that Harry had abused her, too.

Finally, twenty-seven years after the sexual abuse, Daugherty looked straight at her mother: "Why in the hell would I lie about it? What point would there be, at my age, to lie about something like that?"

Her mother had no answer.

It hadn't happened just in her family, she realized now. In an alcohol recovery group, she listened to women she'd gone to school with tell stories similar to her own. Fathers, grandfathers, uncles, brothers: secret incest. Now, thinking back, remembering the talk of her girlfriends, what they knew of sex at a young age—she realized incest had been common.

Patricia had always felt responsible for the sex with Uncle Harry. Her grandmother had spanked *her*. It was her fault.

Now she stumbled, in a driving rain of condemnation, toward her authentic self.

Then she met Al, a math teacher, father of three, who had divorced after sixteen years of marriage. She dated him for a year. They decided to marry.

The bombardment of shaming messages halted. Everyone approved:

"Oh, he'll take care of her and the kids."

"Oh, great, Patricia has found a man. She'll settle down. Things will be fine now. She won't be out drinking."

"Oh, they're going to get married! Isn't this wonderful!"

"Now maybe Al will straighten your mother out," Patricia's mother told her grandsons.

One of her doctor's notes in the medical records she would later read was: "Patricia was divorced, unhappy, and had a period of drinking and partying. But now she has remarried, has a happy marriage, and is doing well." Because she was now hooked up with a man, she was all better. She was no longer that single woman rolling around loose, out of control.

If she had not felt pressured from so many shaming messages, she probably would have taken the time to get to know Al better, she later reflected. She would have felt freer to have other relationships that allowed her to explore who she was. She might not have jumped into marriage. She had been in no hurry to give up that room of her own.

Al, too, was under pressure to marry. The school administrators had made it known to him, he told Patricia, that they would really like to see him marry. He was a single, unattached male and people were beginning to think he was gay. Parents would feel more comfortable about having him around their sons if he were married.

Al had been hired only three years earlier. He didn't have tenure. He could get booted out of his job for anything, he told her. Sooner or later, his single status was going to affect his livelihood.

"I made him look really good," she later reflected. "He had a pretty young wife to marry. I fit the criteria for what he needed. He fit mine."

In the course of a long, intimate talk, he told her that in fact he had had a few sexual encounters with men.

Her therapist's eyebrows rose when Patricia told her.

"He'd better get an AIDS test," she said, perhaps having read the *Time* magazine article that March that mentioned Dr. Dooley Worth's work with HIV-infected women, or some of the articles on women and AIDS that began appearing in women's magazines in 1987.

Patricia asked him to take the test. He was offended, indignant, angry. How dare she ask such a thing! How dare she insult him! She backed down and calmed him with soothing words.

No test.

It was a fairy tale June wedding in 1987. She was a stunningly beautiful princess in a lovely white dress. She invited her parents but, to their annoyance, refused to let them play any role other than guest. When had they ever supported her; *her*, Patricia? Her sixteen-year-old son walked her down the aisle. Her nine-year-old was the ring bearer. She had a good time at her wedding.

But as soon as she walked down that goddamn aisle in that goddamn white dress, the fairy tale ended.

Al changed. Patricia was "his" now. She was "my wife." Possessions were suddenly "ours." During her two years as a "loose" woman, she had cleaned house but if she didn't get to it one week, she just didn't, that's all. Now she began cleaning every Friday without fail. As a loose woman, she had cooked, but if she didn't get home in time for a formal supper, she and the kids ate informally. Now, married, supper became a sacrament again: ritually cooked and served. She didn't want the burden of owning a home. Al did. They built one. She felt her juicy freedom seeping away from her, leaving her dry and astonished.

Three months after the marriage, the family doctor gave Al a routine allergy exam and found that he had low blood platelets, a disorder officially called idiopathic thrombocytopenic purpura or ITP. The doctor referred Al to an oncologist in Portland. Patricia and Al both feared cancer. But he had not been feeling at all bad.

From September until December, the oncologist tested Al exhaustively. His speculations frightened the couple: Maybe it was Hodgkin's disease. Or lupus. Or lymphoma. At the conclusion of the tests, he said he didn't know why Al had low platelets or the enlarged spleen he had found on examination. Perhaps the onset of rheumatoid arthritis, he suggested.

Come back in three months for another checkup, he told Al. Al did. For a year and a half, he returned to the doctor almost monthly. For a year and a half, while newlyweds Patricia and Al had lots of unprotected sex, his ailment went undiagnosed.

They needed to throw a spotlight on women, Linda Lofredo and Lynne MacArthur concluded as they listened at the monthly meetings of the Women and AIDS Project. Women were suffering silently, in darkness. Drag the suffering out into the public light, they figured, and then work for programs, policies, funding that would address women's needs in the epidemic. They decided to organize public hearings in New York State June 12. To get a big audience, they would ask several organizations to cosponsor the hearings. The New York State Division for Women, the Assembly Task Force on Women's Issues, the

Legislative Women's Caucus, and the Women and AIDS Project readily agreed.

The testimony raised a profound and disturbing issue: how to prevent AIDS in women when the inner-city women now being most hit by the epidemic were trapped in an environment in which there was little incentive to live.

"If we are asking them [women] to live," Barbara Gibson of the Urban Health Information Referral Service asked, "what are we asking them to live for?"

Gibson, like most women working on AIDS, emphasized: AIDS is just one crisis among many that women deal with, and it is often not the worst. How to eat tomorrow, where to sleep tonight—these are more urgent problems. The women are living in communities already struggling with poor housing, unemployment, illiteracy, crime, disease, alcoholism, and massive drug addiction.

Gibson pointedly told the hearing that in talking about people with AIDS "we are talking about people who basically live in a culture that does not recognize their being. We look at a society that relegates to a lower standard of living people who are black and brown. When we talk about giving money for AIDS education and prevention, we also have to look at the larger society and recognize that although it is AIDS that we have to address on the surface, the larger issue is the conditions under which these people live."

Testifying at the hearings, Azadeh Khalili of the AIDS Discrimination Unit of the New York City Commission on Human Rights described a common scenario: A woman contracts AIDS. This becomes well known. Soon her healthy children are forced out of school.

"Often there is an attempt to remove children from a mother who has AIDS or who tests HIV-positive," she noted. "In these situations, AIDS or antibody status is used as an indication of unfit parenthood." (In contrast, no one threatened to remove a child from a mother with leukemia.)

Kathleen McMahon, an AIDS nurse clinician at the Memorial Sloan-Kettering Cancer Center, described how she watched and listened to the nurses around her after news broke that three female health care providers had contracted the AIDS virus during routine patient care. Realizing that they, too, had had similar exposures during the past few years and wondering if they could have been infected at work, they suffered insomnia, vivid dreaming, crying jags, and sometimes exploded in anger or shook in fear.

The women testifying at the hearings spoke powerfully, but few heard them. Only two legislators attended. Although MacArthur and Lofredo sent notices to the media, no reports on the hearing were published or broadcast. MacArthur was appalled: the impact of AIDS on women was not important enough to cover. Mainstream women's organizations like the National Organization for Women and the National Women's Political Caucus appeared disinterested, too. They sent no observers.

For Marie St. Cyr of WARN, one of the speakers, the disinterest in women's suffering was so blatant, it was impossible to go into denial. State officials could spare no time even to listen to women's *accounts* of their suffering, let alone do anything to alleviate it.

Lofredo could hardly contain her frustration: "You have to sit back and ask, 'Why is this not being paid attention to?'"

Dr. Dooley Worth, after testifying herself, asked the same question. She was amazed at how little concern or even *interest* there was about what was happening to women in the epidemic, how few resources there were for them. She knew she shouldn't be amazed. When word had come down that the AIDS Institute was going to give $75,000 for women's programs, Worth had told them not to bother. You couldn't even set up one program for that amount and they were going to split it between five!

Now this. Whenever there was a meeting specifically about the problems of women and AIDS, about bringing services to women, those attending would be almost exclusively women. Few men attended. Yet from the beginning of the epidemic, large numbers of women had been volunteering to help male PWAs, to fund-raise, to do whatever was needed.

Male suffering was serious suffering. Female suffering was not worthy of men's notice or attention.

Sitting in her kitchen on Coney Island soon after the Fourth of July, Ada Setal had a strong urge to visit her grandchildren. She had seen them so rarely. Her son Eddie had taken his time introducing his common-law wife to her. Their child, Faith, was already two years old when Ada met her and her mother, Ameda, for the first time.

She hardly knew Ameda. Her impression had been of a sweet, mannerly, intelligent woman. But not a tidy housekeeper. Head-strong, too, judging from the stories Eddie told her. He had been upset when, following the birth of their second child, Jesse, Ameda had aborted a pregnancy. He'd called Ada.

"This girl wants me to marry her," he'd told Ada, "and I'm going to do it but she went ahead and had an abortion without telling me about it. Will you talk to her?"

Ada had called Ameda: "If Eddie loves you and says he wants to marry you and he cares for you and the children, why would you do that without his permission? If you ever get pregnant again, I suggest that you have that baby or you ask his permission to abort, especially if you plan on living the rest of your life with him."

When Ada asked Ameda why she had done it, Ameda had been silent.

Now Ada, in her late fifties, an ordained minister in a Reform Pentecostal church and a mother of eight, got into her car and drove the twenty minutes to Eddie's apartment in Brooklyn, not even know-ing if he were home. Eddie opened the door to her. He was crying. It was the first time she had ever seen him, as an adult, cry. He led her into the bedroom where Ameda, pale, thin, was sitting on the side of the bed, crying. Ada thought someone had died.

As Ada stood, Ameda said police had come that morning and taken the children away. She had given birth to a baby girl, Angela, a month earlier and the doctors had found cocaine in the baby's urine. They had reported this to the Bureau of Child Welfare, which had sent the police. The children were gone, and in a few days Ameda had to go to court to answer a child-neglect charge.

As Ada stood open-mouthed—she had not even known that Ameda had been pregnant again let alone given birth—Ameda asked her to raise the three children. Would she come to court with her, she asked, and offer to raise the children so they would not be placed in foster care?

But there was something more Ada had to know, Ameda said, weeping. She had AIDS. All three children were infected.

It hit Ada like a blow to her body. She looked at Eddie. He, too, was in shock. "What! My God!"

Ameda talked on, breaking her silence for the first time in four years. Before meeting Eddie, she had lived in another common-law marriage, by which she had two children. Her husband's mother was raising those children. Yes, they knew. Her husband had died. Yes, they knew. Of AIDS. Oh, my God.

After his death, when she gave birth to Faith in 1983, the doctors told her that she, too, had been infected and so had the baby. She was afraid to tell Eddie, afraid he would leave her. She did not go for treatment or get pain medications because then he would know. She got pregnant again. Baby Jesse, too, was infected. The next time she became pregnant, she aborted. Her husband was angry and Ada gave her a talking to. Somewhere in all this, silent with her secret and in increasing pain, Ameda began using cocaine. Pregnant again, she did not dare abort.

Ada could hardly speak. They were asking her to raise three infected children! She wanted to say no then and there. But she told them she would think it over. She left Eddie and Ameda weeping on the bed.

Ada wanted to run. This was not her problem. Why was she left to deal with a horror someone else had caused? Alone in her apartment, she wept, prayed, searched her soul, and reproached God: "You're asking me to take the children and now you're telling me they have AIDS? What are you asking me! How could you!"

Later, her face bloated with tears, she prayed: "What would You have me do? I'm telling myself: I don't want to do this. I don't want to have anything to do with AIDS. I didn't bring this on! I didn't make these children sick! So why should I get involved?"

In the night, one word reverberated through her: "The ministry. The ministry. Orphans and widows are the ministry. The children have been abandoned and have no one to care for them and love them. That's where the ministry is."

"I brought my son into the world and let him cause things. So how can I turn my back? I'm part of this because if I had not opened up my womb to conceive him, he would not be here to cause things."

The next morning, she went to see baby Angela in the hospital. That night, she told Eddie and Ameda that she would care for the three children. In August they were hers.

· · ·

Jesse's nosebleeds terrified Ada Setal. Every night he would wake up with blood streaming down his face. It scared him so much, he'd cry and scream and begin choking on the blood, and Ada, rushing to hold the squirming, thrashing child and stop the blood, was petrified both that he'd choke to death and that the blood, infected with the AIDS virus, would contaminate her. She wore gloves. She tried not to get any closer than she had to. But there was a two-year-old in diapers gagging on a heavy stream of blood and she had to do something.

Twice, panicked over the blood he was losing and that she couldn't stem, she called the emergency police number, 911. The police showed her how to hold Jesse in a certain position so he wouldn't choke to death.

After that, she was able to handle him.

His nose bled every night for almost three years.

Ada needed to pick up clothes at the cleaners, a gallon of milk at the store, stamps at the post office. She slung a portable oxygen tank on her shoulder for Angela, who had trouble breathing.

Riding in the car, Faith and Jesse screamed and ducked down when they saw a policeman. They were hiding because they didn't want the policeman to take them away, they told Ada, sobbing. A policeman had grabbed them from their home and brought them to a shelter. They had never seen their mother again.

Ada calmed them. The policeman had not come because Mommy and Daddy were bad but because they were sick and unable to care for their children. Again and again, she would explain, reassure. No policeman was going to take them. They were with her and they were safe.

Each time she stopped the car, opened her door, and set one foot out, Jesse and Faith screamed in terror. They were petrified that Ada was abandoning them. Their terror was so great that Ada would have to take them wherever she was going and keep them close by her side, even when she had a babysitter with her in the car, holding Angela. Walking in with them, she would assure them that she loved them, that they were safe.

"Everything is fine," she would say. "You're never going to be taken. Nobody is going to harm you. You're going to always be with me."

On the street, in stores, at home, their eyes never left her, their ears were alert to every change in her voice tone or volume. It was as if they were determined never to be caught off guard again.

She reassured without cease, without pause: "You're with your grandmother. I'm not going to let anything happen to you. Daddy loves you. Mommy loves you. I love you."

It horrified Ada not to be able to move even from one room to the next without them. They'd grab her legs, clutch her skirts, sobbing, lift their arms up to be held.

It took two years of reassurance before they began to trust that she would not leave them.

She remembers riding through Hamburg, Germany, one day during the war on the back of a bicycle, behind her mother, whom she trusted completely. She was four. To each side of her she saw the heaped ruins of bombed-out houses and fires, small and great. They were leaving the city, her mother had told her. She would return the next day with a car to get their clothes. When Anke Ehrhardt's mother did return the next morning, she found that their home had been bombed during the night.

Her father was away in the war. He'd lost his job because his grandfather had been Jewish. Then the Nazis had drafted him.

As a girl of five, Ehrhardt played with other children in the ruins. It was a forbidden pastime for there could be cave-ins. But it was exciting. She would suddenly make a discovery: a pot, a briefcase, a clock. To adult eyes, relics from another life. Before the war.

As she grew and her country rebuilt, she became an earnest graduate student. Coming to Johns Hopkins on a fellowship in 1964, she decided, in 1969, to live in this country. In 1970 she moved from Baltimore to become an assistant professor in psychiatry and pediatrics at the State University of New York at Buffalo. Within a few years, she had become acting head of the department of child psychiatry at Children's Hospital, an unusual position for a Ph.D. In 1977 she moved to New York City to join the Columbia University faculty and do research in psychoendocrinology at the New York State Psychiatric Institute. By 1980, at forty, she had become a full professor, a rare accomplishment for someone that age and certainly for a woman. Her

blond head and overstuffed briefcase (she seemed to go through briefcases at the same pace as nylon stockings) were a familiar sight on the
walkways and sidewalks between Columbia-Presbyterian Hospital and
the Psychiatric Institute. As her father had, she sprinkled her disci-
plined life with such pleasures as the opera. Smelling the roses, he had
called it.

As homelessness increased throughout the 1980s in her newly
adopted city, it occurred to her that the people living in the streets and
in impoverished inner-city neighborhoods were enduring something
harsher than what she had as a child. She had lived through years of
hunger and hardship after the war but she had had no sense of depri-
vation. Everyone was hungry. Here the homeless saw those around
them living in comfort.

Now the director of the Institute asked Ehrhardt if she'd like to
develop and direct a research center for studies on HIV and AIDS.
The National Institute of Mental Health (NIMH), in conjunction
with the National Institute on Drug Abuse (NIDA), would be funding several centers in the United States. The director urged her to
apply for one of them.

They agreed that another Institute colleague, the South
African–born reproductive epidemiologist Dr. Zena Stein, might be
persuaded to join on as a codirector.

Though Stein's earlier attempts to study women and HIV had
been thwarted by denied grants, she had succeeded in getting funding
for research on children in the HIV epidemic. Throughout her long
career, she had studied congenital and perinatal disability in children.
This new work was a natural for her. A year earlier, with the first
reports of HIV-infected children, she had begun research with her colleagues on what might influence a mother's transmission of HIV to a
fetus, under what circumstances women themselves got this disease,
and how transmission of the disease to women could be prevented.

Stein and Ehrhardt knew each other casually, having served on a
university committee together. Right before Christmas, the director
invited them and a third colleague, psychiatrist Dr. Robert Spitzer, to
a meeting. Within a half hour they had agreed to work together to
build the Center. Its purpose would be to study HIV disease in order
to develop treatments and intervention strategies. They put together
their proposal.

In September 1987, NIMH and NIDA awarded a five-year, multimillion-dollar research grant for the establishment of the HIV Center for Clinical and Behavioral Studies at the New York State Psychiatric Institute and Columbia-Presbyterian Medical Center in New York City, one of three such centers at that time, with more than one hundred researchers and support staff.

One of the Center's first projects was a five-year study of approximately 450 HIV-positive and HIV-negative participants to explore behavioral and neurological factors that were likely to be involved in determining the progression of HIV infection. The central nervous system factors that influence how rapidly infected people develop compromised immune systems and AIDS conditions were largely unknown. Most natural history studies of HIV had been follow-up studies for gay men. But the Center's natural-history-study participants would include drug users as well as gay men. Most notably, women would be included. Ehrhardt and Stein insisted that female as well as male drug users be enrolled. Their scientific colleagues marshaled all their objections to the inclusion of women: Women were too few. Gay men were easy to recruit; women might be difficult. There would be women in one group (drug users) but not in the other (gay men). Any effects or comparison between the gay men and the IV drug users might be diluted.

Stein and Ehrhardt simply closed their ears to problems. No, they said. We are going to recruit women.

They did. They got seventy-five. At this time, there were no natural-history studies of HIV-infected women anywhere in the country.

One-third of their study participants were gay and bisexual men. Two-thirds were male and female IV drug users. In order to make the women comparable to the other samples—the gay men sample and the male IV drug user sample—they used exactly the same kind of measures for the women as for the men.

"We didn't know enough to have a special protocol for women then," Ehrhardt later lamented. There were no pelvic exams for the women, no gynecological measures.

Now, in the midst of long hours of work, she could look back at that October in 1980 when she had walked with three of her friends to see the Halloween parade, dominated in Greenwich Village by exuberant gay men dressed in glitter, spangle, net, and feathers. The friends had walked in leisure, laughed, in retrospect been so carefree and innocent. A memory from another life: Before the Dying Began.

The large doses of AZT Penny Abernathey was taking hit her at work with sudden waves of nausea. The toxic drug got into her bone marrow, disrupting the development of red blood cells, so she was always anemic and fatigued. She kept a trash can in her cubicle for sudden vomiting. She couldn't keep it from her boss, a Christian fundamentalist, any longer. A year after her husband died in Austin, Texas, Penny told him that she had been infected with the AIDS virus.

Her boss felt driven to bring her to the Lord. Her HIV was a by-product of Mark's sinning and she was going to die. People who died without truly knowing the Lord would go to hell.

"You have to be saved," he told her.

So began the evangelizing behind the closed doors of his office. It came in sprints, usually when business was slow and he was bored. He often described how he'd brought other people to the Lord.

"What is this?" Penny asked herself. "Like a conquest thing?"

Penny was an Episcopalian. She had her own beliefs in God but they were not his. She felt that to satisfy him, she had to get down on her knees and confess her conversion before him. Then he'd get a spiritual notch on his belt and be able to say, "Ah, I've brought Penny to the Lord."

She tried to placate him and cruise out of the room fast: "Yes, I thought about what you told me last week. It was really terrific. Well, I'd better get this letter typed."

Her father called it "spiritual rape" and that felt exactly right to her.

What Penny Abernathey told her boss in confidence, he, in the cause of his evangelical work, told her other supervisors.

That's when the humiliating incidents began. Her supervisors had told her that when she felt fatigued, she could go home and lie down for a short time.

"Do what you need to do to be well," they had said. "We care about you."

On occasion, she would do that, always letting them know when she did. A supervisor would then reprimand her on her phone mail—

"We needed you and you weren't here. You're unreliable."—and patch that reprimand onto the phone mail of all her coworkers so that her humiliation was intensified.

Some days, returning home from work, she would cry her eyes out.

She didn't fight back because she felt she was so fortunate to still have her job. She read in the newspapers of people in town who had been fired and thrown out of their apartments when their diagnosis was made public. She was fortunate she was not out on the street.

In 1981 forty-three-year-old Byllye Avery was director for Comprehensive Employment Training Act (CETA) in Gainesville, Florida, training young black women who had dropped out of high school. Avery was surprised at the extreme ill health she was seeing in the women. Just nineteen to twenty-five years old, they were dealing with high blood pressure, diabetes, kidney problems! It was frightening.

That got Avery, a longtime African-American activist in the women's health movement, to thinking about how black women's health issues differed from white women's. It seemed that black women got every "bad" thing—except osteoporosis—worse than white women. According to her research, they were number one with heart problems. They were twice as likely as white women to die from diabetes in middle age, three times as likely to die of cervical cancer. Though they got breast cancer less often than white women, they were more likely to die of it. They had a greater rate of high blood pressure and were more apt to suffer kidney damage from it than white women. The death rate of their infants was twice that of white women's.

Overall, white women were twice as healthy as black women. It costs a lot of money to buy preventive care, Avery learned, and if you don't get that basic health care when you are growing up as a child, the things that go unchecked are dealt with when they've reached acute, body-damaging stages.

And then there's racism—racism that is so pervasive, it affects the assumptions medical workers make. Avery learned that personally:

"I had my teeth pulled and it wasn't until I was in my thirties that I asked a [white] friend, 'Why is it that a lot of white people still have all their teeth?' She said, 'Because they have root canals.' I was never asked, 'Would you rather have a root canal?' It was assumed that I wanted and needed the least expensive thing, which was to have a tooth extracted. Options were never explained. Decisions were made for me and they had to be based solely on my race because when I had these teeth removed, I already had a bachelor's degree. I was working. I could have paid for a root canal. If you multiply that incident by days, if you multiply that by people, if you multiply how pervasive these unconscious racist attitudes are in individuals, you can extend that throughout the whole health care system."

Avery founded the National Black Women's Health Project, based in Atlanta, Georgia, in 1981, with the support of the National Women's Health Network, on whose board she served seven years, and of the Boston Women's Health Book Collective, authors of *Our Bodies, Ourselves*. The Project organized self-help groups in which women shared health information and supported one another.

Now, as the work of Dr. Vickie Mays and others had highlighted, AIDS was hitting black women hard. The National Black Women's Health Project organized a conference on women and AIDS in Washington, D.C. But the organization would not focus its work on AIDS. It made no sense to because *everything* was hitting black women hard.

But Avery believed that if they worked on any one issue the right way, refusing to isolate it from the context of the lives women were living, they would be working simultaneously on all the other issues: education, employment, environmental damage, homelessness, AIDS, the medical care system, drug addiction.

Take drugs. If Avery had to choose one issue to zero in on, that would be it, for there was hardly a family that was not touched by addiction.

"If we worked on drugs and we tried to get our mental well-being straight, we would see that unemployment is a large factor in depression and we would have some appreciation for how bright the children are who are in the drug trade so heavily," she told a journalist. "Most adults don't handle $50,000 or $100,000 a day, but there are little ghetto kids running around doing that all the time. They could learn how to do the stock market but nobody is showing them that way."

Working on drug use, you'd have to examine environmental damage and how that impacts on people's physical and emotional well-being.

"Life has become very painful for a lot of people," Avery observes, "and the way they get through it is by killing the pain, which is by using drugs. You have to look at what people are doing symbolically and whether they need a fast death, which would be what gets them into hard drugs like crack and the violence that comes with it, or whether they take a slower route in dulling the pain. I think that lets you know just how deep the pain is that people are in."

Large numbers of African-Americans were in depression, she saw. It was a hopeless life for a lot of the women and the lights had gone out. Nobody was dealing with the collective depression that was going on.

Dr. Hortensia Amaro of Boston University School of Public Health, a consultant to the National Coalition on Alcohol and Drug Dependent Women and Children, frequently talked with the women Avery spoke of—women in pain and on drugs. Founder of the Mom's Project, a program serving poor and pregnant women with HIV, Amaro encountered many women who were desperate for drug treatment. But a punitive attitude toward drug-using pregnant women reigned, she found. Precious little help in overcoming their addiction was available to these women. In fact, the obstacles women had to surmount to get treatment were formidable. The obstacles were placed by courts, drug treatment programs, social service agencies, medical institutions, and families.

According to many experts, women get little encouragement from their families or partners to seek treatment for drug addiction. One study reported that 23 percent of the women entering treatment experienced opposition from their families and friends, compared to 2 percent of the men. Male addicts are frequently pressured into treatment by their female partners, but a man is less likely to pressure his partner to go into treatment. In fact, the opposite is likely.[14] As Gloria Weissman, deputy chief of the Community Research Branch of the National Institute on Drug Abuse, points out, he'll pressure her to stay home so he doesn't lose her services.

Many male addicts enter treatment with the help of outreach workers who go into the community seeking to recruit them into programs. Women are often missed for recruitment because the strategies of outreach workers have been largely oriented to going where men, not women, gather.

Nor will seeking help from the medical system lead women to treatment for their addiction. Weissman points out that medical and mental health professionals generally know little about substance abuse and tend not to ask patients about it. Women, coping with such problems as keeping themselves and their children fed, sheltered, and safe from assault, may not define their addiction as their main problem but rather as something that helps them through their difficulties. Physicians, not picking up on a woman's addiction, often respond to her nervousness, depression, or anxiety by prescribing psychoactive drugs, including tranquilizers. Not only does she become dually or triply addicted, but the tranquilizers mask her symptoms, thus removing a key motivation for entering treatment.

For women with children—that is, the majority of drug-addicted women—the obstacles to getting help are often insurmountable. In many states, if a woman asks for drug treatment, she will be reported, by law, as an unfit mother and may lose her children. Using drugs is considered presumptive evidence of unfitness as a parent. This is no abstract fear, Weissman points out: "Many women have lost their custody." She adds: "I think women drug users who may want treatment are staying away from drug treatment in droves because they see they will lose their kids."

Hortensia Amaro found that to be the case in managing her NIDA-funded project in Boston. The program was originally based at Boston City Hospital but had to be moved to a community location because women were afraid to come to the hospital and risk losing their children.

If a woman lives in a state where the government does not rush in to take her children away from her as soon as she asks for treatment, and if she is accepted into a program, she will often have no child care available to her. As Amaro points out, there are only a handful of programs around the country that let women come into treatment with their children or help women arrange for child care.

"Imagine a woman, highly motivated to get treatment, who has three or four kids," Amaro asks. "What does she do? The family, by this time, is probably fed up with her. Her friends are not the kind she would want to leave her kids with. So if she wants to go into treatment, she must give her kids up for foster care."

She often fears that if she does that, she will lose them forever—a realistic fear.

So most women go into treatment only after they have lost their children—after they have been arrested on drug charges and the Department of Social Services has investigated and taken the children away.

Punitive actions against pregnant drug-using women seem to be on the rise. In the years 1987 to 1991, fifty-three women were charged with prenatal child abuse or delivering drugs to a minor through the umbilical cord. In these highly publicized cases, courts used drug statutes originally aimed at drug dealers against pregnant women. For example, in 1991 a Florida appeals court upheld the first conviction in the United States of a woman charged with drug-dealing to her minute-old babies. The woman, Jennifer Clarise Johnson, a twenty-five-year-old African-American, *had tried to get drug treatment and been turned away.* Similar charges against women were filed and dismissed in Michigan, Ohio, North Carolina, and Massachusetts. In South Carolina, "child neglect" charges have been used against ten addicted pregnant women. Several have been arrested and handcuffed on the day they gave birth.[15]

Syndicated columnist Charles Krauthammer, as reported in 1990, proposed locking up pregnant drug users en masse to stop the growth of what he termed "a bio-underclass." And in that same year, Ohio considered a bill calling for mandatory sterilization of women who give birth to a second drug-addicted child.[16]

Yet while pregnant women have been hounded, handcuffed, and publicly humiliated for being addicted, they are simultaneously shut out of drug treatment programs. Most refuse pregnant women entry.

In New York City, it was reported in 1990, Dr. Wendy Chavkin, a physician at Beth Israel Medical Center, surveyed seventy-eight drug treatment programs and found that women claiming to be pregnant and drug-addicted were denied service by 54 percent of programs; 67 percent refused treatment to pregnant addicts on Medicaid, and 87 percent shut out pregnant women on Medicaid addicted to crack.[17]

"We have in Boston ten [drug] treatment beds available for pregnant women," Hortensia Amaro notes. "I have in one of my projects more than one hundred women who are pregnant and want to get in treatment."

While women wait for a bed to become available, they may become lost to the system, or even die.

A prerequisite for getting into a resident treatment program is having been through detoxification. But it is a norm among physicians not to detox women past a certain stage of pregnancy because they do not want to be sued if the fetus is damaged. Little research has been done on the best ways to detoxify women during pregnancy so the physicians' practice is based on scant knowledge.

While we are horrified at the sight of drug-addicted newborns, we make it nearly impossible for a pregnant woman to break her addiction.

"On the one hand we say to women, 'Oh, you horrible person, you. Look what you're doing to this baby!'" Hortensia Amaro says. "And when the woman says, 'Okay, get me into treatment,' we say, 'Oh, I'm sorry, we don't have a treatment spot.' It is insane. It is totally insane. No wonder these women go beserk. They are totally desperate. They want to get some treatment.

"We choose not to make treatment available to women, especially pregnant women. And then we blame them for it."

If a woman is lucky enough to get into treatment, there is a high probability that she will enter a program designed by and for men, a program that began admitting women as an afterthought.

Treatment designs in therapeutic communities involve a breaking down of defenses, including denial, through abrasive confrontational methods, and humiliation. The women coming into the programs already have a tremendous amount of shame, Weissman observes. Then they have shame and humiliation loaded onto them as "treatment."

Edith Springer, who finds the entire drug treatment system sadistic, has a friend who, like herself, is also a social worker and a trainer in recovery from drugs, but who, unlike herself, lived in a therapeutic community in an attempt to break her own drug addiction.

"She never talks about it," Springer says. "Never. She said that it took her five years after she got out to feel like a human being again because they had made her feel that she, as a woman, was nothing but slime."

"Many women come into treatment and then leave because they can't take it," Weissman says.

If the women stay in the programs, they may be sexually abused or harassed by drug counselors or by male addicts. There has been a great deal of that abuse, Weissman points out. The vast majority of female drug users—upwards of 80 percent, according to Weissman—already have a history of sexual abuse.

If a woman with a history of abuse by men doesn't want a male counselor, she may be told she's "resisting" treatment. If she stays in the program—despite shaming, sexual abuse, and pressure from her man to return home—the drug program will most likely not deal with the root causes of her addiction such as childhood abandonment and sexual, emotional, and physical abuse.

"When you start taking away people's coping mechanism, their drug use, you have to deal with some of the underlying causes and issues," Weissman observes.

Speaking at a conference in Los Angeles, Weissman said she had been told on several occasions that having to jump over the many hurdles placed in the way of women who want treatment is "good for them." The assumption, Weissman said, was that the woman's desire to stop substance abuse could be measured by her attempts to enter drug treatment. But the many women who did not enter the treatment system, Weissman pointed out, "the so-called hard to reach, were hard to reach only because few had ever tried," and "the 'unmotivated' were unmotivated only because no one had ever offered them hope."[18]

As Hortensia Amaro explains the situation: "We *threaten* to take the kids away. We *threaten* to file a complaint if the child is born with a positive urine toxicology. And yet we're not able to offer her treatment because beds aren't available but we will punish her if—." She breaks off in exasperation. "It's a system that doesn't make any sense if the goal is to help the client."

Indeed.

Information on what women need in drug treatment has been available for more than a decade, as a NIDA training manual points out, but programs have been "lamentably slow" to provide it.[19]

It's time to look at an implicit U.S. policy on drug addiction: keep addicted women drugged.[20]

Dr. Helen Rodriquez believes we need to break out of a moral code that categorizes people with health conditions such as drug addiction as evil.

"In our heart of hearts," she says, "we don't think they deserve treatment. We don't think they deserve the resources."

Drug use is a health, not a moral issue, she says, adding: "But what we, as a society, do about those folks who need vital things that they do not have—*that* is a moral issue. Is it moral to allow people who have a serious health issue to go without treatment? It is immoral."

Angela was the love of Ada Setal's life. She was forever pressing the palms of her hands together and lifting them up, as if in prayer. Catching sight of her, Ada would grin. It made her feel that during their ordeal Angela was in prayer for all of them.

During the day, Ada tended the children and in the evening nursed an elderly patient in her home in Queens. A babysitter stayed with the children.

In November, Faith and Jesse were hospitalized with PCP and Angela with double pneumonia.

Coming home from the hospital one night, Ada found a marijuana cigarette stub under a table. The babysitter had cleaned up after herself but had missed something. Ada stood with the cigarette butt between her fingers, thinking: If the babysitter had invited friends in, and they sat around smoking, they would have had to open all the windows in the tiny apartment to air the smoke out before she, Ada, got home. That cold night air would have blown on the already sick children. Maybe that was how all three had come down with pneumonia at the same time. How else could all three have been struck at once? The children's lives would end soon. How could she leave them with a stranger, not knowing what kind of care they were getting? At least let them not suffer more than they had to during the rest of their short lives. Ada quit her job—losing her own medical insurance when she did so—and stayed home to care for them.

· · ·

Sometimes, in the night, when all three children were sick at the same time, Ada went from one to the other. They had coughs, ran fevers, got infections. Jesse had his nosebleeds and Faith her nightmares. Angela, struggling to breath, had to be put under the croup tent.

Ada was always aware that she was dealing with children who could die at any time, that she could wake up and find them gone.

Too drained and exhausted from nursing the children, she could not even imagine having a social life. Long active in the church, she now walked away from it. The church had not supported her decision to care for the children and would not help her. It disapproved of the activities associated with AIDS transmission—extramarital sexual intercourse and intravenous drug use—and was unwilling to embrace those afflicted by the disease. A support group for AIDS caregivers at Downstate Hospital in Brooklyn provided the only social life she had.

Ada had no time to see her own adult children. Back in July, Ronald, her twenty-three-year-old baby, had telephoned the home where she worked as a health care attendant. Not finding her in, he had left a message that he would come by soon and surprise her. Ada was so busy with the children, she hardly noticed he never did come by. Or maybe he had come when she was at the hospital with the children. If he had called, she had not been there to answer.

During the trying days and nights, Ada thought of Ameda with compassion. How it must have been for her: sick herself, weak, in pain yet too frightened to seek treatment or pain medication, burdened by a terrible secret and a fearful guilt, and caring for sick children she—and she alone of her family—knew would die. And Ada had judged her an untidy housekeeper. She had not known the burden that young woman carried.

Katrina Haslip often talked with her friends in the ACE core group who were intently gathering information on AIDS in newspapers, on television, in pamphlets they wrote away for. Though she tried not to, she couldn't help thinking of her own past and applying the AIDS "risk factors" to herself. The AIDS information she was picking up in the prison was scary. She'd used IV drugs. Yes, but, well, she'd only shared needles a few times. She'd been a prostitute. Yes, but there wasn't that much intercourse. And she'd had that blood transfusion in 1983, before they'd screened the blood supply for HIV.

• • •

Katrina Haslip saw the prison doctor about her recurring vaginitis. The doctor, noting her history—a stomach virus twice in one year— asked her about her drug and sexual history. Listening, she kept shaking her head and looking back over Haslip's charts to see how often she had had recurrent vaginitis. Katrina felt fear in her stomach.

"You've had vaginitis a lot," the doctor commented.

"I thought that was common," Haslip said.

"Sometimes it is, but it could also be early signs of certain things."

"Like what—cancer?"

"Well, you don't have an abnormal pap smear, but with your history, I think you should consider taking the HIV antibody test."

Katrina's heart pounded. "Well, I stopped shooting drugs awhile ago. I don't think I'm infected." Silence. "I'll think about it."

She thought about it a month. The fact that a doctor had suggested the test frightened her.

She decided to be tested. In December her blood was drawn.

In early December, invited, through a physician at Downstate, to speak at a pediatric AIDS conference in White Plains, New York, Ada Setal drove with two other caregivers—Patricia, a foster mother Ada knew from her support group at Downstate, and Lydia, a mother of a child with AIDS. They talked all the way up and all the way back. By the time Ada got out of the car, the three women had decided to form their own support and advocacy group for AIDS caregivers.

They would support each other through crises and when they were exhausted and in despair. They would tell each other: "You can make it. You don't have to lie down and die." They would discuss the things they needed for their children and themselves and then fight collectively to get those things. They would bring each other out of isolation.

Later that month, Ada got a letter from her son Anthony. In it, he wrote her: He had gone to look for a friend one night and someone had told him she was in a crack house. It was a dangerous neighborhood. He took a gun with him for protection. There was a shoot-out in the crack house. The owner was killed. He, Anthony, was arrested, accused of murder. Cleared of the charge, he had pleaded guilty to carrying a weapon. He was writing her from prison.

Holding the letter in her hand, Ada felt like Job. Every time she turned around, someone was bringing news of another tragedy in her family. She did what Job did. Wept. Prayed. She left it in God's hands.

A few days after Christmas, Faith returned to the hospital with PCP and an infection. Afraid to be left alone, she cried. She was five years old. Sometimes Ada stayed with her all day.

Diane Sampson (a pseudonym) was white, married, twenty-seven, lived in a small New Jersey town, had three kids, kept a nice home, went to work, worshiped at the Methodist church Sundays, dressed nicely, attended kids' baseball games with former high school classmates and rooted for her nieces and nephews on the team.

Two years earlier, she had stopped one afternoon to visit her stepfather at work and met Bruce Sampson. He invited her to dinner. Things clicked. They kept seeing each other and soon, in June 1985, a month before Rock Hudson died of AIDS, they married.

No one Diane Sampson knew had spoken much about AIDS before then. But with Hudson's illness and death all over the newspapers, everyone suddenly paid attention to it.

"Because he was somebody," she recalled later. "He wasn't a junkie dying in the street or a queer down on the corner."

The attitude of most people around her toward the AIDS epidemic at that time, she recalled, was: "Let them die. If a woman gets it, she deserves it because she's a junkie."

Her husband had told Diane he had used drugs in the past. She didn't think much about it. Then was then and now was now.

Diane conceived quickly and bore a son. She had brought two children from a previous relationship into the marriage. Now there were three.

One autumn night in 1987, she watched "A Current Affair" television report on attempts by people of Arcadia, Florida, to bar three HIV-positive young hemophiliacs from the public elementary school. The school board had offered the three boys tutoring at home. The boys' parents, Clifford and Louise Ray, thought the three hours of tutoring a week offered was inadequate compared to the twenty-five weekly learning hours available in the schools. They sued the school board and won. A spokesman for a new community group, Citizens Against AIDS in Schools, expressed outrage, as did a school spokesman and local parents. Chronic threats against the Ray family increased in severity and frequency. Under protection of a court order, the Ray children went to school Monday, August 24. That Friday, when the Rays were out visiting friends, their small house was doused with gasoline and torched. A few days after the fire, the Rays moved out of town.[21]

Watching the television report, Diane Sampson immediately sided with the townspeople who wanted the HIV-infected children barred from the school. God forbid the Ray boys played football or soccer—contact sports where kids got cut and bled. She wouldn't want *her* kids in school with them! The townspeople were right to protest. Clifford and Louise Ray were sick and demented, she thought. Why subject their own children to all the nonsense they were going through? Wouldn't it be easier just to get a tutor? Why be so insistent that their children were normal when they clearly were not?

As she thought her thoughts, the HIV virus was most likely already running through Diane Sampson's veins. But she would not know it for another two years.

"Have you ever been raped or forced to have sex?"

Epidemiologist Dr. Sally Zierler wanted this query included on the questionnaire she and her colleagues at Brown University were developing for their study on heterosexual transmission of the HIV virus in Rhode Island and southeastern Massachusetts. It would help them discover the prevalence of sexual assault in childhood. Were sexual assault survivors at increased risk of HIV? That sexual abuse affected public health, Zierler knew. But the medical system had not yet recognized this. Bringing in solid numbers might compel recognition.

The middle of five children, Zierler grew up and attended college in Baltimore. In the 1960s, studying at Goucher College, she demonstrated against the Vietnam War and for civil rights, involved in what she later called "the New Left/white boys' movement."

Long before the then-emerging feminist movement touched her,

Zierler had known the reality of sexual assaults against females. But the feminist movement, whose literature she read in the 1970s during graduate school, gave her words to say what she knew.

In her recovery work, Zierler had sat in groups of women, told her own story, and listened to other women telling theirs. She had been struck by the lifelong spiritual damage to women that led them to continue childhood assaults on their bodies through a variety of means. Women's sexuality, Zierler came to believe, is a powerful spiritual energy. In rape, men assault, not just a woman's body, but her spirit as well, injuring to the core her ability to esteem and love herself and others. That injury felt permanent. It never fully healed.

In the course of AIDS-prevention work among women in the Rhode Island prison system, Zierler had listened to female inmates talking about their assaults as well. One day in prison, every one of the eight women she interviewed reported a history of sexual assault. It was hard for them to talk about their experiences. It could have happened twenty years before, but they still cried about it.

Millions of women in the country were sexual assault survivors. What, then, were the public health implications of such a large community of people who could not love or nurture themselves and those around them, who did not feel that they deserved anything or could create anything? Zierler asked herself.

On a physical level, it could lead women to neglect their bodies by, for example, contemptuously refusing themselves needed sleep or exercise. Or worse, it led to women continuing the assault on their own bodies, cooperating with their own victimization: through abuse of alcohol and other drugs; by accepting health-ravaging conditions on the job with no sense of outrage at yet another bodily violation; by punishing their bodies through cycles of dieting and starving, gorging and purging.

This whole area of women's reality needed to be looked at more systematically.

Zierler did not explicitly make the link between childhood sexual assault and impairment of public health until 1980, when she was teaching her first epidemiology section at the Harvard School of Public Health in Boston, Massachusetts.

She was teaching the mathematical concept of incidence rates. The example she used was rape. She stood before this class of graduate students, most of whom were white male physicians older than her-self, and unexpectedly heard herself say: "Rape is a major public health problem." She pronounced the words matter-of-factly but as she did so, a rush, a release, a power she did not know she had flowed through her.

Rape was never *ever* discussed at Harvard as a public health prob-lem. But now, there sat all the conscientious students, diligently writ-ing the instructor's words in their notebooks: "Rape is a major public health problem."

Watching them, exhilaration rushed through her. This was a math problem she was teaching!

She turned her back and wrote problems on the blackboard to show the students how to come up with incidence rate ratios and inci-dence rate differences: "We say among women ages fifteen to nineteen, fifty per thousand women per year in this community are raped . . . " Then on to the next age group: how many per year are raped?

That was her first explicit linking of sexual assault and public health.

Now, in 1987, Zierler was an epidemiologist, an associate profes-sor of medical science in the Department of Community Health at Brown University and coprincipal investigator of the New England Behavioral Health Study. In designing a study of heterosexual trans-mission of HIV, she wanted a certain question included: "Have you ever been raped or forced to have sex?"

Sister Eileen Hogan had spent nine years working closely with female prisoners. When she left Riker's Island in 1987, her superior offered her a year to study and pray. Reflecting, she found she had learned this in her years as a jail chaplain: that women in prison knew no way to heal their battered psyches.

That, to Hogan, was the real cause of crime. People like Donna, Joanna, and Mary grow up in disaster. They block out their pain, "for-get" the injuries done to them. They numb feelings with food, drugs, alcohol, sex. They never confront their losses: the father who knew his friends were sexually abusing them, but offered no protection; the father who walked out on them; the mother who was always drunk; the kindergarten teacher who shamed them; the beatings; the birthdays never celebrated; the "merry" Christmases that ended in shouts, slaps, and sobs. If the losses are not faced, they build up, almost in the body itself. The connection between the body and soul is real, Hogan came to understand.

The subconscious can only absorb so many hurts before those hurts take their toll somewhere. They are taken out in the way people act. They commit crimes. Then they blame themselves.

If they get a little sober, they say, "I don't want to go back to alcohol" or heroin, sugary foods, or crack. But they don't have the skills not to go back.

They heap contempt upon themselves. They get angry, bitter. They seem powerless to change the way they behave.

We know a good deal about healing our bodies, Hogan reflected. We learn how to exercise, eat good food, rest. But we were never taught how to access our psychic energies to heal our spirits.

To heal, Hogan found, people need help in looking at their lives piece by piece, deeper and deeper. They must look at the hurts they have endured, thaw the frozen pain, feel it and let it go.

They need to confront and grieve all those losses. Then they can begin to reconstruct their lives and look at themselves the way God perhaps looks at them: with love and forgiveness. Only when people feel good about themselves, Hogan reflected, can they do good things for themselves.

This is one way Hogan would work with a woman on healing. As the woman closed her eyes and relaxed, Hogan would encourage her to find a safe spot within herself: a memory of a time when she felt secure—perhaps one afternoon spent in the kitchen with a grand-mother. Every week she would close her eyes and go back to that safe spot within herself. Then Hogan would ask the woman to bring in a healing light—she could call the light whatever she liked: love, the God-dess, the Great Spirit, God. She would just sit and let that light pene-trate the wall around her. Later, the woman would talk about how she felt there, the things she remembered. She would take her pain in her hands, look at it, and let that light heal the pain. The pain is separate from you, Hogan would remind her. You are not what happened to you.

It's a long process. Women come to treat themselves differently afterward. They treat themselves as, Hogan believed, God would treat them. With compassion, love, care, respect.

···

The first results from the studies on HIV prevalence in babies born in New York State came out in December, and Dr. Helen Rodriquez-Trias at Newark's Beth Israel Hospital was one of the many health officials and professionals shocked by the results: on the order of one out of ninety babies in New York State and one out of every sixty babies in New York City carried HIV in its blood.

Horrendous, Rodriquez thought.

All states have mandated examination of baby's blood to screen for various diseases. But in New York State, beginning in 1986, HIV was added to the conditions tested for in the babies' blood. For this test, the bloods are sent to the state laboratories identified only by the hospital they were sent from. (So this was a "blind" study.) Although blood was taken from the baby, the tests were actually revealing the HIV status of the mothers, since, in the first fifteen to eighteen months of life, babies carry their mothers' antibodies in their blood. Some of those babies will themselves turn out to actually have the virus but others, after initially testing positive, will, when their blood supply is cleared of the mothers' antibodies, test negative.

What also was stunning to Rodriquez was that the obvious conclusion from this study didn't hit people: "Hey, these are infected *women!*" It took awhile for it to dawn on epidemiologists and other professionals that these results reflected what was happening to *women*. The focus of their perception was off. It wasn't that the epidemiologists didn't understand that it was the antibodies from the *woman* that were being picked up in the test. On a scientific level, everyone understood that. But what did not come was the realization. "How has this happened—that so many women have become infected? What do we have to do to keep this rate from becoming even greater?" Officials raised no immediate alarm. Nor, Rodriquez saw, were resources and prevention programs focused, as they should have been, on women.

"Policy," as Rodriquez defined it, was "what's coming down on us," and here she recognized another implicit AIDS policy: insufficient weight is assigned to the growing epidemiological evidence, from the beginning of the epidemic, that women are involved.

Government reaction to the results of the blind seroprevalence study in New York showed how evidence of women's involvement in the epidemic was ignored. But even earlier, physicians and public health officials did not connect the severe illnesses in women, particularly in IV drug-using women, with possible HIV infection.

Scientific thinking didn't occur in a vacuum, Rodriquez knew. Somewhere along the line, unconscious value judgments were made. They came out in the phrases so often heard when the epidemiology of AIDS was discussed: "It's not spreading to *the general population.*" "This is only in *specific* populations that have *specific* behaviors."

The CDC's creation of "risk groups" (these *specific* populations) helped obscure the evidence from the very beginning that women were being hit in the AIDS epidemic. The effect of delineating "risk groups"—"homosexual males," "IV drug users," "Haitians," "blood recipients," "people with multiple sex partners"—was to totally obscure the heterosexual transmission of AIDS, Rodriquez believed.

Not that she much liked the phrase "heterosexual transmission" either; it obscured the fact that the risk for women in having sex with men is much greater than the risk for men in having sex with women. Even that fact had not come clearly into focus, though the data seemed to suggest that for any one risk encounter, the risk for the woman was ten times higher than for the man. If people talked simply about "heterosexual transmission," it made it seem as though the risk were posed equally to men and women.

"Risk groups" were perhaps necessary at the beginning of the epidemic, Rodriquez believed, but they were always arbitrary and artificial and when enough was known about AIDS, those categories should have been discarded. According to Rodriquez, everyone who is sexually active and everyone who injects anything at any time with any equipment is at risk of HIV.

Rather than putting resources into HIV prevention activities for women, the initial public health emphasis was placed on women as prostitutes and as pregnant women spreading HIV to the "innocent." These entrenched biases, including the racial ones as the majority of women with HIV began to be identified as black and Latino, led to the notion that the afflicted were "not the general population" (i.e., not "us") and also led to a failure to study the disease in women. That there had been to date no prospective studies on how HIV disease manifested and progressed in women was an example of implicit policy, Rodriquez believed. That resources for studying women and for providing services to women were withheld was implicit policy.

1988

The January 1988 cover of *Cosmopolitan* magazine proclaimed an important message: "Reassuring News About AIDS: A Doctor Tells Why *You* May Not Be at Risk." The tease for the inside article was directed at *Cosmo*'s eleven million readers between the ages of eighteen and thirty-four.

The doctor was not an AIDS specialist but a psychiatrist, Robert E. Gould, with a practice on wealthy East End Avenue in Manhattan. He told women in his article that repeated, unprotected vaginal intercourse, even with a man who was HIV-positive, was safe as long as their vaginas were "healthy."

Many AIDS experts were outraged. Knowing Gould was wrong, they were shocked at the publication of such dangerous, divisive misinformation.

Women in ACT UP were equally appalled at the risks women would be exposed to if they believed Gould. They vowed to take him on.

The harm in advising women to be cautious about engaging in vaginal intercourse, Gould wrote, "exists in the continually mounting fear and false alarm that may make it difficult for any of us to enjoy sex. . . . We are once again being persuaded that sex is wrong, dirty, bad for us, even deadly. . . . This killing of our sexual selves, I feel, may prove more destructive in the long run than the AIDS virus itself."

"We," he wrote to *Cosmo's* women readers, need to hold on to the "enlightenment" of the sexual "revolution" of the 1970s: that sex is "a natural part of being alive."

"We need to believe we can enjoy sex without fearing that our life is in danger with every sexual encounter."

The article seemed fueled by an anxiety that the "sexual revolution" was being threatened: women frightened of AIDS were just not going to be so readily accessible for sex.

Gould was so much more protective of men than of women, ACT UP activist Maxine Wolfe thought and soon told him. To protect men from having to wear condoms, he was willing to let women die.

Within four days, ACT UP women mobilized a demonstration. But first, they wanted to meet with Helen Gurley Brown, editor of *Cosmopolitan,* and with Gould. If the two were just ignorant and were willing to repair the damage without ACT UP having to take direct action against them, why not?

Brown refused to meet with them. Gould agreed to a meeting and allowed videographer Jean Carlomusto to film it. The meeting between Gould and eight ACT UP women, including Maria Magenti, became part of a video Carlomusto and Magenti produced, *Women, Doctors and Liars.*

Seated in his office, the women asked the white-haired psychiatrist what his expertise in AIDS was.

"I became concerned because as a psychiatrist, all of my patients were talking about AIDS and their fear of AIDS and what risk are they at and should they be changing their sexual habits and so on." He got interested in the topic, he explained, in order to be able to advise his clients on their sexual practices.

Why had he chosen *Cosmopolitan* as the place to make his assertions, Magenti asked him, when he knew that in a magazine article, he couldn't substantiate his claims with the necessary footnoting and bibliography?

"It was purely fortuitous," he replied, noting that an editor at the magazine was a good friend of his. "She knows my thinking. We've talked about things at dinner—one thing and another. And she said, 'You know, I think this would be a good piece for our readers.'"

He thought about it, he said, and concluded: "If what I'm saying is correct, it would be very useful for a lot of scared people whose lives are being compromised. *If* I'm correct."

Denise Ribble, a nurse caring for HIV-infected women, read to him from his article: "'Can recurrent sexual activity with a person who does carry the AIDS virus cause you to develop AIDS? Not if you subscribe to the theory, supported by considerable fact which I have just put forward, that you don't get AIDS from sexual activity with a man who has the disease or carries the virus unless you engage in anal sex or there is an open lesion in the vagina when you are having vaginal intercourse.'"

Ribble looked up from the magazine, directly at Gould.

"That's wrong," she said quietly.

"How many women in the United States do you think have a healthy vagina?" Wolfe followed up. "That is, one that has no cuts, no abrasions, no internal lesions, no mild yeast infection, no vaginitis, no chlamydia?"

Many women *did* have small lesions, Gould replied, but he didn't really think that lesions were involved in transmitting the HIV virus. If they were, he asserted, there would be many more cases of heterosexually transmitted AIDS in women.

The women challenged him on this. The data he had cited in his article was fully one year out of date, and in that one year there had been approximately one thousand new recorded cases.

While there were allegedly more women getting AIDS, he replied, he knew, from his own patients, that the women's reports of their sexual activity weren't necessarily trustworthy.

"I do know that there are women who have had anal sex who have not acknowledged it or admitted it."

In other words, he was implying that if a woman had AIDS and said she had had only vaginal intercourse, she was lying. The virus must have been transmitted through anal intercourse.

In fact, just the year before, Dr. Mary Guinan and Ann Hardy of the CDC had written in a medical journal that in various studies of heterosexually acquired AIDS in women, vaginal intercourse appeared to be the primary mode of transmission.[1]

Quoting from Gould's article, the activists challenged the racism of the following statement: ". . . too many men in Africa take their women in a brutal way so that some heterosexual activity regarded as normal by them would be closer to rape by our standards."

Many African nurses had described such brutality to him, Gould said, defending his statement.

That statement, Wolfe noted, "implies that men in the United States do not do that."

"In less numbers," Gould asserted.

"We don't know that," Wolfe replied, "since one-third of women will be raped in their lifetime and we don't know what happens to the other two-thirds."

Gould stuck by the assertions in his article. The women decided to hold a demonstration.

It seemed to Anke Ehrhardt, director of the HIV Center in New York City, that anger about the article was mounting within the AIDS community. She felt the article implied that all white middle-class women who have regular sex don't have anything to worry about and that "other" women get sick because they do sexually bizarre things or live in Africa where men aren't as nice to women as they are here! It was breathtakingly racist.

January 15 was a freezing day. At noon, three hundred ACT UP activists formed a chanting picket line on the sidewalk outside the *Cosmopolitan* offices on West Fifty-seventh Street while others handed out leaflets to the lunchtime crowd.

"For every *Cosmo* lie, more women die!" the activists chanted.

Guards were placed at the entrances to the building and, with women continually trying to enter, those entrances were eventually all closed. After forty-five minutes of chanting, the demonstrators moved to *Cosmo*'s parent corporation, Hearst, three blocks away, backing up traffic as they walked slowly across two major intersections.

Throughout 1988, women read little to alert them to their risk of HIV. Gould's assurance that women could safely have vaginal intercourse with men with AIDS—not to worry!—was an extreme example of the lulling of women, but other media, like *The New York Times,* were also downplaying the heterosexual spread of AIDS and risk to women.

In a series of editorials beginning in 1987, the *Times* had repeatedly argued that "fears that [AIDS] is spreading into the heterosexual population are just that, fears," as journalist Chris Norwood found in a study of print media coverage of women and AIDS centering on 1988. Yet in New York City at that time, almost 25 percent of women's cases were attributed to heterosexual transmission. Norwood pointed to a term the *Times* used that obscured the danger hetero-sex presented to women: in the "pie charts" and graphs illustrating risk factors for AIDS, women infected heterosexually are called "others."[2]

Much reporting presented heterosexual AIDS as "confined" to poorer black and Hispanic women, while a number of studies finding HIV infection among white women and among middle-class women of all races were generally not reported, Norwood found.

While women were being reassured that they had nothing to fear, in fact Norwood was picking up disturbing indications that in the previous years, some women may well have been dying of AIDS without ever having been given that diagnosis.

Between 1981 and 1986, total deaths for women in states and cities with heavy concentrations of AIDS grew at staggering rates, she found and reported on in the July issue of *Ms.* magazine and in the newsletter of the National Women's Health Network. Excluding traffic accidents, deaths from all causes for young and middle-aged women rose by 21 percent in New York, 18 percent in New Jersey, 30 percent in Connecticut, 8 percent in Maryland, and 17 percent in Washington, D.C.

In major AIDS areas, the numbers of women dying from a variety of respiratory and infectious diseases thought to be AIDS-related dramatically increased, Norwood found. For example, in New York City, pneumonia and influenza deaths among women aged fifteen to forty-four increased from fifty to 127, a 154 percent jump, between 1981 and 1986. During this same period in Maryland, these deaths increased by 267 percent; in Washington, D.C., by 225 percent; in Connecticut, by 133 percent; and in New Jersey, by 38 percent. In the states and cities hard hit by AIDS during this period, deaths among women aged fifteen to forty-four rose significantly for other diseases and causes such as tuberculosis, septicemia, rare parasitic infections, chronic obstructive pulmonary disease, and nephritis and nephrotic syndrome, Norwood reported. The women's deaths were almost never attributed to AIDS.

In Idaho, a state that had not yet had a single female death attributed to AIDS, no increase in infectious, parasitic, or respiratory disease mortality was reported among women of this same age group.

While women were being reassured that they were at little risk of getting AIDS, they were expected to prevent the spread of it. It was their job to get men to wear condoms. In response to the epidemic, manufacturers produced "feminine" condom packaging—pastel colors and flowery designs—for women who were now instructed to carry condoms in their purses. Women are the real "Centers for Disease Control," Dr. Janice Raymond, a medical ethicist and professor of Women's Studies at the University of Massachusetts, noted, commenting on this situation.

Press coverage simply ignored the role of men in AIDS prevention. Norwood couldn't find a single major article in 1988 examining heterosexual HIV prevention strategies that included men. ACT UP women would challenge that status quo this year with a creative demonstration at a baseball game.

While 1988 marched on, women (as prostitutes and "pregnants") continued to be blamed for spreading a disease that women were being reassured, on the other hand, they could hardly get. A neat trick, Sandra Elkin would note dryly.

What was happening to women in the epidemic was going largely unreported: Ada Setal cared for her grandchildren and began organizing AIDS caretakers without media attention; women were infected and infected women were excluded from clinical trials of AIDS drugs largely without press notice.

Leadership in addressing the AIDS epidemic, a crucial threat to the security and well-being of the United States, did not come, in 1988, from the federal government or from the President himself, Ronald Reagan, who, in an astonishing example of pussy-footing, signed a bill proclaiming October "AIDS Awareness Month" on October 28, three days before the month ended.[3] No, in 1988 the moral leadership in dealing with the AIDS epidemic, as we will see, came from convicts in New York State's maximum-security prison for women.

Katrina had a bad cold and made an appointment with the doctor for February 11.

"What's the problem?" Dr. Child asked when Haslip sat down in the chair before her.

"I can't shake this cold. I knew I had to see a doctor if I wanted antibiotics."

The doctor flipped through her chart.

"You know you're HIV-positive?"

Katrina's heart stopped. "Excuse me?"

"You know you're HIV-positive?"

"My test results came back?"

The doctor showed them to Katrina.

Katrina stood up. The doctor said she would give her a prescription for her cold. Katrina walked out, the doctor making no attempt to stop her.

Katrina walked up the hill to her unit in a daze, crying. If there had been a bridge, she would have jumped from it. Back inside, her sister inmates looked at her:

"Are you okay? What's wrong? What happened?"

"Somebody died," she said.

Katrina Haslip.

She went into her cell and asked the guards to lock her door.

She cried for two weeks. She'd lie on her bed wondering what was going to happen to her, how she would tell her family, whether she would die in prison.

She spoke to nobody. Each time she heard someone say something about AIDS, she went to her cell and cried.

No one has to know, she thought. I'll never have sex again so I'll never have to tell anybody. She didn't want to think about treatment.

Something was happening to her and she couldn't control it. It was living inside her body every day. It was growing. She couldn't spit it out or cough it up or outsleep it. She felt dirty. Something had invaded her body.

She felt angry at herself for allowing this violation. She wanted to know: Who gave me AIDS? Who made me experience this pain? She needed a face. The guy who stabbed her? Eight pints of blood transfused into her before blood was screened for HIV. No one would believe that's how she, an ex-prostitute and an ex–IV drug user, got HIV.

She didn't feel like herself anymore.

• • •

It was April, two months after Katrina Haslip learned she was HIV-infected. She decided to visit the women with AIDS at IPC. She wanted to contribute something before she got too sick to do so. So she planned to spend time at IPC and read the women a book, hold their hands, whatever they needed.

When she walked in, she found one of the young women, Margaret (pseudonym), suffering from toxoplasmosis, an infection affecting the brain. She was paralyzed on one side. Ugly skin irritations had erupted on her body. Katrina, remembering Margaret's vibrancy, was horrified: was this what lay before her?

She entered the room, greeted Margaret. Impossible to read a book or hold a hand. She felt suffocated. She had to get out of there. In a few minutes, Katrina told Margaret she had something else to do and left.

For Penny Abernathey, an attractive, dark-haired twenty-nine-year-old widow in Austin, Texas, being stood up on a date had become a regular event. It was two years since her husband's death from AIDS. She knew HIV could not be transmitted through kissing, but she never let a date kiss her before telling him she had the virus.

She had learned to create safe daytime dates so the need to tell would not arise so quickly: feeding the ducks in the park, going on a picnic. But eventually, she would have to say the words: "I need to let you know something about me."

Sometimes they'd bring her home in the middle of the date. One man, insistently trying to kiss her in the car before they went into a movie theater, abruptly stopped when she told him she had HIV, drove her home, let her out at the curb, and left in a screech of burned rubber.

Others she told would ask her out again. Fine, she'd say. Then she would wait and wait. No one came.

After uncounted slams, she said to herself: "This is my hovel. This is my life. This is my shit hole. This is it. This is how I'm going to live—alone forever. I'll raise my son and it's going to be him and me against the world."

But later her self-respect rose up in rage: "No, damn it! I didn't do anything wrong! Why do I have to be treated like this? Why can't I have companionship? No, damn it! This isn't the way it has to be."

Women in this male-dominated society sometimes have the sensation that they are invisible, that they exist in the shadows while men take center stage—at work, in politics, in science, in the media, and even in our minds. Women speak and it is as if no words had been uttered, as if no one had even been there.

During crucial years of the epidemic, it appeared that women didn't get AIDS because for many medical professionals women are dark shapes in dark shadows who don't come into focus unless they are seen as endangering either men or fetuses.

In the late 1960s and early 1970s, thousands of women, galvanized by the re-emerged women's movement, stepped out of the shadows and sat together in small consciousness-raising (CR) groups and at political meetings in every part of the country. Among them were four women, unknown to each other, who would join together in the 1980s to shine a light on women, help making women visible in the AIDS epidemic.

One, an Englishwoman, had had every privilege. Rachel Fruchter had studied at England's Oxford University on grounds calm, green, well-cared for, in halls of solid, century-weathered stone. Short, gray-eyed, brown-haired, she had gotten in, done well. There were ten men to every woman at Oxford in the 1950s, when she was a student. Science. She wanted to be a scientist.

She married an American in 1962 immediately after Oxford, moved to New York, and entered graduate school at the elite Rockefeller Institute, where students were expected to have, if not greatness, at least the potential for it.

Rachel felt out of place at Rockefeller. Despite the privileges given her, she agonized, look at how inadequate she was! And she hadn't a prayer of ever being great. She believed the conventional elite wisdom: a scientist does his best work young, or not at all. Yet she wanted children and wanted to spend the years of her youth raising them.

She had her first child in 1967, a year after getting her Ph.D. in biochemistry, and continued in laboratory science. In the last months of pregnancy with her daughter, the following year, she joined her first feminist group.

Women were in an intellectual ferment, an emotional upheaval as they talked with one another and made sense of their lives. Sitting in a circle in one of their living rooms, they talked about their experiences as girls growing up, as women on the job, in relationships with men. They talked of sex, faking orgasms, illegal abortions. For most, it was the first time they had ever spoken of their abortion in a space so public as a living room. The panic trying to find the name of someone who would do it, the cryptic conversations on the telephone with cold strangers ("Be sure the money is in cash"), the terror of walking up those stairs, opening that door . . . the fear of sharp instruments, pain, blood, death. Telling, they cried. This talk opened the women up—to themselves and to one another.

Rachel was reading all the feminist pamphlets churning out of mimeograph machines. Finally she understood why she was conflicted: there were all sorts of things in the structure of society and in her family upbringing that militated against women feeling any self-confidence.

She began to understand how, despite her elite education, despite thinking she was different, privileged, in fact she wasn't different. She was deeply affected by the male-dominated structure. No wonder it was a constant struggle for her to feel that she was as good as the others, as the men. She stopped blaming herself for her supposed defectiveness. She began to see her life in the context of institutionalized sexism.

These insights brought Fruchter tremendous relief. Her sense of inadequacy evaporated.

She joined women from HealthPac, a collective of intellectuals that published a radical critique of the U.S. medical system. They met regularly to discuss women, health, and medicine. (At the same time in Boston, feminists got together around the same issues and became the Boston Women's Health Book Collective, writing a thirty-five cent booklet on newsprint, *Our Bodies, Ourselves,* precursor of the landmark book published in 1973.)

Fruchter's group discussed contraceptives like the Pill, vaginal infections, gynecological surgery, why doctors didn't explain things to patients, how afraid women were to ask the doctor questions.

None of these issues were abstract to Rachel or the other women. There were women in the group who had had abortions under horrendous conditions; one who'd developed life-threatening thrombophlebitis from the Pill; another who'd had trouble with an IUD. The IUD had been associated in the 1930s and 1940s with such high rates of infection and complications that physicians had condemned it as dangerous but, under the auspices of population control advocates, it was resurrected in the late 1950s and early 1960s without any convincing new evidence of its safety.[4] Rachel herself, pregnant with her second child, was attending the one hospital clinic open to her that allowed women to give birth naturally. She feared, because of her payment scheme, that she'd be thrown out of that clinic and forced to give birth at Bellevue Hospital, where they still tied birthing women down and drugged them.

Meeting week after week, the group decided to put together a women's issue of *HealthPac Bulletin* and begin political activism on legalizing abortion. There were demonstrations, press conferences, speak-outs.

In 1972 she, her husband, and children moved into a three-family commune where they lived for the next thirteen years. Her concern aroused by her work in the women's health movement, she got a master's degree in public health in 1973. The next year, she joined the faculty of the medical school associated with Kings County Hospital—the State University of New York (SUNY) Health Science Center in Brooklyn—where she was to remain for many years, working in community outreach and cancer prevention, and where she eventually would come face-to-face with the AIDS epidemic.

In 1969, as twenty-nine-year-old Rachel Fruchter was marching in feminist demonstrations, chanting down broad avenues in New York City, most likely seventeen-year-old Mardge Cohen was marching along with her.

A freshman at Barnard College, Cohen would graduate in the usual four years though it seemed to her, looking back, that classes were peripheral to her real life. All her energy poured into the political meetings of the ragtag Students for a Democratic Society, her weekly CR group, demonstrations for legalized abortion, and an end to the Vietnam War.

It was an exciting, turbulent time, suffused with the conviction that they could end racism, abolish sexism, and change the world.

College over, Cohen left New York in 1973, entering medical school in Chicago where she planned to specialize in women's health care. But she found she hated ob/gyn. She just couldn't stand the way women were treated. She specialized in internal medicine instead.

As a medical student, active in groups such as the Reproductive Rights National Network (R2N2), she worked to make abortion available to the poor. Though legal since the 1973 *Roe* v. *Wade* Supreme Court decision, access to abortion for the poor was curtailed in 1976 through the Hyde Amendment, which barred Medicaid payment for the procedure. Cohen, along with other feminist nursing and medical students, also went into the jails to provide health education and some services to incarcerated women.

Committed to working in a public hospital with the poor, she joined the Cook County Hospital staff in 1976, stayed on, married, had two children.

In 1986 the Women's Health Taskforce she belonged to transformed itself into Women Organized for Reproductive Choice. Drawing few members, it metamorphosed again into the Chicago Women's AIDS Project. Activists in the group believed that issues around AIDS were ones women of all races could work on. As more women were becoming infected, the Project aimed to improve the environment for those women who'd be coming to places like Cook County Hospital.

Cohen stayed with the group through its changes. As a physician at County, she had long been working with people affected by the conditions related to the HIV epidemic (poverty, drug use). Now, in the Women's AIDS Project, as she began seeing gynecological manifestations of AIDS that, judging from the medical literature, did not exist, she would come back to the specialty she had turned from in medical school.

In 1969, while Mardge Cohen and Rachel Fruchter were immersed in the intellectual and emotional intensity of the burgeoning feminist movement, Patricia Kelly, a twenty-year-old sophomore at Baltimore's Notre Dame College, glimpsed the movement swirling around her but could not jump in and move with it. She had a baby daughter to care for. She'd gotten pregnant out of wedlock. After fourteen years of Catholic school, she had known nothing about contraception and had no one to go to for information or help. So she and her boyfriend had used rhythm. She thought that contraceptive method would be okay. But no. The marriage was sudden and, for Kelly, miserable.

When her husband graduated, they moved to Albany, New York, for his career. Kelly went to college and here she did join a CR group. After speaking at her second or third meeting, someone sitting in the circle of women said:

"It looks like Pat is having a hard time and needs special attention tonight."

They all turned to her and let her talk at length. Someone suggested she didn't have to stay in the misery of her marriage all her life. One woman said Pat could come live with her if she needed a place to go. Pat was stunned: women helping other women they did not even know! In three weeks, with the women's help, she had left her husband.

Kelly's life had been changed and shaped by her early pregnancy. Now, as she joined the women's liberation movement, she knew—as Rachel Fruchter also had—that health issues were hers. Moving to Brooklyn, she joined a small women's health group. They did street theater, including a piece she loved about a pregnant man. They also helped women get access to the abortions that were now legal. Bookkeeping earned her income. She and her daughter joined one of the many burgeoning communes and lived there happily for seven years.

In 1978 Kelly returned to college and became a nurse practitioner. For many years she had felt inadequate, stupid, wrong, too much, not enough—and now back in school, she discovered something: she was intelligent.

After graduating, she, along with other nurse practitioners and midwives, provided prenatal care to poor women in upstate New York who otherwise would have had none at all. There were *no* private physicians in her area who would give that care to women on Medicaid.

Returning to Brooklyn in the summer of 1988, Kelly joined Kings County Hospital, after consulting the friend of a friend, Rachel Fruchter, on employment possibilities. Later, Kelly would meet Fruchter in person at a Healthpac conference for activists.

Founded in 1831 as a one-room infirmary, Kings County's complex of antiquated buildings was now the third largest public hospital in the country. Here Ada Setal brought Faith and Jesse for medical care. Here, where Kelly began caring for HIV-infected women, she saw the same familiar scene: physicians ignoring the health care needs of poor women while ringing their hands over the women's sick babies, victims of their nasty, evil mothers.

It was all so depressingly familiar.

Carola Marte, a graduate student in classics at Columbia University in New York when Kelly, Fruchter, and Cohen were marching in demonstrations, discussed feminist issues with her women friends as she began to teach Greek classics and conduct research.

In the 1970s, as her academic career drew her more deeply into research and administration, she found herself uncomfortably isolated from social justice issues. A career in medicine could involve her with those issues. And she knew from the experiences of family and friends that women's problems were often trivialized by medicine. That was enough to motivate her to work in women's health.

In 1978, at the age of forty, Marte entered Yale Medical School. The pelvic exam was then not being taught as a part of the physical exam. Until recently, medical schools across the nation had hired women in prostitution or used anesthetized female patients as models for their students. In the early 1970s, under the influence of feminism, students at Yale challenged the appropriateness of a training in women's health care grounded in medicalized rape and prostitution.

Some of the women medical students offered to be the subjects for ethical pelvic exam training. That proposal was blocked by the Ob-Gyn Department with remarks indicating that they thought the volunteers were seeking thrills.

A standoff. The upshot was that pelvic exams were just not taught at all. Anyone interested in learning would go over to the nursing school where the nursing students practiced on each other.[5]

So this was one context for the neglect of women's health issues. It was still true, by 1988, that there was a gross underemphasis on the pelvic exam. In many cases, hospitals continued to neglect the pelvic as part of the physical exam. Basically, a woman's genitals and pelvic organs, except when she is pregnant or giving birth, are considered something that is not, and should not be, a part of real medicine, Marte learned. So what was happening inside women's bodies was not looked for. And what was not looked for was not seen.

Soon Marte would come together with Rachel Fruchter, Pat Kelly, and Mardge Cohen. Four more who, like Eileen Hogan, would notice: something was happening to women.

In her apartment building, Ada Setal met a reliable elderly woman, Miss Lily (pseudonym), who agreed to babysit for the three grandchildren Ada had taken in six months earlier. Ada didn't know how to tell her the children were infected. Without telling her, she let her look after the children twice but felt terribly guilty and then worried for Miss Lily's safety. "Oh, my God, what if Jesse's nose got in a bleed and she handled him and happened to have a cut on her finger and got that blood on her!" So she sat Miss Lily down and told her she had found out that the children were infected with the AIDS virus. Oh, my God! said Miss Lily. Ada thought Miss Lily would run. She was afraid she would tell the other people in the building. But Miss Lily did not run. She did not tell the other people in the building. From then on, when Ada was at the hospital with one child or out running errands, Miss Lily cared for the children.

Ada dialed her son Eddie's number periodically so Faith and Jesse could talk with their parents. After each call, the children threw things at Ada, screamed at her, and tore around the house smashing things. Faith yelled, "I want to go home! I want to be with Daddy! I want to be with Mama! I want to see my dog! I want to see my cat! I want to be home!" They both cried.

The house was in an uproar for hours after a telephone call. Ada thought: I can't handle this. I've got so much to deal with.

She told the children they could not talk on the phone with their parents anymore. She would show them pictures of Mama and Daddy and they could dictate letters to her for them, but they could not call anymore.

It was heartbreaking, Ada thought. But she could not handle their explosions of grief and rage over their lost parents.

* * *

Ada Setal knew that she, as a caregiver, needed things she didn't have and she knew if that were true for her, it must be true for others. She and her two friends from the caregivers' support group at Downstate Medical Center in Brooklyn, Lydia and Pat, decided to fight for themselves and others. Almost all caregivers they knew were women. Some were too sick to fight, or too tied up going to clinics. Others did not know where to go or what to do to get help. They needed an advocate.

At the beginning of 1988, the three women met and brainstormed a name for their advocacy group: AIDS Children Teaching Us About Love (ACTUAL). Because the children gave and looked for love—reaching out for a hug, a loving word—they taught caregivers how to respond with compassion rather than fear.

The women talked about what they wanted and would agitate for:

- Better service in the clinics. The drained mothers and restless, sick children were sitting four or five hours in the waiting rooms.
- Time off. They needed someone to come occasionally and say, "I'll take the children for a day or two and let you get some rest." Because Faith and Jesse were in the foster care system, Ada had respite services. But many natural mothers did not.
- Health insurance for caregivers provided by the state.

"If you're caring for a dying child, and then when you get sick, there's nothing for you, that's wrong," Ada argued.

In her late fifties, Ada had lost her health insurance when she gave up her job to care for the children. If she got sick herself, she was in trouble.

At the end of April, baby Angela was hospitalized for a month. She had anemia, a heart murmur, thrush, body tremors, difficulty breathing. She would hardly eat and was losing weight.

Rushing around caring for the children, one day Ada stopped as a thought hit her: "Hey, where's Ronald? He said he was going to come surprise me but I haven't seen or heard from him in months."

She began to search for him, calmly at first, then, when someone told her she had heard Ronald had died, frantically. She went to the morgue. There she learned that five months earlier, he had collapsed on Forty-second Street, been taken to a hospital, and fifteen minutes later died. His heart stopped, the doctors said. He had had no identification on him. No one tried to find his family. He had been buried in Potter's Field. Her baby. Ada wept again. Maybe, she thought, before he died, he had come by to see her, but she, sitting in the clinic waiting room with the children, had not been home to open the door to him.

The community she had built with other caregivers in ACTUAL was a comfort to her now. Shut out of normal social life, their children put out of day-care centers and schools, sometimes shunned by their families and churches, the women had felt isolated, unable to speak openly of AIDS in their family and ask for and receive help.

Through ACTUAL, which soon had eighty members, they created their own community. They met at amusement parks on a Saturday with the children. The children played and then they'd have a picnic lunch. They went to the circus. They had potluck suppers just to get together, laugh, and talk. They celebrated each other's birthdays. When one of their children or companions died, they gathered to grieve. Now, with Ronald dead, Ada Setal's community grieved with her.

In July one-year-old Angela began to bleed from the rectum and was hospitalized. Three days later, she died.

It's better for Angela to sleep and be with God, Ada explained to five-year-old Faith and three-year-old Jesse. You wouldn't want Angela to suffer through all her pain. You know how she cried.

At the wake, Faith and Jesse each put a toy in Angela's casket. They wanted her to have company, something she liked to play with.

It rained July 17, the funeral day. There was no cover over the dug-out grave and the hole filled with rain. The men couldn't put the casket in the ground after the ceremony because the water first had to be dipped. Ada, Faith, and Jesse walked away from the grave, leaving the casket by the side.

Faith kept stopping and turning around to look at the little casket left by the open grave. "She's all by herself," she said to Ada. "She's left alone. Nobody to be with her. Why do we have to leave her there? Why do we have to leave her there like that? She's all alone."

Both children were upset, but especially Faith. This was what Faith feared about death: being isolated and alone and away from everybody.

Ada stooped down and peered in Faith's eyes. "Look across the cemetery," she said. "See all the headstones. There are so many people in all the graves. Angela's not alone. She has company all around her."

Ada talked with the children many times at home and told them that Angela could always be alive in their hearts. They could remember how she was and put those memories in their hearts and walk with her spirit inside them.

In the months after the funeral, Faith would put a bottle in her doll's mouth, carry it around, and make-believe it was Angela. She'd put the doll in her bed sometimes and say, "When I die, I want my doll to be with me so I can have company."

Faith was hospitalized for PCP in November. When the doctors discovered she had renal problems, they biopsied her kidneys and found a malignancy.

Rachel Fruchter had been doing a routine follow-up of the cancer patients at University Hospital (SUNY), where she worked in the division of gynecologic oncology, and at neighboring Kings County Hospital one day in 1983. She telephoned the home of a woman diagnosed with cervical cancer three years earlier. How was the woman doing? she asked her family. She was dead, they replied. She had died of AIDS the previous year. That fact plunked itself down in Fruchter's mind and held on, waiting.

Then, in 1985, Fruchter and others in the gynecologic cancer division began to suspect a relationship between HIV in women and cervical dysplasia, a condition of abnormal cells on the cervix (the neck of the uterus) that have the potential to develop into cancer. There are three grades of severity of cervical dysplasia.[6] None is invasive or life-threatening. Physicians pay attention to dysplasia because of its potential for progressing to invasive cancer if not treated. With pap smear screening, abnormalities are picked up at a stage when they can be treated on an out-patient basis at minimum cost and with little risk to the patient.

What first alerted Fruchter to a possible connection between HIV and cervical dysplasia was the work of a colleague in her division at University Hospital, Dr. Frederick Stillman. Back in the 1970s, Stillman had begun encountering abnormal pap smears and cervical cancer in young women. He had several young patients who died of a disease—cervical cancer—that should have been completely curable. In a couple of cases, a young woman came in, had a procedure (cryotherapy or laser therapy) that typically would remove and cure the cervical dysplasia. But in these cases, after the treatment, the disease spread, not only into the cervix but also to the vulva and the anus. One woman had operation after operation—a hysterectomy and vaginectomy among them—and finally died.

The women in these few early cases had something in common: they were immunodeficient. Physicians had made the women immunodeficient by giving them steroids to suppress their immune systems. In some cases, physicians had done this because the women had an autoimmune disease. In others, physicians were treating female kidney (renal) transplant patients and they had to prevent the women's immune system from rejecting a transplanted kidney.

That was the first alert to a connection between immunodeficiency and cervical dysplasia and cancer. Stillman was publishing and lecturing about his work, so people in the division were familiar with it. When Fruchter first heard about AIDS, the new immunodeficiency disease, she, like her colleagues, thought: "Oh, my goodness. HIV-associated immunodeficiency might have the same problems."

An additional alert: It had already been established in the 1970s that renal transplant patients who are immunosuppressed have three kinds of cancer at a very high rate: non-Hodgkin's lymphoma, Kaposi's sarcoma, and squamous cell carcinomas of the skin and—in the case of women—of the genital/anal area. Since HIV-infected people were also immunocompromised, gynecologic cancer specialists at Kings County knew these cancers could show up in them, too.

Then Fruchter and the other specialists began hearing of actual cases.

This was sobering news. Fruchter knew, as did her colleagues, that HIV disease could totally change the professional lives of everyone who worked in gynecology at Kings County. Brooklyn had one of the highest rates of cervical cancer in the country. Kings County had a vast population of patients with the disease. It was the primary cancer they dealt with. It was a disease associated with poverty[7] and this was an impoverished area. All public hospitals in Brooklyn referred their cervical cancer patients to Kings County.

Fruchter ran the Kings County and University Hospital registries for gynecological cancer. The department had been trying to prevent cervical cancer by early detection and treatment so she had done many epidemiological studies of their patients since 1974, when she worked on research and evaluation for the Division of Gynecologic Oncology.

In doing those epidemiological studies, Fruchter knew that, over the years, one or two admitted drug addicts a year would develop cervical cancer. They tended to come in for treatment at an advanced stage of the disease, not follow through on all the treatments, and die rapidly. Now, hearing that HIV could be spread through sharing needles, she realized, as did her colleagues, that some of these patients might actually have had HIV. It was her guess that they had. Not knowing of the disease early on in the epidemic, they hadn't looked for or diagnosed it.

The first thing Fruchter did was review the records of a couple of women drug addicts. One had oral candidiasis—thrush—and the other had a note in the chart from someone in the Department of Medicine: "Tested for HIV."

In 1987 physicians in the gynecologic cancer department faced a difficult treatment decision. What if a woman with cervical cancer spread throughout the pelvis was HIV-infected? If they gave her a typical therapy—radiation and various chemotherapy drugs that suppress the immune system—would they be doing more harm than good? Giving such an immunosuppressive treatment might kill her faster than if they had treated her only with surgery. They didn't know what to do.

To make treatment decisions, they had to know whether the women had HIV. So they began asking women under fifty with invasive cervical cancer if they would be willing to be tested for HIV.[8] Between 70 and 80 percent of the women agreed.

The results shocked them: Twenty to 25 percent of their Kings County patients under fifty with cervical cancer had HIV infection.

They had been sure they'd find a few, but 25 percent? Never! It really upset them.

That same year, another finding shocked physicians in the gynecologic cancer division for it held terrifying implications for their own safety. Their colleagues in obstetrics had shown a 2 to 3 percent HIV infection rate among their childbearing patients. That was pretty bad. The gynecologic cancer specialists were afraid they'd find a similar rate among their own patients in the Kings County colposcopy clinic where women with abnormal pap smears came for further investigation. They did a blood survey for syphilis—an increasing epidemic— on the clinic's patients, then took all identifiers off the blood samples and tested for HIV. Not 2 or 3 percent, but a full 10 percent of the women at the colposcopy clinic were HIV-infected. The entire department was stunned.

The physicians among them had been doing surgery three or four times a week. The radical surgery they did in cancer patients could be time-consuming and bloody. They were getting needle sticks and cutting themselves all the time. They had been risking their lives weekly without knowing it.

The high rate of HIV infection among their patients threw them for a loop. Younger physicians had to rethink their career plans: did they really want to spend their work life doing surgery in a community that had a lot of HIV?

Fruchter was ready to keep going. So was a young physician colleague, Mitchell Maiman. They launched collaborative studies of HIV and cervical disease.

Fruchter began collecting data in preparation for writing a research proposal for the National Cancer Institute of NIH. In the gynecologic cancer division at that time, in addition to seeing the staggeringly high rate of HIV infection, they were also seeing a number of young women who eventually died of cervical cancer. This was upsetting and worrying all of them. With early treatment, cervical cancer was highly curable. Fruchter had worked on evaluations of mortality rates. They had excellent records on all their cervical cancer patients going back to 1967. Why was there still so much cervical cancer in Brooklyn even though women throughout the borough were getting pap smears as fast as they could give them out? It worried them.

At the end of 1987, Fruchter and Maiman wrote a grant for the

National Cancer Institute hypothesizing that cervical cancer would be more common and more aggressive in women with HIV disease. They proposed to look at the characteristics of cervical dysplasia, and of invasive cancer, in HIV-negative and HIV-positive women, and to follow up each group after treatment and see how the women survived.

Establishing a connection between HIV and cervical cancer would not be easy.[9] For one thing, nobody looking at death certificates or at the cancer registry would be able to detect such a connection. The deaths of almost all the HIV-infected women in Brooklyn who had died with cervical cancer had been attributed to that cancer. If the women had had HIV or AIDS, that fact would not be noted on the women's death certificates. Fruchter knew; she ran the cancer registry. She and Maiman expected there to be a connection and started looking for it, offering women who came in with cervical cancer HIV counseling and testing.

NIH did not fund their study. Maybe it was too early in the game, Fruchter thought. Next, they submitted a proposal to the American Cancer Society. That, too, was turned down. They persevered and got a small grant ($500) from the faculty union. With another proposal to the American Cancer Society to look at HIV and cervical cancer, Maiman won a three-year award earmarked for a physician.[10]

Fruchter, who was personally involved in the follow-up of women with severe dysplasia (carcinoma in situ) went back to the Tumor Registry and reviewed the history of all the young patients. Many had died. Looking up the causes of death, she repeatedly found HIV disease, pneumococcal pneumonia, or drug-related conditions.

Fruchter had no real epidemiologic evidence that this rate of death in young women had been increasing since the 1970s. A homeless woman who had carcinoma in situ five years earlier and died on a sidewalk one winter night could have died from exposure, or from a drug addiction–related condition, or from HIV disease. So there was no proof.

But there was a box. Fruchter began keeping a whole file in her office of young women with carcinoma in situ whom she would have expected to be completely cured but who had died young. She was keeping the file because she thought that at some point she would be able to use the evidence as part of the data supporting an association between HIV and cervical cancer.[11]

···

Probation officer Richard Brooks went to the county jail in Syracuse to interview Helen Cover, the woman who had abandoned her dream of nursing and now stood accused of cutting another woman in a fight. Brooks had the right to see her in the private client/attorney room where they could converse through bars. But knowing she had AIDS, he insisted on interviewing her in the crowded visiting room where a Plexiglas partition stood between them. In order for him to hear her, Cover had to yell out personal details about her disease and her life.

In his report, Brooks recommended prison for Cover. To counter that recommendation, Cover's court-appointed attorney, Jack Lynch, asked the National Center on Institutions and Alternatives to propose an alternative to prison for Helen. The Center's director, Marsha Weissman, agreed. In preparation for the sentencing memorandum, she sent Lesley Noble to interview Helen.

Helen was very ill. She was given no ongoing medical care in the jail. She received treatment only when she was ill enough to be hospitalized. It was in the hospital that Noble interviewed Cover.

Noble liked her. Warm and generous, Cover put her at her ease immediately.

"Gee, you look pretty young," she said.

Weissman and Noble talked with Helen's longtime companion, Tim, and he agreed to take her back. Then they tried to find a drug treatment program for Cover. It was difficult. None would provide child care for her two children.

The Center wanted a halfway house for her. But when they told the programs that she was HIV-infected, most shied away. They were unequipped to handle someone with that problem, they said.

Finally, the Center found an out-patient clinic that would take her.

In one of many conversations, Helen told Noble that she was terrified she would meet the same fate as her mother: die a drug-related death young, leaving her children motherless. She knew what it meant to be left unprotected. She did not want her children to suffer as she had.

Helen Cover was arraigned before County Court Judge J. Kevin Mulroy April 26.

The next day, probation officer Brooks recommended imprisonment, concluding that Cover "represents a high risk to the community's safety and to herself."

Helen Cover was a first-time offender with no history of violence. Pointing these facts out, Weissman and Noble noted in a sentencing memorandum the big discrepancy in life expectancy between people with AIDS living in prison (5.5 months) and in the community (two years).

They recommended that in addition to out-patient drug treatment she receive counseling to help her cope with the prospect of death.

Noble explained to Helen that they were going to ask the judge for probation with drug counseling and that one condition of probation was "no drinking." Helen was taken aback. She didn't drink much, she said, but did love a glass of white wine once in a while.

"I know, but you can't do it!" Lesley told her.

In July Judge Mulroy sentenced Cover to six months in jail and four and a half years on probation. He ordered her to get treatment for her drug and health problems. Helen stood before him at the bench.

"Has your lawyer explained the conditions of probation?" he asked her.

Most prisoners answered by rote, as their lawyers advised: "Yes, I understand." But Helen said, "Well, yeah, you know, but I got this question, Judge, about the wine."

Lynch began biting his nails while Noble silently screamed, *Don't bring that up!*

But Noble had to laugh. Helen was charming. Here she was facing severe hardships, a prison term, and death, and she was still bringing up the wine question.

"I don't know, Judge," she was saying. "It's pretty hard to accept."

It was as if Helen were weighing a prison term on one hand and the absence of an occasional glass of white wine on the other and was having trouble deciding which was worse.

Finally: "Well, okay. Give me the probation."

Even Judge Mulroy laughed.

Leaving the courtroom, Marsha Weissman thought that part of

the reason they got Cover probation was that they had explained to the judge that Helen was likely to die very soon. That was reassuring. Their argument had been, she felt, a little bizarre: Yep, she really is going to die. I swear and promise, she is going to die.

Route 26 in rural Maine wound past country stores with signs on their windows, "Game Inspection Station," and rifles and moose heads mounted on the walls. One night, down one of the muddy dirt roads off the route, newlyweds Al and Patricia made love in the home they had just built. Then Patricia passed a blood clot. She was fevered, in pain. Al bundled her in the car and delivered her to the emergency room of the small one-story hospital. The physician, a woman, took a culture, told Patricia she had an infection she couldn't identify, gave her penicillin, and advised her to see her family doctor the next day.

Al drove her there the next morning. After examining her, the doctor looked sternly at her across his desk.

"Patricia," he said, "all women pass a clot now and then. It's nothing. Ever since I've known you, you've had trouble with your period. Always. I think you just don't like being a woman."

His words felt like a punch to her stomach. The red heat of a blush spread over her face.

"I'm thirty-five years old," she told him, defensively. "No, I don't enjoy my periods, but I'm used to them. It's a part of my life."

She felt so humiliated, his saying such a thing in front of her new husband. Yet she believed him. She was having this gynecological trouble because there was something terribly wrong about her. She didn't like having her period and therefore didn't like being a woman and that's why she felt so sick.

She continued to feel terrible, but convinced herself that it was all in her head.

In fact, she had an infection from August to October. She believes the HIV infected her then, that August.

Surgeon General Everett Koop and other public health officials were giving women advice on how to protect themselves from HIV infection: Find out your partner's sexual and drug-taking past, they said.

Know with certainty whether your sexual partner is at risk for AIDS. Interview him. Ask him if he has used IV drugs and shared needles. Ask him if he has been exposed to the virus by having sex with someone who was infected. Has he ever had sex with men? In the anal-receptive position?

Interview your partner. Was this good advice?

Dr. Vickie Mays and her colleague, Dr. Susan Cochran, were about to find out. In 1986, their research group, the Black CARE (Community AIDS Research and Education) Project, had begun studying relationship behaviors of young adults in southern California. The subjects, who included women and men aged eighteen to twenty-four, were all in college or trade school. Mays and Cochran collected data on sexual behavior and the young adults' perception of their risk of AIDS. To pick up changes in attitude over time, the researchers planned to go back into the same community every two years.

For this 1988 round, they would focus on the current advice being disseminated by public health officials.

There were public service announcements showing "If you slept with this one, that means you slept with this and this and this one," and stressing the importance of talking to your partner. It was one of those nice thirty-second sound bites that did well for public service announcements, Mays thought. Young adults heard the sound bite that got their attention so they did ask the questions. But the Public Health Service did not couple that with what they should *do* with the information: continue to use condoms until they had some objective information.

As social scientists, Mays and her colleagues realized that early on in relationships, particularly when people are dating and trying to get to know each other well, they put their best foot forward. They don't necessarily lie, but they may not instantly give a history of their sexual pasts.

Before revealing intimate details of their lives, most people want to feel intimate. They want to know that they're accepted, that they'll be listened to, that they'll be able to explain why they did something. After all, Mays thought—this was very intimate data people were being asked to come across with: how many sexual partners they'd had; what kinds of sexual acts they'd engaged in; whether or not they'd been shooting drugs. That kind of information isn't usually shared until *after* there has been intimacy. For some people, that intimacy occurred *after* sex.

In their interviews, Mays and Cochran found that 52 percent said that asking such questions about sexual and drug histories was one of their main precautions.

But the study also found that men lie to women in order to have sex with them. So many of the men had lied about their sexual past and drug use that it seemed pointless for the women dating them to ask.

Thirty-five percent of the men questioned admitted they had lied in some form or another to a woman to get her into bed, an estimate Mays and Cochran considered low. Sixty percent of the women said they thought a man had lied to them. Common lies the men reported telling a woman were that they felt more for her than they really did, that they had no other sexual relationships, and that they had fewer sexual partners than they really did. Twenty percent of the men said they would lie to a woman who asked if they had had an AIDS test. They'd tell her that they had, everything was fine, they were HIV-negative.

Fully two-thirds of the men at higher risk for HIV (that is, men who had had sex with other men or with intravenous drug users or with multiple partners or had had STDs) did not think they needed to use condoms. They relied on women to be using some form of contraception, they reported.

Mays did not see the lying as malicious. If people don't understand all the ways they might have been exposed, if they associate AIDS with the faces of IV drug users and gay men, and they're asked if they've been exposed to HIV, they may think: "So how would I get it? That's a dumb question! No, I'm sure if they gave me the test right now, I'd be negative." And then say: "I had the HIV test and I'm negative."

Deception may be a contributing factor in the spread of AIDS, particularly among women, Cochran and Mays concluded.

As other researchers had found, women disclose intimate information earlier in a relationship than men do. Women who followed the Public Health Service advice to interview their partner would be at more risk of HIV infection than men who followed that advice because women would not get the honest disclosures as early as men would, Mays knew.[12]

··· ·

"Education of those who risk infecting themselves or infecting other people is the only way we can stop the spread of AIDS," the Surgeon General would tell the U.S. public in pamphlets sent to every U.S. household. He was echoing the assertion of public health officials since the early years of the epidemic.

Now Sandra Elkin, a former PBS producer, was charged by the HIV Center in New York City with producing an educational video on AIDS. She had asked Anke Ehrhardt, director of the HIV Center, and psychiatrist Dr. Rafael Tavares, who was directing the Center's collaborations with community organizations, to see some of the videos people were then using. She was appalled.

"They're racist, sexist, incompetent, low-budget, poor quality, flat, boring, rampant with white male doctors in white coats lecturing into a camera about what people should and should not do and talking about viruses in ways nobody could understand," she told them. "For starters."

"Be frank now," Tavares said. They all laughed.

"We can't do it like that," Elkin asserted. "Even with a low budget, we can do better than this."

All three knew, as research had shown, that information doesn't change behavior. Neither do scare tactics. Despite this, the videos kept throwing information at people and scaring them. Women were told to get men to wear condoms or die. It wasn't such a hot idea to base the whole strategy for preventing HIV transmission to women on instructing women to do something they didn't have the power to do.

Education was being censored. The federal government barred the CDC from funding AIDS education, information, or prevention materials that could be interpreted as promoting or encouraging homosexuality or drug use.[13]

Elkin, Ehrhardt, Tavares, and colleagues set about developing a model for producing health educational materials that would actually reach people. Elkin had the freedom to do whatever needed to be done to reach the women only because the HIV Center, in arranging financing of the video, found a way to avoid governmental control of the content.

The first thing the video team did was ask people from inner-city communities what AIDS education materials they most needed. In

August, in sweltering rooms in the Bronx and Brooklyn, Dr. Rafael Tavares met with residents. They had nothing adequate for female partners of IV drug users who were being hard hit by the epidemic, they told him.

Okay, they'd make a video for that group.

The AIDS prevention message had to come from someone viewers would find credible. White male doctors were not necessarily credible for women of any race or for women and men of color. They were out. Women were in; the women's movement had demonstrated that women like to get information from one another.

The script would be based on the experiences of actual women and written by a professional scriptwriter, Deborah Cavanaugh. Through Dooley Worth, whom Ehrhardt had met at a NIDA meeting in Washington, D.C., in January, the writer spoke with some of the women the video would be designed to reach. Worth later talked extensively to Cavenaugh and arranged for her to meet with women at a methadone maintenance clinic. She listened to the women's life stories and what they said about the men in their lives.

She was especially struck by the woman who emerged naturally as the leader of the support group: an HIV-infected prostitute whose children had been taken from her. As the women in the group talked, the leader (soon to be "Nicole" in the video) identified the behavior of the men in their lives, even when they themselves could not. That's controlling behavior, she'd say. That's manipulation. He's sleeping around and lying about it. He's hammering away at you.

And she not only talked about the behavior of her own husband, she told the women what she was doing to counteract it. When she threw him out, she said: If I stayed with him, he'd only drag me down. I'd never see my kids again because the city won't allow them back into a home where there are drugs. I'm clean. He won't get clean. I've got to think about myself and my kids.

She'd tell the other women: I want to get out of prostitution, go to night school, develop a skill I can use to earn a living. I don't know how to do it but I'm going to find a way.

Over a period of time, as she found ways, she'd share them with the group: "I start school next week. This is how I'm going to do it."

"Nicole" gave the other women a new perspective on their lives, courage to act on their own behalf, a role model. Through her leadership, nine other women in the group gave up drugs.

It became clear that if the video were going to help stop the spread of a virus that was transmitted sexually, it had to deal with how men treat women in sexual encounters and how that affects women's ability to protect themselves. They could deal with that if they scripted the story like a soap opera, the video team decided. The writer translated the experiences of four African-American women into a script that did for viewers what Nicole did for the other female characters: named male behavior.

The one authority figure in the video became then not a doctor in a white coat but a woman in prostitution. She led, got angry, made intelligent commentary, and delivered the important message in the video.[14]

The team entitled the video *AIDS Is About Secrets,* the secrets including those women keep from one another about how the men in their lives treat them—for example, that women cannot discuss certain things with men without making them angry.

(Patricia Daugherty in rural Maine never confided to her women friends that she'd asked Al to take an AIDS test because he'd had sex with men; that he got angry so she was afraid to push; that now she was marrying him not knowing whether or not he was infected with a fatal, sexually transmitted virus. The bullying Daugherty was subjected to when she tried to protect herself remained a secret.)

In the opening scene of *Secrets,* the character Sly, a young African-American man, comes home very late. His wife, Jaleen, doesn't believe his account of where he's been—moving furniture with his brother Clinton. Sly wants to have sex with her because he thinks it will shut her up. Jaleen wants him to wear a condom. She wiggles it in front of his nose, trying to make her request playful. He takes the condom out of her hand and throws it away. It's clear she can't press that anymore. So that scene shows: you can only go so far.

Jaleen brings up her suspicion that Sly's brother Clinton is using drugs. This worries her because she fears he'll suck Sly back into drugs. They fight. He begins to get loud. His body language—the way he holds his hands and arms and clenches his fists—says: I'm trying not to knock her around. She yells at him but in the end, she lets him sweet-talk her into giving up the argument because she knows he's holding back and in a few minutes, he's not going to hold back anymore. There will be violence and it will land on her.

Watching *Secrets* opened the floodgates for some women at Riker's jail. Jeri Woodhouse, a member of Manhattan borough president Ruth Messinger's staff, had designed an AIDS prevention education program for the women. In eight or nine consecutive meetings, she and her partner continually tried to get a discussion going on AIDS-related topics but the women did not want to talk about it. There was tremendous denial, Woodhouse thought. She couldn't get anywhere. The women chatted with one another during presentations and walked about. Then she brought in *Secrets*. The women were riveted to the video, relating to the characters.

"Right on, sister!" they'd cheer at the television screen. "You tell them!"

When the video was over, a floodgate opened that did not close for the remainder of the Project. The women talked about how hard it was to get a man to wear a condom; what the consequences were of trying; how men treated them. They talked of their worries about AIDS, of people in their families who were ill or had died of the disease. At the next meeting, they wanted to see the video again. Correction officers providing security in the area were hanging over the partition, watching the film, and later asked if it could be shown to the officers.

Secrets sparked the women's ability to talk more openly about something that was frightening, worrying, and, for some, already personally painful, Woodhouse found.

Even though the video team had targeted African-American inner-city partners of male drug users as their audience, it subsequently found that the video reached women across a wide range of races, classes, nationalities, and cultures because the behavior the film named was *gender* behavior. *Secrets* was shown on national television throughout blond, blue-eyed Sweden. It was shown in South Africa, Canada, Austria, the Netherlands. One of the secrets AIDS was about was that gender behavior—how men treat women—is a major factor in the spread of AIDS.

When the film was completed, Elkin soon learned that if she and her crew had been subject to government regulations, *Secrets* would never have been made. An executive from the government agency that had funded the video called Elkin's office and said the agency would have nothing to do with the video. It would not distribute thousands of copies of *Secrets* free to clinics throughout the United States as it had the power to do. Nor would it recommend the film.

The official objected to the language in the script, was displeased that the prostitute delivered the message, and thought that the soap opera character Tamara risked losing her man if she told him, *before* she'd had the test, that she had been exposed to HIV. Best to keep mum till after the test results came in, the official thought. That wasn't all.

"Do you know there are six 'fucks' in that script?" she asked Elkin, irate.

Elkin had never actually counted them. After hanging up, she did. The official was wrong. There were seven.

Elkin couldn't believe it. Dollars were being poured down the drain making AIDS education videos that didn't work, that gave people no help in protecting themselves from the virus, because some government officials were concerned about language and propriety.

Secrets, a video that went on to win several awards in film and video festivals, now had to be quietly distributed underground since the government was turning its nose up at it.

As she screened the video for groups doing AIDS education in various communities, Elkin's anger heated to fury. Time after time, she showed it to health educators who said, "The characters and incidents in the video are so realistic. How did you do that?"

At first, Elkin thought they were asking her about the production process. But what they really wanted to know was: how did Elkin get away with making a video like that? They would tell her they needed an educational video for this or that group but then added, "But of course we can't do it because we can't say those things or show those things or write that language."

"Why not?" Elkin would ask.

The answer was always the same: the money they got from city, state, or federal governmental agencies came with strings attached. They couldn't use real street language. They couldn't appear to be condoning nongovernmentally sanctioned sexual relations: gay relationships, any outside of marriage. They couldn't show how to put on a condom.

If they couldn't go as far as they needed to go to reach people, showing their lives accurately and thereby winning their trust, then the AIDS prevention materials were going to be as ineffective as most already were.

Elkin would sit at the screenings, the breath knocked out of her with the enormity of their statement: we are spending money on AIDS education tools that we all know are not going to work.

After Elkin showed *Secrets* at a city family planning agency, one official took her to a file cabinet in her office.

"We get videos from the state and the city and they're so useless, we just put them here," she said, pulling out a file drawer. Elkin saw how many videos were resting in peace. The official pushed the drawer back and it slammed, leaving a sound in Elkin's head that would not go away.

Government and public health people kept saying, "Education is the only vaccine we have for HIV and AIDS." If that's so, Elkin thought angrily, why are we being so blatantly sloppy about the way we plan and produce it? Why are we letting people who have little or no expertise make decisions about it? We need to treat the development of education in the same careful way we would treat the development of a vaccine. We wouldn't pick the lowest bidder for a surgeon to save somebody's life. The video makers should be chosen as carefully as we'd choose the surgeon who would do open-heart surgery on us—our lives could depend on that decision.

While the U.S. government's explicit policy on AIDS may be that it wants to protect its citizens from the disease and is taking action to do so, Sandra Elkin got a vivid education on the country's implicit public policy on AIDS, the policy implemented through regulations, budgets, hiring decisions, and the sloppy, halfhearted development and production of AIDS education materials. That policy was: let 'em die.

Carola Marte, the physician treating HIV patients at the Community Health Project in Manhattan, had met Mardge Cohen in 1987 when Cohen, the activist-physician from Chicago, rose at the women's caucus of a meeting of Society for General Internal Medicine (SGIM) and asked the caucus to support a resolution opposing mandatory HIV testing of women. The resolution, proposed by Dr. Helen Rodriquez at an earlier meeting of the American Public Health Association, stipulated that HIV prevention and education measures should be available, but no forced testing. After the meeting, the two women discussed the political issues raised for women in the epidemic. Spending more time together at other conferences that year, they became friends.

In July 1988, at Cook County Hospital in Chicago, Dr. Mardge Cohen, working with other women in the Chicago Women's AIDS Project, opened a clinic in which HIV-infected women and children were seen at the same time. There was only one other clinic in the country—in Miami—that was doing that. Soon, their HIV service delivery and prevention and education program received three-year funding from the Robert Wood Johnson Foundation.

The need for the clinic was clear to them: pediatric and gynecological services were fragmented, placing an exhausting burden on ill women who had to get themselves and their children to different clinics in different locations at different times. In providing pediatric services for HIV-infected children, it had not occurred to service planners—except in a blaming way—that if a child were infected, in most cases the mother would be as well. A dark shape in dark shadows, she was no human being who herself needed care for the disease. In the service delivery model feminists from the women's health movement devised, women themselves were taken seriously, not just their children.

They put together a team (entirely female as it turned out) that coordinated the care offered women: case managers (African-American, Spanish-speaking, and white), internists, obstetrician-gynecologists, psychologists, pediatricians, health educators.

The ob/gyn department at the hospital had pretty much avoided dealing with the HIV crisis in women. But the ob/gyn on their team, an African-American long committed to the women of the community, buffered them from that reality. Rather than treating only conditions in the women's pelvic organs, she acted as the women's primary-care physician.

From the beginning, a support group for women was part of the standard of care at County. It should be everywhere, Cohen maintained, because the women live in a terrible, debilitating isolation, unable to talk with anyone else about what they are going through. Twenty women met at the clinic every week. They were not the *same* twenty women throughout those three years. As women in the group died, newly diagnosed women took their places.

The clinic cared for the children and served the women lunch while they met. With a health educator facilitating, the women talked about what it meant for them to be infected.

The facilitators came to name what happened in the group "the evolution of dignity." The women were expected to sit for hours with ill children in the packed waiting rooms of large and unresponsive institutions. In the group, the women strengthened one another. They modeled for each other assertive behavior in getting aid, entitlements, child care, and in dealing with Cook County Hospital itself.

The support group gave the health team feedback on what issues the women were facing, medically and socially, so that the providers could figure out which programs should be discontinued, which should go on, what needed to be created.

Interested women in the group were trained as paid peer HIV-prevention educators in a six-week program. They then went out and talked about HIV in various community settings.

At the clinic, they routinely did pap smears on the women. One day, they would look closely at those pap smears and see that in their clinic the rate of abnormality was five to eight times greater than the baseline rate at Cook County.

Charlotte married Steven in 1988. They had met three years earlier at Columbia University where both were undergraduates. Early in their relationship, he told her that in his past, he had been in a long-term homosexual union.

Caring relationships were important to Charlotte Schafer (a pseudonym), not the sex of the partners. She accepted his past.

Before marrying, they had talked about AIDS. He had reassured her that that was no problem for them. She never thought of asking him to get an HIV test. She and a friend discussed what she would do if ever he turned out to have AIDS. That would make no difference in her affection for him, Charlotte said. AIDS fell under the category "for better or for worse."

She thought of AIDS in terms of supporting Steven as he went through it. It hadn't occurred to her that *she* could be infected. Never. It was never a part of any discussion she had with Steven or with the three friends who knew of his past. She didn't remember hearing of any woman ever getting it back then. When they were dating in 1985, 1986, and 1987, there had not been much information out there about women and AIDS. Maybe the information existed, but if it did, you had to dig for it. Charlotte had not dug.

After college, Charlotte worked as a paralegal in the district attorney's office in New York, Steven in an investment bank.

In the first autumn after their marriage, when they walked the dogs at night, she noticed that Steven was very slow and bowlegged and walked as if he were a little drunk. In November he told Charlotte he would check out his walking and balance problems with a doctor after the new year.

Helen Cover, on probation, was reunited with her boyfriend Tim and her two children. At first, Lesley Noble, a young woman from the National Center on Institutions and Alternatives who had helped her win probation, was happy for her. Maybe now her life would turn around.

But Helen missed some of her drug counseling appointments. The program provided no child care and she had trouble finding babysitters. Without a car, she had to arrange rides to the clinic and then get herself from site to site when she was weak and in pain.

When Cover began to have problems, she called Lesley Noble and Noble's boss, Marsha Weissman. A substance abuse counselor she was seeing was out sick and her appointment had been rescheduled for three weeks later. For an addict, three weeks without support can be critical, Weissman knew.

Helen kept using drugs. The probation department never helped her, she later pointed out. "They just sent me right back out there to be back around drug people. They knew I had nowhere to go." The same probation officer who had already demonstrated his hostility to her and his ignorance of her disease was assigned to supervise her. Helen had been set up to fail, Noble thought.

A few months later, Noble saw Helen in the Marine Midland Bank shivering in jeans and a denim jacket. She looked bad. Helen told her Tim had thrown her out of the house in October and she had nowhere to go. She was trying to stay with friends on the South Side.

Oh, boy, Noble thought. The South Side is bad territory for anyone trying to get off drugs.

Later, Helen called Noble from a friend's house where she was so sick she could not move. She needed to get to a hospital. Noble sent someone for her from the AIDS Task Force.

From October to December, Helen lived in the streets, except when she was in the hospital. Sometimes—hungry, tired, cold, wheezing—she would kneel down and draw pictures on the sidewalk. She had always loved to draw.

She slept in abandoned buildings when she could. Sometimes she would not sleep for three or four nights in a row, walking the streets continually, hustling, looking for a stranger to take her in for the night or get her high. She offered men blow jobs for cocaine.

Once she told Noble, "The johns, the junkies, are the only people who will take me in."

She was desperate. She knew she had failed. She had given up doing what she had to do to survive. Those lovely things the National Center on Institutions and Alternatives had recommended for her—a residential setting with constant supervision, counseling to help her cope with the prospect of death—had not become real in this world.

To help her cope with the prospect of death, Helen Cover had cocaine—high, numb, and homeless in the face of death.

In Brooklyn, Pat Kelly, the activist nurse practitioner, had heard scattered reports that cervical carcinomas were much more virulent in HIV-positive women, though those informal reports hadn't been checked out in any systematic way. Right there in Brooklyn, she'd heard, a few HIV-infected adolescents had died of cervical cancer. Adolescents dying of a disease that appeared, not in teenagers, but in older women! That was astonishing.

Kelly, who had started work at Downstate just this summer, knew that many HIV-infected women were using the Infectious Disease Clinic for their primary care. But they weren't getting pelvic exams there. Instead, the docs would refer them to the gyn clinic. The whole setup was so complicated for the women to master that they might or might not ever end up jumping all the hurdles in the maze to actually get a pelvic exam and pap smear.

Kelly started raising a ruckus at the clinic in December 1988. They ought to be doing paps on the women, she said. They had an obligation.

None of the infectious disease docs wanted to do gyn exams. Those exams were gross. Besides, some commented, "Women are going to die from their HIV disease before they'll die from any cervical problems so why should we bother to do this?" They expressed such repugnance at the proposal, rejected it so wholeheartedly, were so upfront in expressing their distaste to Kelly that she had moments of self-doubt: Was she really on the right track here? Or was there something weird about her wanting to do this?

In 1988, no pelvic exams were done on HIV-infected women coming into the Infectious Disease Clinic.

Each woman in the core group of those concerned about AIDS at Bedford Hills prison sought out other inmates who might help break the silence around the disease. When they reached thirty-five, they called a meeting.

It was a warm day in early autumn. The thirty-five inmates in prison greens entered the second-floor room, grabbed chairs, and sat around a table. Through the windows, they could see the parking lot outside and the tall metal fences.

To Katrina Haslip, many of the women were strangers. They were a mixed group: black women, white, Latinas from a variety of Spanish-speaking cultures; young (eighteen), older (forty-five), some from the street life like Lady T herself, some from leftist politics, others from homes where they had been battered. While some could not read, others, like Kathy Boudin, had master's degrees.

This was the first time women who wanted to change the prison environment around AIDS sat down together to talk about the disease in such a public forum. Women were being stigmatized. Women were dying. They needed to talk about it. But they didn't know what would come out of this meeting. Every woman knew that just by sitting in that room, she risked being stigmatized as a Person With AIDS (PWA) herself and shunned.

Kathy Boudin called the meeting to order and introduced herself. The atmosphere was tense. Everyone stared at her, waiting for each word to leave her mouth. She suggested they go around the room, introduce themselves, and say why they'd come.

Several inmates said they wanted to do something about the way they were all living with AIDS in the prison. One had a friend who died of AIDS. Others said they were there to learn more about the disease. Then the tenth woman spoke in a Puerto Rican accent: "My name is Sonia and I have AIDS. I think we need a group like this here."

Stunned silence exploded in the room. No one at Bedford Hills had ever said out loud in a group that she had AIDS. Sonia knew what the attitudes toward AIDS were in the prison. She challenged them earlier when she'd pushed to rejoin the lawn crew. She knew how much fear was there and how punishing that fear could be to anyone who aroused it. But she spoke out among strangers. Without shame. Katrina trembled: how could she have the courage to tell? Then she felt admiration well up in her: Sonia took a chance and had faith that friends and strangers in that room would react to her illness without cruelty. She looked around the room. How many other women sitting there was Sonia speaking for? How many other healthy-looking women, like herself, were infected with HIV but afraid to say it aloud?

Many rose from their chairs, walked to Sonia, and embraced her. Some cried. What did she need from them? one woman asked Sonia.

She said she wanted attitudes to change. She wanted women with AIDS to be able to move around the prison and relate to other inmates. She wanted people not to be afraid of her. She wanted people to learn how you could catch AIDS and how you could not.

"I'm *Sonia*," she kept telling the women, as if, Katrina thought, they had all forgotten that. "Remember, I'm Sonia. The same person you knew before I got sick. I didn't change. I'm *Sonia*."

Katrina was amazed that the women, many of whom had never met Sonia before, did not run from her. Rather, they were smothering her in their hugs and asking what they could do for her. Katrina could not believe it.

She herself would never have the courage to say it out loud, Katrina thought, but Sonia gave her hope. Maybe she would find a few women willing to listen to her.

Women who had come to the meeting merely out of curiosity began to slip out of the room. Katrina, observing them, thought, "This is too real for them." She could feel the weeding-out process. The room became warmer. Women reached out and touched the hand or the shoulder of the woman next to them, not knowing and not caring whether she were HIV-infected.

Sonia's words emboldened other secretly positive women in the room.

"I just took the test and it turned out positive," one said tearfully, putting her arm around the friend sitting beside her. "If she hadn't been here for me, I don't know how I would have gotten through the last days."

Then a third woman revealed she had AIDS.

Katrina had never experienced anything like this. In a tense, fear-filled room, a woman spoke with courage, shame-free, calling forth from the others a strength and a caring so real you could feel the temperature in the room rise and your skin prickle with it. You could touch courage. Cup it in your hands. Pass some to the woman next to you. Breathe it in. It was that palpable.

When the meeting broke up, Katrina, who had spent years of her life so anesthetized with drugs she had seldom known what she was feeling, left the room in tears. In tears and elated. She knew, they all knew: They were going to make a difference. They were going to be there for the women struck with the disease. They were going to challenge the stigma of AIDS. They were going to take care of one another.

When they looked back on that meeting a few years later, the women called it "Breaking Silence."

Marie Tulman of Brooklyn gave blood to the blood bank through her job. A few weeks later, she got a letter asking her to come in. As she entered the nurse-clinician's office, she noticed a tall, muscle-bound man in a white uniform sitting outside it.

The nurse told her gently that her blood had tested positive for HIV.

So I didn't escape it after all, Tulman thought. After thirteen years in recovery from alcohol addiction, her mind immediately went to the serenity prayer she had prayed thousands of times: God, grant me the serenity to accept the things I cannot change, the courage to change the things I can, and the wisdom to know the difference. This was one of the things she could not change and had to accept.

"What do I do next?" she asked the nurse.

After the woman had given her information, Tulman asked why the man in the white uniform had been sitting outside the office. Some people didn't handle the news that they were HIV-positive well, the nurse explained. They became enraged and lashed out at her. Sometimes they overturned her desk. The man was outside in case the client had to be restrained. The smelling salts on the table—that was for those who fainted.

Marie Tulman called her husband, Lamont, a former drug user who had been clean for two years when she had met him in 1982, and gave him the bad news. He hoped she was joking. He soon went for an HIV test. Positive. A few days later, sitting at a meeting of his drug recovery group, he dropped dead.

Maybe I shouldn't have told him, Tulman thought.

A friend told her about a new group in Brooklyn, Lifeforce, that was training women to serve as HIV educators in the community. Marie decided to work with Lifeforce simply because women needed it. Women were such underdogs. We women feel so unworthy, Tulman thought, we take little breaths.

CDC decided to turn some of its "prostitute" studies into longitudinal studies to see what happened over time: Did the women become infected? Did they change their behavior? Did they use condoms more? Cohen's group, which had been conducting one of the studies of women, bid on the new study, got it, and began work in the fall. They had already enrolled more than six hundred women in the earlier study and were following them to see what happened to their blood and their behavior over time. They knew of no other study like this.

Cohen and Dr. Connie Wofsy had earlier received funding from the CDC, as part of a study conducted by different teams of researchers in several cities, to look at HIV infection among prostitutes. CDC wasn't interested in other women, Cohen noted dryly. As originally proposed, this CDC study would not have provided the women with counseling or medical referrals. The researchers would just draw blood and ask questions. Cohen's group had written to CDC stating it refused to respond to its proposal and explained at length why it found the proposal to be both bad science and bad ethics. CDC invited Cohen and Wofsy to present their views to those who had bid on the proposal and work out with them a study design that would yield comparable information from the various study sites. They did so, gladly taking the CDC money.

The two women swayed researchers in some cities but others did test prostitutes in jail.

After conducting their research, Cohen and Wofsy reported that prostitutes were not at excess risk of HIV. The problem was primarily drug use, they found. Drug treatment programs were needed for women, not incarceration.

ACT UP women went to a Mets ball game at Shea Stadium May 4, the evening of Women and AIDS Day. They'd ordered four hundred tickets—one-third of them in each of the top three sections of the U-shaped stadium—left end, right end, and center. Then they sold the seats to ACT UP members and supporters.

As the opposing club came up to bat, the activists opened their banners, one strip at a time, one section at a time in call-and-response fashion.

DONT BALK

AT

SAFER SEX

Holding the banners up, they swayed back and forth, keeping them visible for ten minutes each time. Then they sat, cheered the game, talked with their neighbors, ate peanuts. Again they rose.

AIDS
KILLS
WOMEN

More shouts, cheers, hisses, smack of ball against bat, stolen bases, crowds jumping to their feet, home runs, soda pop, and, again on their feet, the activists in two rows of seats unfurled their part:

NO GLOVE

and activists in the next two rows unfurled theirs:

NO LOVE

Almost all campaigning on safer sex placed responsibility on women: women were supposed to "just say no" and carry condoms in their purses. The women wanted to point out male responsibility for safer sex. They needed a male-identified arena. They wanted to alert women to their risk of AIDS. They wanted to reach out to people they didn't know. At Shea Stadium, they directly reached twenty thousand in the ball park, and many more through national media coverage, including a story on Sports Network Cable.

As crowds entered the stadium, they had passed out three thousand condoms and ten thousand leaflets:

AIDS IS NOT A BALL GAME

Men! Don't endanger the women you love. (And if you can't be with the one you love, protect the one you're with.) AIDS is the leading cause of death among women between the ages of 25 and 34 in New York City. Here's the score:

Single: Only *one* woman has been included in government-sponsored tests for new drugs for AIDS.

Double: Women diagnosed with AIDS die *twice* as fast as men.

Triple: The number of women with AIDS has *tripled* as a result of sexual contact with men in New York City since the 1984 World Series.

The Grand Slam: MOST MEN STILL DON'T USE CONDOMS.

1989

Off Route 26 in Maine, the muddy dirt road that led to Al and Patricia's house in the woods froze in February, making the drive in and out effortless. Patricia Daugherty drove it often, on her way to and from the family doctor's. She was very ill with a virus that gave her flu symptoms. Her fever was high, her lymph nodes enlarged.

Her family doctor admitted her to the hospital, did every test under the sun on her, and couldn't find out what was wrong.

"I think you have mononucleosis," he'd tell her one day. And the next, "No, I think it's hepatitis."

"No," he'd report after another test, "your liver is enlarged so you must have—it must be that flu that's killing old people."

He sent her to a gastroenterologist, a specialist in diseases of the stomach and intestine, for her enlarged liver.

Both physicians told her that she had a prolonged viral illness and they didn't know what the virus was. Patricia knew that AIDS involved a virus.

"I think I need an AIDS test," she told the gastroenterologist.

"Patricia," he told her sternly. "You do *not* need an AIDS test. You're too healthy. You have no AIDS infection."

Daugherty thought of AIDS as a gay disease and assumed that if someone had it, it would be evident. Something would happen—like red spots sprouting on a kid with measles—and you'd know it. But this *was* a prolonged viral illness she had. That's why she kept bringing it up. Just to rule it out.

She came back three more times, asking for an AIDS test, in the back of her mind knowing Al had had a few homosexual encounters. Finally, her persistence exasperated the doctor: "You do not need an AIDS test! Now cut that out, Patricia! You've got the flu. You'll get over it!"

And the doctor was right: she did get over it. She returned to work, feeling better. The fever receded, and the enlarged lymph nodes and liver eventually went down. She didn't have to see the gastroenterologist any more. Everything seemed fine.

Except that Patricia knew she was never going to be the same again.

She became obsessed with finding out what hit her. All the doctors had told her was that she had a prolonged viral infection. It had left her with extreme fatigue, body aches, and mouth ulcers that did not heal. Something was very wrong with her.

She checked medical books out of the public library, pored over them, and began telephoning physicians with questions. She just couldn't figure it out. One day in March she opened the telephone book and there was a number for the AIDS hotline.

She decided to call it. Not that she thought she had AIDS; the doctors had told her she couldn't possibly have it and they must know what AIDS symptoms are. No, she called simply because her eyes fell on the words in the telephone book.

"What are the specific symptoms of AIDS?" she asked the man who answered the hotline.

The symptoms were common, he told her, and could be expressions of many other diseases.

"My husband's been followed by a cancer doctor for a year and a half," she said. "Wouldn't he know if my husband had AIDS?"

"No, not necessarily."

Patricia felt panic rising in her.

"Oh, my God," she thought. "This could be it."

She began asking Al how many relationships he had had. With men or women. He had had many one-night stands with women, he told her. Especially right after his divorce. And some homosexual encounters.

"Al," she told him. "I think we need to have an AIDS test."

Just to check. Just to rule it out. Al's oncologist tested Al first.

That week, Al became deathly ill. He went to the family doctor, who examined him and said: "Oh, you've got what Patricia had—that flu. Take a leave from school because you're going to be sick for three months."

When Al got a bad cough and ran a high fever, the doctor put him on antibiotics. They didn't help. Al got worse.

Sitting on a kitchen stool while Patricia stood nearby, Al called the oncologist's office to learn if the results were in. They were. Al was positive for HIV. He began shaking and sobbing uncontrollably. He couldn't complete the telephone conversation. Patricia hung up the phone for him.

They were both terrified, shocked, angry. They couldn't believe it. They didn't know what to do. Patricia walked over to the wall, leaned against it, and slid to the floor as Al sobbed.

What to do? Patricia got herself to the telephone and called the local mental health clinic. Come in, they said. Patricia drove Al down the frozen dirt road, out to the clinic off Route 26. In shock, her eyes fixed, walking like a zombie, she helped Al put one foot in front of the other to get into the clinic. The therapist put them in touch with an AIDS specialist in Portland. Make an appointment *now*, he said, from *here*.

The next week, Al's health plummeted. He had PCP and a temperature of 106. He must have been infected with HIV anywhere from seven to ten years earlier, the AIDS specialist figured. When Patricia was tested, she, too, was positive.

Even though they had had a year and a half of unprotected sex, Patricia had probably not been infected until August 1988, when a pelvic infection provided a hospitable entry to the virus. That was when she had had the painful symptoms her family doctor had attributed to her inability to accept her womanhood. She had seroconverted (produced antibodies to HIV) six months later, the AIDS specialist believed. What her doctor diagnosed as a "flu" was likely acute HIV infection.

Patricia had to accept the fact that her husband would soon die and that she had a fatal illness. Still in shock, she began caring for Al through one ailment after another.

From the day she slumped against the kitchen wall and slid to the floor, she rode a terrifyingly fast roller coaster of powerful emotions. She couldn't be angry with Al immediately because he was sick. But some months later, she did furiously blame him, calling him a "queer" and he, feeling guilty, took all reproaches and accusations without defending himself, and she, still later, was filled with pity and sorrow for him, and regret for her reproaches.

Shame. That arrived immediately, with the diagnosis. She wasn't going to tell anyone what they had. She had to keep it secret. It was a sexual shame. Uncle Harry in the barn. The incest. Again. In another form.

Despite the contradiction, she came to feel both that there should *be* no shame at having AIDS, and that the shame was Al's. All her life she had carried the shame for the men around her: Uncle Harry's shame. Her father's shame as he openly cheated on her mother. Now Al's? No! She'd tell people Al got it through a blood transfusion. Why did her sons have to be shamed because of something Al did? Even now, she felt more indignant at her three sons carrying Al's shame than she herself carrying it.

Fear. She and Al both feared that if people knew, they would throw rocks at them. Or—the more terrifying prospect—they'd be fired from their jobs.

Grief. Now she would never watch her children grow up. She grieved that loss. And she grieved the loss of her marriage.

Within a week, Al, very ill, was hospitalized. The physicians, knowing Patricia had nursing training, sent him home earlier than they ordinarily would, expecting her to administer his IV antibiotic therapy, shots, and chemotherapy drugs. That established a pattern that continued almost to Al's death: Patricia nursed him at home, saving the insurance company money. Patricia had to tell the children Al had AIDS. Al didn't want her to but she couldn't keep it from them— not when, with all the medical equipment, their house was transformed overnight into a hospital. The three boys—aged seventeen, thirteen, and seven—were shocked, angry, frightened.

Throughout the many haggard days and sleep-disturbed nights of Al's illness, Patricia, her fury at Al spent, worked hard not to focus on *how* he got the virus. They just didn't know and never would. He had had a blood transfusion in the later 1970s. After his divorce, he had slept with many women. One of the nights they stayed up talking intimately until 4:00 A.M., he revealed that he had had not just a few homosexual experiences but many.

Some doctors who saw him assumed he was gay and that he had been infected through anal intercourse.

Oh, what did it matter whether he had relationships with men or women, Patricia soon came to think in exasperation. It didn't. Not in any way. The damn disease was spread sexually. Period. Heterosexually. Homosexually. Bisexually. *Sexually!*

This was what now infuriated her: They had each been divorced, he for five years, she for two. Neither of them had been celibate during their single life for the simple damn fact that they were human beings and humans are sexual. HIV is spread sexually. Yet none of the doctors they consulted picked up on that reality and thought of HIV.

Look at the medical care they had gotten! Because she and Al were a heterosexual couple, not one of the doctors they'd seen repeatedly from September 1987 to March 1989 had ever suggested an HIV test. Not one. Not ever. Al had seen the oncologist almost monthly for a year and a half. When Patricia had been to her family doctor, he had explained her severe pelvic pain with the assertion that she didn't like being a woman.

Why is it that men's stuff isn't all in their heads? Patricia asked herself, enraged. Why isn't all this colon cancer men get in their heads? If men go to the doctor because they have cramps, how come doctors actually run tests on them and find out what it is?

Her doctor had referred her to a gynecologist for a laparoscopy and the gynecologist also failed to diagnose the HIV.

They misdiagnosed Al. Now the AIDS specialists they were seeing were pretty certain that at the time Al's low blood platelets (ITP) had been detected and physicians began testing and treating him, Patricia was not yet infected with HIV. If they had diagnosed his HIV promptly, she would almost certainly not be infected now.

When Patricia herself *was* infected, the doctors had ridiculed her concerns about AIDS, telling her they were unnecessary.

"Not me!" she thought now. "Not me! I'm white. I'm female. I'm married and in nursing school. Not Al! He's married, a math teacher going to graduate school nights. 'No,' they told me, 'this only happens to prostitutes, drug addicts, and gay men and you're none of those.' No, AIDS did not affect me at all."

She was Mom, driving her kids to their basketball games and music lessons, and he was Dad at the PTA meetings. In rural Maine, Mom and Dad don't get AIDS.

If they had diagnosed Al sooner, if they hadn't acted on their belief that this was just a disease that people they didn't like got—fags, junkies, whores—she would not be infected, she thought.

She directed some anger at herself: I should have seen it coming. I should have *demanded* that Al be tested before the wedding, no matter how angry he got. I should have *insisted* the doctors test us for AIDS. Why didn't I put my foot down?! Why didn't I . . . ?

The self-hating voices tormented her most cruelly when one of her kids had a problem—like a bad report card. The voices said: "You ruined your kids' lives. First by getting divorced. Then by getting married. And ultimately by getting AIDS."

She *did* tell their friends the news. They were shocked. They'd only heard of gay men getting the disease. Or drug users. Occasionally, a hemophiliac like Ryan White, whom they considered "innocent." But the others were "guilty" and should be put away.

Patricia answered their questions about the disease. To her surprise, most friends were loving and supportive. A few couldn't deal with it; they stayed away.

Patricia's parents showed little emotion when she told them. They had always used denial to deal with unpleasantness and they now reached automatically to pull it up around them, comforting themselves in the warm blanket of "it-isn't-so." They never talked with her about it. As Al got sicker and she begged for help in caring for him, they stayed away.

Al's parents told their friends Al had cancer. When Al died the following year, their friends gave donations to a cancer research society.

Anguished in the middle of a sleepless night, Patricia recalled all the shaming messages that had bombarded her during the only two years of her life she had been "free," under the roofs of neither her parents nor her husband, a "loose" woman unattached to any man, living in a trailer with her three children. Recalled how she had been pulled back into the magnetic field of marriage. Recalled that day in June 1987 when a lovely princess in a white gown married a dashing prince with whom she was to live happily ever after.

· · ·

While unknown numbers of women in rural America, like Patricia Daugherty, were being infected in the invisible epidemic, little notice of this was taken publicly. Within ACT UP, an overwhelmingly white, male organization with many professionals—physicians, lawyers, university professors—as participants and fifty-seven chapters nationwide, small numbers of feminist activists were doing their best to make women visible. Buoyed by the success of their early demonstrations at Cosmo and at Shea Stadium in 1988, they accelerated their organizing and activism in 1989. Part of their activism involved research and study. In investigating the governmental response to the AIDS epidemic, they had already, in 1987, identified the exclusion of women from drug treatment trials as an issue.

It would become a central focus of their protests, though it was an issue they embraced with considerable ambivalence. Like Dr. Helen Rodriquez, who had learned how her countrywomen in Puerto Rico had been used to test the Pill, they knew the history of brutal medical experimentation on women with drugs and devices, including not only the Pill, but DES, Depo-Provera and the Dalkon Shield IUD.[1] Nonetheless, they believed, women with a life-threatening illness should decide for themselves whether they wanted to participate in an experimental treatment trial that might provide their only access to treatment.

In 1989 at New York University, the site of one government-funded trial, ACT UP women protested the exclusion of women.

The tiny core group of women at Bedford Hills addressing the AIDS issue, expanding after the meeting in 1988, had developed into a formal prison organization: AIDS Counseling and Education (ACE). A group of inmates now sat at an ACE seminar, listening to Katrina Haslip, one of the seminar leaders. As she spoke, Katrina felt cold fear in the pit of her stomach.

She had kept her HIV infection a secret for the entire year she had known of it. Now she was going to tell. It would be a shock, she knew, for she was hardly the image of a fatally ill woman. She jogged around the yard every day. Full of energy, she competently held not one job, but two—in ACE and as a law clerk in the prison library.

"We've been talking a lot about AIDS," Katrina said, standing in her prison greens. "We talked about HIV testing, about what AIDS is, how you get it. But we haven't really talked about people living with AIDS. We're all living with AIDS in the sense that we're all either *af*fected or *in*fected. I'm living with AIDS from the *in*fected perspective."

The women were stunned, silent.

Katrina told them this was the first time she had ever said it out loud. It felt good, she said. Keeping her silence, covering up one lie with another, had taken so much energy. Suddenly, she found herself weeping in the otherwise silent room. When she regained her composure, she went on:

"I want to break that silence because it is that silence that is killing people. I'm tired of standing by and watching it. I'm willing to challenge the stigma. I know that once I say it out loud, I can't take it back. I know that I might be identified as someone with AIDS because the stigma doesn't distinguish between AIDS and HIV infection. I hope I'm ready for that."

As she looked around the audience, Katrina saw that jaws had dropped open and eyes stared. The women were beginning to whisper among themselves. Then, another dead silence. Her friends dropped their heads and covered them with their hands in movements that said to Katrina, "This isn't real!"

"Okay," she told them. "You can close your mouths now."

Some women approached and embraced her. After that seminar, some were supportive of her and others not. To her friends, her HIV status made no difference.

Katrina thought about the day Sonia Perez had spoken openly of her AIDS at that meeting a year earlier. Katrina had felt Sonia was speaking for her, too. Sonia had given her hope and peace. Before deciding to break her silence, every time she had thought about keeping her infection hidden, she had remembered Sonia's courage.

Helen Cover had to lie down. She was sick. She went to the home of another junkie, and lay on a mattress on the floor, fevered, for three days. By January 12 she had not eaten for four days. It was a bitterly cold night. She went out to get money for food. There was a man on Holland Street in Syracuse. She told him she'd give him a blow job for twenty-five dollars. An undercover cop, he arrested her.

They put her in jail. She was just about to get out—Jail Ministry posted bond—when she was charged with breaking probation. She pled guilty to two charges: she "failed to keep out of further trouble" and "failed to notify Probation of change of address," i.e., from the hospital into the street.

There was an arraignment. Judge Mulroy castigated her for soliciting when she had AIDS.

"I need the food," she replied. "I didn't have no food."

Attorney Jack Lynch tried to get her out on bail January 26. But Assistant District Attorney Terence Langan said Helen was a "danger to the community" because of her AIDS and the prostitution allegation. The prosecution wanted to see if it could charge Helen with something more serious than prostitution, he said. Like attempted murder.

Lynch made his case: there had not been one proven instance in the United States of a man getting AIDS as a consequence of fellatio. Female-to-male sexual transmission of HIV in the United States was much less common than the reverse, etc.[2]

No one seemed to hear him. The judge denied the bail request, citing her medical problems and protection of the community.

The front page of the *Syracuse Herald-Journal* January 29 proclaimed "Prostitution Suspect Has AIDS; Officials Try to Keep Her Jailed."

They locked Helen up without bail. Treatment for her disease was abruptly cut off because the sheriff's deputies couldn't take Cover for weekly experimental drug treatments.

Lesley Noble visited Helen in jail where masked and gloved jail personnel brought her her food. Few spoke with Helen. She couldn't use the phone. She did not have the strength to write.

"You're the only person who comes to see me," she told Noble.

She was so alone! When you have even a cold, you want someone to just be there with you, Noble thought.

Assistant D.A. Terence Langan gave up on charging Helen with attempted murder. It would be hard to build the case against her, since there was no medical evidence that AIDS could be transmitted through saliva, he explained. But neither he, the judge, nor television reporters concluded from this that their "plague dog" view of her had been wrong. Langan, noting that she faced a maximum of up to seven prison years for violating probation, told the press: "The bottom line is to protect the public. I don't think she's going to get out for a while."

Cover pled guilty March 1 to failing to stay out of further trouble. Television cameras followed her down the hall. "She's so upset," Lynch told Noble. "She doesn't want to go on camera and have her children see her on the evening news. They don't know she has AIDS."

"Jack, here!" Noble said, handing him her multicolored scarf and sunglasses. Helen hid her face with them.

Weissman and Noble canvassed the state for a twenty-four-hour residential drug program that they could propose as a prison alternative. Nobody would take Helen. One agency told Noble: "We have found that oftentimes persons with illnesses will use their illness to get out of doing work in the group."

"Yeah, yeah," Noble thought, crossing the agency off her dwindling list. "I guess when someone's missing a lung, that might impede their dishwashing."

There was nothing that could help a woman with a substance abuse problem compounded by HIV. There were only two or three programs in New York State, all with a waiting list a mile long.

Finally Noble found one residential program that was willing to interview Helen.

Talk of protecting the community from the threat posed by Helen Cover permeated the court proceedings. The phrase "the community" sounded solid, sacred even. Yet the "community" that was being protected was the community of men. More specifically, it was the community of johns.

In contrast, it was standard practice not to protect the community of women. When women appealed to police for protection from mates who battered them in the home, the police frequently left the women alone with their assailants. Although battery was the leading cause of injury to women in the late 1980s, only ten states legally mandate arrest for domestic violence.[3]

While men were outraged over the mere *suggestion* that the community of johns might be harmed, there was no judicial outrage over the *fact* that men did assault and sometimes kill women in the home. As Susan Faludi points out in her searing book *Backlash,* domestic violence shelters recorded an increase of more than 100 percent in the numbers of women taking refuge in their facilities between 1983 and 1987; reported rapes more than doubled from the early 1970s; while the homicide rate declined, sex-related murders rose 160 percent between 1976 and 1984, and at least one-third of the women were killed by their husbands or boyfriends.

Male judges, newspaper owners, prosecutors never named johns a "menace to society" though johns frequently attacked the community of women in the streets. (Sally shot. Carol strangled. Katrina stabbed.)

In his handling of Helen Cover, Judge Mulroy was continuing an historical trend: the male blaming of women for sexually transmitted diseases.[4]

To male physicians of the nineteenth century in both the United States and England, women did not themselves suffer from venereal diseases; they just infected men with them. They described women as "hosts" and "disease distributors." (Then, as now with AIDS, women were accused of spreading a disease they were told they couldn't get.)

Acting from the belief that VD was something women gave to men, New York State legislators in 1910 passed a law requiring medical examination of women convicted of soliciting. Venereally infected women would be detained during treatment until they were noncontagious. One male public health educator objected, noting that the law "is directed against a particular class of women for the protection of a particular class of men. . . . The licentious. . . . The fatal defect of every sanitary scheme to control venereal disease has been that the masculine spreader of contagion has been entirely ignored as mythical or practically nonexistent. . . ."

In both World Wars, male government and civic officials in the United States urged the quarantine and internment of women arrested for prostitution to protect soldiers' health and therefore their "military efficiency." Many states passed laws requiring examinations of women for VD, and most courts upheld those laws. In *all* cases of such legislation for the prevention of VD, the laws were directed against women and women alone. Through the decades, through the centuries, "the masculine spreader of contagion" continued to be "entirely ignored as mythical or practically nonexistent."

In both world wars, American women were interned on American soil in detention camps—many secured with guards and barbed wire—as a medical/military measure for the prevention of venereal disease. In 1918 the National Security and Defense Fund constructed and maintained detention buildings for women arrested for prostitution. In World War II some thirty detention camps were built and thousands of women were imprisoned in them.[5] In recent years, we in the United States have begun to feel a most appropriate shame for having interned Japanese-Americans during World War II. But there is no shame about—or even knowledge of—the extensive internment of women during the war.

The strategy of mandating pelvic exams, quarantine, and internment of women during the world wars kept the system of prostitution—that made women sexually accessible to men—intact. In Helen Cover's case, men replicated this strategy. But here, they went a step further in the medicalization of prostitution. Dr. Janice Raymond, medical ethicist and associate director of the Massachusetts-based Institute on Women and Technology, explains: "Here, the woman is actually made a kind of contagious criminal just as women are being made reproductive criminals in fetal abuse cases where there is an alcohol or drug passage from the woman to the fetus."[6]

The sheriff's deputies, gloved and masked, brought Cover, who was wheezing and coughing, into the courtroom March 3 for the sentencing. She was handcuffed, the chains wrapped around once in front. As if she could escape. She had been hospitalized with pneumonia the week before.

To cover her face, Jack Lynch had found a gray ski mask with three slits for eyes and mouth. He didn't know what else to do to prevent Helen's children from seeing her on the evening news. But it was horrible. She looked like a sniper.

"Here she comes! Here she comes!" the television crews cried, rushing after her, pointing huge lights in her face as the cameras rolled. Helen sobbed.

Twenty students from Syracuse Law School had been brought in to observe the proceedings. They sat chatting, snapping gum, holding notebooks. A television reporter stood in her full-length fur coat talking with the attorneys.

"Jesus Christ," Noble thought, disgusted, "Helen's dying. She's facing two to four years in state penitentiary. She's in pain and we're all donning our best fur coats, and bringing in the kids to watch the circus."

The court admitted a letter from Helen's physician stating that her life expectancy was less than two years.

Noble was called to testify. She told Judge Mulroy she had found a residential program interested in Cover. It could deal with both her substance abuse and AIDS. Mulroy refused to release her to it because it was not a twenty-four-hour lockup.

Helen did not pose a threat to the community, Lynch was arguing.

Whoa! the judge cried. You're telling me a drug abuser with a communicable disease arrested for prostitution isn't a threat to the community? AIDS was not easily transmitted, Lynch responded, especially from oral sex. Helen didn't pose a greater threat to the community than a drunken driver. She should not bear the full blame for not getting drug treatment. She needed an in-patient drug program and Probation had not found a program that would take her. Probation officer Brooks admitted that Cover had trouble finding addiction treatment.

Listening to the judge's assertion that he was sentencing Helen not for having AIDS, but because she "did not address [her] drug problems," Noble remembered Helen telling her once, "You know, my doctor said to me the cocaine is going to kill me before the AIDS does."

"Yeah?" Noble had said. "What do you think about that?"

"I don't know," she'd responded. "Maybe he's right. But to tell you the truth, sometimes I just do it because it helps the pain."

"Then who are we to judge this woman and to call her a drug addict when she goes through indescribable pain every day?" Noble now fumed from her seat in the courtroom. "What judge in this country wouldn't be pumping himself full of morphine if he had contracted a disease like this?"

Here was the judge defining the issue as Cover's threat to the community, she thought. But that was not the issue. The issue was that the community had failed Cover. There was nothing there to help her. The community had left her to die on the streets, medicating her pain with an illegal drug. (Nor, for that matter, had it helped Helen's mother free herself from her drug addiction and stay with her children. When Helen's grandmother became too ill to care for the children, the community didn't come in with housekeeping or child care so that Helen and her sisters could stay with a woman who deeply loved them and wanted to protect them.) As for the charges, the assault—the one and only time Helen had ever been charged with a violent act—was two screwed-up women fighting over a boom box. It just happened that the other woman got to the cops first. If Helen had, the other woman would have been behind bars.

Noble listened to the judge describe how magnanimous he had been to Cover: he had generously offered her probation. And she was throwing this generosity and kindness back in his face!

Helen did not need more punishment, Lynch was saying. "The stigma, the humiliation she faces, the fact that she stands here today with a mask on her face—isn't that punishment enough?" What she needed, he said, "is an opportunity to live out what's left of her life in a facility that just isn't so certain of bleakness and death as a prison would be for this woman."

Then Helen spoke and what you could see of her was her eyes and her mouth through the slits in the ski mask and here she was standing in a court in Syracuse—Syracuse that she'd come to because it was the country to her and it was fresh air and she'd been there as a child and she remembered it as a clean place and not full of crime and ugliness and she wanted something out of life, she wanted to be a nurse and she remembered Syracuse and Syracuse was where she was going to get that something out of life and here she was, wheezing and sobbing, saying:

"I realize I violated my probation, but to me at the time, I had no choice. I was homeless, and I was hungry, and I had no help and no one to turn to. Only people I did know was the drug addicts. My boyfriend kicked me out. I have no family here at all. I was only wearing the clothes on my back when I was arrested. That's all I owned, and it's very difficult to survive when you have no one to help you. I did what I thought was right to survive. And I would never intentionally go out to use drugs or to hurt anyone. I wasn't—that wasn't what

I was about. I always wanted to be a nurse, and my life is ruined now. I have no future. It was me that I was hurting, because I gave up.

"All I want is my kids—I don't want to use drugs. I feel at the time, what did [I] have to live for any longer? Why suffer? I'm in pain every day. That wasn't my choice in life. It just happened that way. My dreams are all gone and shattered. I don't want my kids to see me go like this. I want maybe to leave something more in life for them. That's all I got left to live for is my family and my kids. And I wanted to do something positive for them before my time comes."

She sobbed loudly, "her tears hidden by her mask," *Syracuse Herald-Journal* reporter Jim O'Hara wrote that afternoon.

Judge Mulroy, knowing her life expectancy was less than two years, sentenced her to one and one-third to four years at Bedford Hills. A life sentence for offering to give a twenty-five-dollar blow job.

"The Probation Department stood there with open arms . . . ," the judge told her. "There is nothing else that can be done with you."

Open arms? When her probation officer would talk with her only with a plastic partition keeping her at a distance from him?

In an interview with reporter Jim O'Brien some days after court, Helen said the judge was imprisoning her because she had AIDS, not for her offense. Judge Mulroy, responding to Cover's charge, told O'Brien he didn't sentence her to prison to punish her for having AIDS but that AIDS was a factor in his decision to have her locked up:

"I wasn't going to run the risk of her giving a death sentence to someone else. Helen Cover got treated differently. She did. But the circumstances were different. Not only did she have AIDS, but her inability to control her drug habit sent her out to the streets."

In the law library at Bedford Hills, Katrina Haslip saw a newspaper photograph of Helen, masked and sobbing in the courtroom. What was the point of humiliating Helen so cruelly, she thought. She felt protective. She wished she could befriend Helen.[7]

The Helen Cover case exemplified cases that occurred in many areas of the country, including, as we have seen, New Haven and San Francisco. As in Cover's case, most received regional, rather than national, news coverage.

The news media had tried to portray Helen as a hooker-on-the-loose, Lesley Noble reflected. The case was almost riot-inciting. "Here's this prostitute with AIDS and she's running around on the street. She's coming to get you! Lock your doors! The plague! The plague!" But even though media people had started out wanting to blame her, Lesley thought that as they just let their cameras roll and let her speak and looked into the record of her painful life, hearts turned. You had to be a stone not to be moved by the TV film footage of Helen.

Remembering Helen, Lesley pictured her not in the courtroom but as she was when she was being mischievous. ("Can you smuggle me in a candy bar?") Helen had a presence. She was funny, kind, highly intelligent. In the end all Lesley could do for her was give her a scarf and a pair of dark glasses.

Many clients Marsha Weissman worked with had been so beaten down you could hardly connect with them. But not Helen Cover. She had a spark. She had dignity. Pride. To Weissman, the spirit that shone through Helen made her fate even sadder. If she'd had half a break, what this woman might have been!

Jack Lynch, too, was left to reflect on the client he had not saved from prison. What the judge had done was legal. But Lynch knew that had Helen been suffering from cancer or any other disease, she would not have been sentenced to state prison for a minor probation violation. He couldn't prove it, but in his heart he knew it.

Helen Cover was sent to Bedford Hills Correctional Facility.

In 1912 the Bureau of Social Hygiene, formed by three prominent white men—John D. Rockefeller, Jr., Paul Warburg, and Starr Murphy—to study prostitution and venereal disease "scientifically," operated a Laboratory of Social Hygiene at Bedford Hills. There, the laboratory conducted research to develop rehabilitation methods for female offenders. Women sentenced to Bedford Hills Correctional Facility had been subjected to a battery of physical and psychological tests in order to isolate the factors that contributed to prostitution.

Eugenicists eager to demonstrate that prostitution was genetically caused—that women in prostitution had a genetic predisposition to promiscuity—soon influenced the laboratory's research. The eugenics movement, widespread and respected, advocated improvement of the human race by curtailing births among "inferior" classes of people and increasing births among the "better" classes.

Charles B. Davenport, leader of the American eugenics movement, endorsed reports circulating that more than half the women in prostitution were feebleminded and needed lifelong imprisonment, or, more delicately put, "custodial care."

Davenport explained: "Evidence is accumulating to show that the primary factor is an inherited predisposition toward an exceptionally active sexual life. . . . The heightened licentiousness is favored by an additional germinal determinant that less licentious persons do not have."

While various "vice commissions" had presented social and economic explanations for prostitution (one commission member went so far as to advocate better economic opportunities for women as a method of contracting the supply of prostitutes), the eugenicists' use of Bureau of Social Hygiene research signaled a change to notions of hereditary criminal behavior.[8]

Helen Cover was now imprisoned in an institution where, seventy-seven years earlier, her foremothers had been minutely and scientifically examined and found to carry prostitution in their genes.

Cover wanted to see her children again before she died. She would appeal the judge's sentence. Prisoners' Legal Services told her to check out the prison law library when she arrived at Bedford. One of the inmates there, trained as a law clerk, would help her with her appeal.

The law clerk was Katrina Haslip. It wasn't until after her first meeting with Helen that Katrina put this new prisoner together with the stories she had read earlier of the masked woman in Syracuse. She went back to look at that story. The next time they met, she pointed to the photograph and asked Helen, "Is this you?"

With the photograph of the masked Helen on the table between them, Helen told Katrina how humiliated and isolated she had felt in court. She had wanted to crawl into the floor and hide, she told Katrina. She would just stare ahead and try to block everything out because she could not bear the humiliation.

As Katrina listened and later read the court transcripts and worked on the appeal, she became increasingly enraged at what the court had done to Helen.

Helen, too, was angry at the judge. Katrina and she spoke often of using her anger positively: by outliving Mulroy's sentence, she could revenge the judge who wanted her to die in prison.

In the months that followed, Helen often laughed. "I'm living out of stubbornness. He gave me a year to four. I'm going to show him that I can do those years."

When Helen moved to IPC, Katrina visited her, as well as the other HIV-infected women, Gladys and Kathy, often. Helen soon became "the baby." The convicts' faces softened when they spoke to her, of her. Even Kathy, sick as she was herself, pampered Helen.

Katrina would do Helen's hair. Helen wanted hundreds of tiny plaits and Katrina would braid them for her, insisting that she wasn't going to be the one to take all those plaits down later. But she always was.

As Katrina massaged Helen's scalp, as she brushed and braided, they talked about how they had survived on the street. Helen spoke often of her need to see her ten-year-old daughter and three-year-old son. Tim, who had been her companion for almost a decade, kept promising to bring the children to see her. Once he did. The fact that he brought them gave her hope that he would do it again. But each time he came, despite his promises, he came alone.

"I want him to bring them before I die," Helen would tell Katrina.

Sometimes Katrina would stand and brush Helen's hair and their talking would gradually peter off and Helen would fall asleep. Sometimes they would watch soap operas together. Or movies. Helen liked Katrina to read the Bible to her and Katrina obliged even though she was, as she described herself, "Islamically inclined." Helen read the Bible every day. To Katrina, Helen was spiritual—kindhearted and generous.

Helen often drew. Katrina, seeing her drawings, would exclaim, "Helen, you're really good."

"Am I?" Helen would ask, surprised. She was uncertain of her talent but kept drawing because she loved it, had always loved it.

One spring day Scott Porter, the Syracuse lawyer handling Helen's appeal, came to Bedford Hills. He didn't usually make the trek out to the state penitentiary but Helen was a special case. He had read about her before he became her lawyer, seen the newspaper photographs of the gloved guards and Helen sobbing in her mask. He had felt outraged over the undignified way she had been treated.

Helen was very sick by the time Porter met her in IPC. She was coughing and in pain.

At Bedford, Porter met Katrina, the law clerk, and was impressed by her extraordinary competence. He felt perplexed by the fact that she was wearing prison greens and so must be an inmate. How could someone that intelligent, articulate, and caring have done anything bad enough to be imprisoned? It seemed incongruous. Maybe she was really a state employee hired to help the inmates.

Helen's appeal came up in July. Porter made yet another stab at getting through to the judge the point Lynch had made: there wasn't much chance a woman could pass HIV to a man through oral sex. In fact, Porter's research turned up only one possible case and that, reported in a letter to the *New England Journal of Medicine*, was by no means proven.[9]

But Porter found it tough making his arguments to the judge. There he was before the bench talking about blow jobs, AIDS, prostitution, drug addicts—and he was met with a bristling anger.

Many times, Porter pointed out, terminally ill defendants accused of violent crimes—the overwhelming majority of whom are male—have requested and received dismissals of their cases at the trial level in the interest of justice. He cited eight specific cases to support this. The indictments in these cases generally involved harsher crimes than what Helen ultimately pled guilty to. In four of these cases, the defendants were repeat offenders.

"The relief requested [in Cover's case] is essentially the same—that a terminally ill person be allowed to die in dignity, outside of prison walls."

Porter pointed out that PWAs often experience intense psychological effects such as anxiety, sadness, hopelessness, and worthlessness. This, added with the factor that Helen had no stable home, made the judge's condemnation of Helen "especially ruthless and unfair. It recalls Justice Douglas's words in *Robinson:* 'We would forget the teachings of the Eighth Amendment if we allowed sickness to be made a crime and permitted sick people to be punished for being sick. This age of enlightenment cannot tolerate such barbarous action."

But it could. The appeal was denied.

· · ·

Attorney Scott Parker succeeded in getting all the time Helen Cover had spent in jail locally credited to her prison time. Then he brought a lawsuit to move up her parole date. So in December, having served her time, Helen Cover came up before the Parole Board. She had made it through. She had lived longer than those men in the court thought she could. She would see her children before she died.

In preparing for her hearing, Helen's parole officer from the Department of Corrections showed her the information that would be available to the board. Helen later told Katrina that the district attorney and judge were recommending that she be denied parole and that the D.A. had letters from johns saying they had been intimate with her and had not known she had AIDS and now they were worried that they might be infected and Helen was a menace, a hazard to society.[10]

The Parole Board denied Cover parole. She could apply again in eighteen months, it informed her.

It knew she was not expected to live eighteen months.

Helen gave up. Less than a month later, she died in prison. She did not see her children one last time. She left unfinished the portrait of her father she had been drawing. The convicts of Bedford Hills placed that portrait, along with their farewells ("Helen, your life enriched mine") on the quilt square they sewed to commemorate her life. They claimed Helen Cover as one of their own in the community of women.

In January 1989, Steven Schafer, married less than a year to a coed he had met as an undergraduate at Columbia University, saw a doctor about his difficulty walking.

"AIDS-related neuropathy," the doctor pronounced.

Steven's bride, Charlotte, was dumbfounded. She found it hard to believe. Now she was being told that *she* had to be tested for HIV! Result: negative. But on a retest in November, the virus was there.

But they hadn't had that much sex! And they always used condoms when they did! Except for maybe four times.

Now, reeling from the news, she just couldn't get a grip on why, before the marriage, she had never asked Steven to be tested.

She was scared. And angry. Because, though Steven had told her of his past gay relationship, he had not told her that fidelity had been no part of it. He'd had relations with many. She had no objections to homosexuality but she did object to substituting sex for caring in a relationship. It was stupid, foolish. It didn't do anything for anybody and to get sick for that reason! That was—that was idiotic!

She was angry. She said it. And it was over.

Charlotte told her parents and three sisters that Steven had AIDS. What about her, they asked. No, she lied. She had tested negative.

If she told them the truth, she'd have to run around fetching smelling salts for them for the next year. She didn't have the energy to take care of them emotionally. She had too much to deal with now.

Near the small New Jersey town where he lived with Diane, his wife of four years, Bruce Sampson donated blood. Soon after, the Central Blood Bank of New Jersey wrote, asking him to come in. He stopped by on his thirtieth birthday, January 17. He had the HIV virus, they told him.

Shattered, Bruce brought the news back to Diane. She had just delivered their youngest child, Elizabeth, a month earlier. They had five children now.

Diane couldn't take it in. AIDS happened to junkies in the city, gay men, people who do jail time. It couldn't touch her small-town Methodist life. AIDS was for people who did bad things. She hadn't done anything wrong. All she did was fall in love, she thought. She didn't get high. She was petrified of needles.

She and the children needed to be tested, the people at the blood bank said. Waiting for the children's test results to come back, she was filled with fear and dread. But they were lucky. All the children were fine—no HIV infection.

Diane herself was HIV-positive.

So, she thought, she would be dead soon. The dying part—she had no problem with that. The burning question for her was: how much time did she have to get everything in order, to get the children provided for? She did not want the five children split up. Her brothers and sisters themselves had large families. Which of them would be able—emotionally, financially, spatially—to take on the care of an additional five children?

She made her will.

When her husband told his family the news, several brothers

soon spread it around the small town. Hearing it, people did not think "HIV." The news was: Bruce and Diane had AIDS.

Diane had to tell her parents. She did not want them learning the news on the street.

"But Diane," her mother said, unbelieving, "you can't have this! You're not gay and you're afraid of needles. So how could this happen to you?"

When the news finally sank in, she cried.

"Let the children come to us for a week," her father suggested. "That will give you time to cry. If you want to beat the walls, beat the walls. You're not sure how it's going to set in in the next couple of days."

That week, Diane stared at ceilings, sobbed.

Bruce was no support to her. Straight and sober until he heard the news from the blood bank, he now dove into a bottle and stayed there.

The frost set over Diane's world. People she had known for years turned their heads, raised their noses. Many friends pulled away. People she'd gone to school with, and, as an adult, rooted with in noisy baseball stands on school playing fields stayed away.

Townspeople talked about her. Some would not serve her when she entered their shops. Their attitude, it felt to her, was "Get an island and put Diane and the other AIDS lepers on it." She felt like a witch the townspeople wanted to burn.

"People can be cold," she thought. "So cold."

She recalled the Ray children, hounded out of Arcadia, Florida, two years earlier. How indignant she herself had been at the boys' parents. How easy it had been then to throw stones, she thought. Now that she was infected and taking a crash course in HIV, she could understand why the Rays had been so persistent. There had been no reason for their children to have been shut out. They had posed no threat to the other schoolchildren.

For the first time, she sympathized with the Rays: "Now that I have my own cross to carry, I can feel the weight. The cross never looks heavy when someone else is carrying it."

Dr. Zena Stein, responsible for the HIV Center's international work, had received her first reports in 1982 from her contacts in Africa that women on the continent were getting AIDS. Now there were slightly more women than men falling ill.

Women needed a way to protect themselves. Public health strategies focused on reducing the number of sexual partners, interviewing potential partners on their sexual and drug use histories, using condoms, and avoiding risky sexual practices such as anal intercourse and vaginal intercourse during menstruation. These strategies might help in some circumstances and to some degree, but from a worldwide perspective, Stein felt, they were woefully inadequate.

Condoms were efficacious—they did prevent HIV transmission—but not effective because they were not used consistently enough. Condoms would never be enough to protect women either in the United States or Africa. In Africa large numbers of men had never, ever used a condom, or even seen one.

Mobile men were a chief cause of the spread of AIDS in Africa, in Stein's analysis. They had sex on the road and then brought the disease back to their wives. Stein would say men were the vectors of the disease, an idiosyncratic framing of reality in a male-supremacist world.

It was clear in Africa that women needed special attention because in many communities women ran everything. They, the main agricultural producers, worked in the fields, bore and raised the children, nursed the men who came home sick, and contracted the disease themselves. Hospitals in Africa did not have the resources to cope with AIDS. The family coped. But the family *was* the woman. The young women died and the grandmothers or great-aunts took over, caring for the orphans.

Many men wanted children, the more the better. If the condom were used to prevent HIV infection, it would also make it impossible for the women to get pregnant. Given the economic and social pressure on women to produce children, that was just not going to be acceptable to large numbers of people.[11]

Methods women could use to prevent HIV transmission claimed very little of national or international research budgets, Stein knew. That needed to change.

In January Stein asked herself, What can be done? She and Anke Ehrhardt, her codirector at the HIV Center, discussed the problem often. Stein read up on spermicides and diaphragms, finding that barrier contraceptive methods and spermicides might protect women against STDs. That, in itself, could be helpful in preventing HIV since there did seem to be a connection between other STDs and infection with HIV. But maybe the spermicides would also directly prevent HIV.

At the HIV Center, Ehrhardt and Stein developed focus groups of women to discuss with them what they needed to protect themselves: Could they get their men to use a condom? If not, what could they see themselves using?

After listening to the women, Stein and Ehrhardt became convinced that women must have preventive methods under their own control. A wider range of chemical and physicial barriers that blocked HIV transmission through the vaginal route would have to be developed and tested. A few potential candidates were already available: nonoxynol 9, sodium oxychlorosene, and benzalkonium chloride. These had already been used as gels, suppositories, ovules, or sponges. They might be used immediately before or after intercourse.

Or a virucide might be incorporated into a vaginal ring or an intracervical device. The diaphragm, as well as a so-called female condom, needed evaluation as HIV prophylactics.

Stein had noticed that at the international AIDS meeting in Stockholm the previous year, remarkably few of the thousands of presentations and abstracts dealt with the prevention of transmission by a means that did not involve the man's participation.

In the spring, Ehrhardt and Stein flew to Miami for a meeting of researchers at all five U.S. HIV centers.

For the first time, Stein, making her presentation, forcefully argued that condoms were not going to work for women and that they needed to develop virucides. Ehrhardt was struck by the extreme contrast in the way male and female researchers responded to Stein. The men lackadaisically commented that yes, the development of virucides was important, but in the meantime, it was necessary to concentrate on condoms. The women researchers crowded around Stein and herself, excited, urgent, immediately understanding the problem, and saying, "Yes, of course! *Of course* we know condoms aren't going to work. We need something new."

Ameda was in the hospital again. Ada wanted to bring Faith and Jesse to visit her but Ameda objected. She did not want them to see her emaciated and disfigured. So Ada brought her photographs of the children.

At the next hospitalization, Ada found Ameda's face dropped as after a stroke, her mouth cocked open, head tilted back, a tube down her nose. Ameda could not talk; only her eyes could move. Ada, remembering how pretty she had been, hated to see her like that. Ameda was twenty-seven.

In October Ameda died. Ada gathered Faith and Jesse in her arms. "You know your mommy was very sick," she reminded them. "Now she is no longer here. She's gone just like Angela."

The children wanted to see her at the funeral. That morning, Ada asked Faith if she would like to put something in her mother's casket.

"Yes," Faith said, "I want to put a ring in."

"A ring?" Ada asked. "Why a ring?"

"'Cause Mommy always said she and Daddy was going to get married. She always said, 'Daddy's going to put a diamond ring on my finger.'"

Ada went to her room and found a ring. Not a diamond ring but a pretty nice ring nonetheless. She took Eddie aside and handed it to him.

"When you go up to the casket, you take your daughter with you and you put this ring on Ameda's finger."

Eddie took Faith and Jesse with him. When he placed the ring on Ameda's finger, Faith smiled.

Jesse, looking at his mother in the casket, began saying "Mama 'Meda." Ada was stunned. He had never spoken of her before, never mentioned her name.

"'Meda, my mama's dead. 'Meda give me bottle. My mommy. I want to go where my mommy is."

Ada stood behind the child. "We all goin' to go one day," she told him. "But not just yet."

In the weeks that followed, Jesse recounted incidents from his babyhood with Ameda, incidents Faith could verify. Ada couldn't believe it. Maybe that, then, was why he had cried so much, why he'd had such tantrums. He was frustrated. He wanted to be with 'Meda Mama. He couldn't even say it because he had not yet learned to speak.

He had had all those memories inside him all during his long silence.

. . .

The Stuyvesant Polyclinic on New York City's Lower East Side changed administrators. The new director was unsympathetic to the support group for women affected by AIDS. One by one, she dismissed the personnel responsible for the group, including Dooley Worth.

The women's group survived by meeting after hours. The director did not know the women were there. They tiptoed around. They couldn't advertise the support group in the community for fear that the clinic director would know it still existed. One night she stayed late, ran into the women, and threw them out.

That was the kind of help available to women in the U.S. city where they were hardest hit by the AIDS epidemic.

A woman telephoned Marie-Lucie Brutus at the WARN offices, now moved to Brooklyn, explaining that her husband had had an affair with a woman who had AIDS. The wife feared he was infected and was terrified that she would be, too. She wanted him to go for the HIV test. He refused. She wanted support—someone to talk with as she struggled to protect herself.

Brutus had managed to see her a few times outside her home. The woman called her when she could. But if her husband was around and heard her talking, he took the phone from his wife's hand and hung it up. He felt threatened. He didn't want her to tell anyone outside what was going on with them.

The woman had thought of leaving him. She realized he had abused her. But she felt she loved him and feared being alone. During the many years of her marriage, she had lost any confidence that she could take care of herself.

Penny Abernathey joined the Austin Travis County HIV Commission in Texas, a group of citizens banded together to deal with the HIV epidemic. People with HIV should not be scorned, they'd say, speaking to community and business groups. HIV is a disease much like leukemia. A person who has leukemia doesn't get treated like garbage and neither should a person with HIV.

Penny talked in schools, churches, to teachers, sororities—anybody who would listen to her: protect yourself, she'd say, and don't hurt people who have it. AIDS is a tragedy. It's not about fault. It's not wrong. It's a virus and it can get into any body on this planet. It doesn't matter where you come from. Doesn't matter if your father is an Episcopal priest, as mine is. It's not anything you have to be ashamed or embarrassed about. People with HIV deserve to get on with their lives and people who don't have it need to let them.

She told her story over and over. Told it on TV. Told it to the newspapers. Still, she had to tell it again.

Every time she went in front of a group, she left thinking, "God, again! Didn't anybody listen before? There are still so many people out here thinking, 'Oh, well, I'm not black. I'm not gay. I'm not a junkie. I don't have anything to do with AIDS.'"

She'd go with other commission members to PTA meetings and say, "We implore you to put HIV education in the schools. Too many teenagers are getting infected. We implore you to listen to us."

"Yes, thank you for your presentation. Next, please?"

It was an uphill battle.

It infuriated Penny that people with HIV were often condemned as "promiscuous." She detested the word. Marriages planned don't happen, relationships begun do not work out. How can someone be faulted for exploring themselves and their relationships? People did not need to be made to feel guilty for living their lives.

Time after time, the pap smear Dr. Carola Marte took on an HIV-infected client at the Community Health Project (CHP) in Manhattan would come back abnormal. She would refer the woman to the gynecology clinic of the project's backup hospital, Bellevue, where clients would get lost in the shuffle. These women were kept waiting hours, examined slapdash and given an appointment for six months later. Sometimes their charts would be lost. Often Marte couldn't find out what had happened with the women. It wasn't that care at Bellevue was exceptionally bad; it was typical of the medical care in clinics in public hospitals. It was one reason, Marte thought, why the United States needed a National Health Service such as the one that benefited Canadians.

To enable her to follow up on her clients with abnormal paps, Marte needed one specific gynecologist at Bellevue to whom she could refer them all. In the spring, Dr. Machelle Allen, new on the Bellevue staff, agreed to cooperate.

The attitude of many physicians—and Marte heard it over and over again from gynecologists around the country at meetings, in private conversations, in clinics—was that HIV-infected women were going to die of AIDS soon anyway. So why bother treating them for cervical abnormalities? Once you're infected, they erroneously believed, you're cooked. The news that there was an average ten-year latency period for HIV had not yet reached many physicians. It was depressing, Marte felt. To not take care of cervical cancer and let the woman die of that much earlier than she would have died of HIV—it was just awful!

At that point, Carola Marte and Machelle Allen, securing the support of the ob/gyn chair at Bellevue, worked together to develop a protocol (standard procedure) for the gynecology and medical clinics.

To alert physicians treating HIV-infected women to the need for a gynecological protocol for them, Marte put together a poster for the Fifth International AIDS Conference in Montreal in June. It included her dysplasia rates at the Community Health Project. She had handed out a brief questionnaire to her women clients, asking them if they had had basic gynecological complaints, previous abnormal paps, etc., to get some handle on what their history had been. It was not a scientific research tool but a useful seat-of-the-pants survey of symptoms. She had found a high proportion of women with histories of gynecological abnormalities, as well as a large number—roughly a third of the women—who had had abnormal pap smears. That was about eight times the comparison rate. With Fruchter's permission, she also included data from Downstate in Brooklyn.

In Montreal, at the sessions when researchers stood by their posters and discussed their findings with those who stopped by, Marte, somewhere between amusement and chagrin, found herself surrounded by posters showing penile ulcers and lesions. The conference organizers had not placed her poster in the ob/gyn section with several others on cervical dysplasia. Someone had decided to classify her poster by organ systems. Perhaps because it dealt not with one specific issue that's often researched and published about, but with something broader—a gynecological protocol that included STDs and other conditions as well as cervical dysplasia. Marte's poster seemed to be about female genitalia, so they put it next to male genitalia in the urology section. The poster was in the back of the room, not easily seen. Marte figured that was part of the usual saga in women's health care.

Some people concerned with HIV-positive women had managed to spot her poster in the abstract book that briefly described each paper and poster presented at the conference. They tracked it down to the back of the room. Among them was Pat Kelly who, just that spring, had begun doing pelvic exams on all the HIV-infected women coming into the Infectious Diseases Clinic at Kings County. She'd given up her fruitless campaign to get the docs at the clinic to do pelvics on their female patients.

"All right," she'd told them, independently taking the same approach Marte had at the Community Health Project. "I'll do pelvics on all the patients."

Kelly was thrilled to meet Marte, someone else who cared what was happening to women in the HIV epidemic. Talking, they found they had a friend in common, Rachel Fruchter.

As Marte was arriving at Montreal with her poster, ACT UP activists, including Maxine Wolfe, were already in the city.

ACT UP registered one person for the Fifth International AIDS Conference in Montreal to get a conference badge. Within forty minutes, the activists had learned where, in Montreal, they could photocopy in color and buy plastic badge cases. Within another half hour, they had forty counterfeit congress badges. ACT UP entered the conference.

In this action, they threw a spotlight on women who were even more invisible than most: lesbians. If a lesbian were not bearing children or threatening to infect men with AIDS, there was apparently no reason to pay any attention to her at all.

Out of seven thousand papers being presented at the conference, ACT UP charged in a leaflet, only one concerned lesbians and AIDS. There were no papers on the incidence of woman-to-woman HIV transmission. There was a simple way to resolve a debate about whether HIV could be transmitted from woman to woman, they pointed out. Study it. But no one was. Why not? Why did researchers simply *presume* that all women in their studies were heterosexual?

Lesbians, the activists argued, should be targeted in all safer sex campaigns, including those for adolescents, worldwide.

The next month, in New York City, ACT UP's Women's Caucus held a "safer sex" forum for lesbians at which they pointed out that, according to the CDC, at least 164 women, self-identified as having had sex with women, had been diagnosed with AIDS nationwide. Of these 164, half of them had had sex *only* with other women since 1977. This statistic could not represent the total number of lesbians with AIDS because the CDC does not ask women for sexual identification or about cunnilingus as a sexual practice. The CDC puts all women in one category. So the total number of HIV-infected lesbians and bisexual women is unknown.

The rate of unknown transmission of HIV was four to five times higher for women than for men, they pointed out. In women, that rate was 8 percent nationally and 10 percent in New York City, while in men it was only 2.3 percent. Is women-to-women sexual transmission hidden in that "unknown" area, they questioned?

In the summer of 1989, Sandra Elkin urgently felt that those who saw what was happening to women needed to come together and act to protect women in this epidemic.

"A lunch at the faculty club at the HIV Center," she told Ehrhardt.

"You're on," the scientist replied.

Linda Lofredo, Lynne MacArthur, and Anna Marie Lewis came from the Women and AIDS project; from the National Women's Political Caucus, Barbara Van Buren; Jeri Woodhouse from the staff of Manhattan borough president Ruth Messinger; Pauline Miles from Empire Blue Cross/Blue Shield; Stein and Ehrhardt from the HIV Center; Elkin herself from the Media Group.

All were disheartened and frustrated by the way women were— or rather, were not—treated in the AIDS epidemic.

How could they make AIDS an issue for women? They had to raise consciousness, assemble the information and analysis they had, and present that to leaders in the community of women so those leaders could put "AIDS epidemic" on the agendas of their organizations. A series of breakfast meetings—that would be a start, each meeting targeted to different groups of key women who could spread the word further, using their influence in their networks to effect change.

At each breakfast, a panel of speakers would lay out the issues for women. They planned and held breakfasts for leaders of women's organizations; women in government; in community-based organizations; in print and broadcast journalism.

Carola Marte, Pat Kelly, and Rachel Fruchter, all working in New York, discussed the cervical dysplasias they were seeing in HIV-infected women at their clinics. They decided to do a study together, pooling their data. They would enlist Mardge Cohen in their effort.

At the American Public Health Association meeting in Chicago in November on a brisk fall day, the three women sat down with Cohen. They compared notes on what they were seeing in women, and in effect said: "We have this information that seems important. People should know about it. If it takes an article to convince people on our staffs to do gyn exams and pap smears, then that's what we have to do."

By pooling their data, and having more clinics and higher numbers of women represented in their study, they had a better shot at convincing medical providers that there was a problem. Kelly, Marte, and Cohen, who were all taking care of HIV-infected women, felt that women's needs, and all the ob/gyn problems, were being ignored by the infectious disease specialists. Fruchter worried that HIV-positive women were going to have cervical cancer and all sorts of additional problems including other viral infections, and they wouldn't respond to standard therapies.

For the joint study, the three caregivers would take the pap smears. Fruchter would help structure the study, write the data collection instruments, and put the data together.

Their study was unusual. A research project typically is the next step in a larger investigation already in existence. It is designed to provide a new piece of information that, combined with pieces provided by other researchers, will answer a larger question that has already been posed. Research tends to be a series of small incremental steps, based on what has already been done, attempting to answer a question already posed.

But in this case, the women did not start on some already defined research problem but rather with what they were actually observing in women. Nobody, they realized, was even asking a question about a phenomenon they were actually seeing.

Why had the question not been asked and therefore, until they came along, never researched? Marte believed it was because gynecology had been segregated out from the field of medicine. Internal medicine is one field and gynecology, a surgical specialty, an entirely different one. Which just didn't make sense. Not when it came to such matters as sexually transmitted diseases and the general health of the mucous membranes. There was no good reason why the organs unique to women should not be a part of medicine along with all the other parts of the human body. Because women's organs were cast out of internal medicine, the very first research step thinking about what was going on with gynecological problems had never been taken. If the first step isn't taken, none of the subsequent ones are either.

The same old story played out wherever you looked: women's health, women's medicine, women's bodies had been cut off and defined as "other," put out into a separate territory for specialization or for neglect as the case might be. It was phenomenal, Marte thought. Phenomenal.

The four women collaborated not only to raise the number of women studied but also out of a politics of women's health. What they hoped to do, as women, was important research *for* women. They were also aware that working collaboratively rather than competitively was more in line with feminist than with medical politics. By working together, they would be saying: "Okay, here is us, on our own time, in our own way, doing this with no research tools and no research money. But this is important and you need to sit up and take notice."

JANUARY–JUNE 1990

A Kleenex box sat by Sandra Elkin's computer, along with a cup of hot water, honey, and lemon juice, and a bottle of Vitamin C. Only her sneezes broke the 2:00 A.M. stillness. Despite her miserable March cold, she had to get her speech for the Women and AIDS breakfast in Albany two days later written that night. She was scheduled to shoot a video the next day at 7:30 A.M. The shoot would leave her no other time to work on the speech.

She was going to describe how prevention messages for women had been politicized in the same ways the AIDS virus had. The messages were rooted in sexism, racism, and disregard for the reality of women's lives. She had the speech title—"Sex, Lies, and No Good Video Tapes"—but the speech itself wouldn't come. She wanted to find a way to characterize the utterly absurd prevention messages directed to women, messages that would not protect women from AIDS. But how? Saying it straight out didn't seem to work. Frustrated, she tried approach after approach, sneezing, crossing out failed lines, looking at the clock, grabbing Kleenex, swallowing vitamin C tablets, feeling horrible.

Suddenly, it popped into her mind the way the Kleenex was popping out of the box. What if we treated the common cold virus in the same way that we treat the AIDS virus! How would it be for women if the cold virus were politicized in the same way the AIDS virus had been?

"Then this Kleenex wouldn't fit on my nose," Elkin thought. "And I wouldn't be allowed to see a Kleenex until I was thirty-five years old."

Laughing, she began writing a tale set in the United States some years after it is discovered that sneezing and sharing Kleenex can spread the cold virus:

A government panel of white-coated experts convenes to educate women about preventing infection from the deadly cold virus. They tell the women that they can become infected if they allow a man with the virus to sneeze in their presence without using a Kleenex.

"Do not engage in unprotected sneezing," they tell the women.

The women look at one another in puzzlement. Then one raises her hand: "How do we make sure a man doesn't sneeze around us without using a Kleenex?"

The experts put their heads together, whispering, and one explains: "You ask him if he has ever sneezed around a woman before, or if he has ever shared a Kleenex. Then you will be able to make a decision about your risk."

The women laugh. One points out that a study in California found that men lie to women under such circumstances.

"There are two ways you can protect yourselves," another panelist replies. "You could either never ever leave your houses so that no man could sneeze on you. Sneezing abstinence. Or, if you must go out of your houses, you bring lots of Kleenex in your purses and the minute a man sneezes, a—"

One woman yells out, "Sometimes it doesn't even take a minute!"

While the women roar with laughter, the expert, annoyed at the interruption, continues: "—if you think a man might sneeze, you whip out a Kleenex and convince him to use it before he sneezes."

The women protest that it's impossible for all women to convince all men to do that every single time they sneeze. That's just not the way it works between men and women.

The experts look at one another, puzzled. The chairman asks, "Any more questions?"

"Are there Kleenex for us to use?" one woman asks.

"No. The Kleenex only fit on men's noses."

An older woman stands: "Then why are you telling *us* to use Kleenex? If you can send a man to the moon and much of the world can watch CNN, why haven't you developed Kleenex women can use?"

The women applaud. A young woman shyly raises her hand: "But I've never been allowed to even see a Kleenex. My father told me that only bad girls use Kleenex. My parents think that if they let me see a Kleenex, I'll want to hang around sneezing men."

An expert responds: "At your age, we are advising you to stay in your house."

A woman asks: "My man won't do it. He'll split. And then where will I be? I have four children."

Another asks: "What about women who love women? Are they at risk?"

The experts stare blankly. While the women wait for an answer, the chairman clears his throat and adjourns the session of Deadly Cold Virus Education.

By the time Elkin finished writing her speech, she was no longer chuckling: "In spite of all the panel's efforts to educate women about the cold virus and how to protect themselves from it, some women started to sneeze. When women began to ask questions, they were told not to worry: only other women were sneezing and it had nothing to do with them. The women believed that. And more and more women began to sneeze."

The women looked around the hall in Albany, New York, angrily: not even the food or coffee had been delivered. Despite all assurances to the organizers that everything was ready for the breakfast meeting to educate New York legislators on women and AIDS, nothing had been prepared.

"Well, folks," Pauline Miles of Empire Blue Cross/Blue Shield, one of the breakfast sponsors, said with determination. "We have a breakfast in half an hour."

The women—Marie St. Cyr, Linda Lofredo, Lynne MacArthur, Sandra Elkin, Zena Stein, and Anke Ehrhardt—took off their suit jackets and began pulling the heavy tables into a horseshoe shape.

Newly arriving women—state officials, physicians, research scientists—lent their hands to the task. Floor-to-ceiling windows at one end of the large hall gave all the light that the overcast day could provide. As the women pulled and tugged and laughed about it, all formality was broken. Later, it struck Lofredo as a fitting symbolic gesture: women literally "pulling together."

The food finally arrived. The women spread it out on a buffet table near the door. A news crew from a local television station arrived, too, and then, in a prison van, in an air of excitement, the featured speakers, Bedford Hills superintendent Elaine Lord and five women from ACE. Three of the inmates, ineligible for furloughs, were in green prison uniforms and, until they entered the hall, shackled. Katrina Haslip wore "civilian" clothes.

When the audience was seated, the ACE women talked about what the organization did and what it meant to them. They held up the quilt square they had made for "the baby" among them, Helen Cover, twenty-seven, who had died two months earlier.

Katrina Haslip told how central ACE had been in building her self-esteem: "All of us in prison were labeled the outcasts of society. Yet we so-called misfits were doing something constructive that some people outside—the elite of society—were not doing. I got a charge from that. I'm supposed to be this criminal and yet I'm concerned about humanity here and I'm trying to bring about behavior changes and educate. I'm trying to extend myself to the next person. I'm not seeing that happen outside. So what is so bad about me?"

Renée Scott, an African-American woman who, like Katrina, discovered in prison that she was infected with HIV, spoke of the support ACE women gave her when, terrified, she went to learn her test results:

"These were *convicts!* Women felons! The support they gave me—it was like I jumped from the Empire State Building and landed in cotton. A cushioned fall. That's how ACE was there for me. It's hard to say without its sounding phony, but it's real."

Now it was Kathy Selzer's turn. She had recently lost one hundred pounds, getting a food addiction under control as she dealt with a past shaped by childhood abuse and sexual assault. HIV-negative, she had joined ACE and played a quiet role, handling correspondence with outside agencies. But other ACE women had been encouraging her to stretch herself by doing public speaking, an urging she, terrified, had finally yielded to today.

She asked Katrina to come up with her and hold her hand as she spoke. They walked to the podium together.

"I'm really nervous," Selzer told the huge room, "and Katrina is here to support me."

The audience laughed warmly.

Watching Haslip, an African-American woman, holding the hand of a white woman through her ordeal, Elkin thought: Here is the answer to the whole thing. If people could respond this way to the epidemic and the people affected by it, it would be an entirely different epidemic.

Anke Ehrhardt, moved and impressed by the presentation of the ACE women, invited them to speak at the HIV Center in Manhattan soon after. During the lunch break, she sat next to Katrina Haslip. Why was she in prison? Ehrhardt asked her.

"Well, I was a thief," Haslip replied. "A pickpocket."

She paused and smiled.

"I was a very *good* thief."

The two women laughed.

In all three centers of their ongoing study—Cook County in Chicago, Community Health Project in Manhattan, and Kings County in Brooklyn—HIV-infected women had a much higher rate of abnormal pap smears than the general population of women living in those communities.

Carola Marte, Pat Kelly, Mardge Cohen, and Rachel Fruchter knew something worrisome was going on. They felt women infected with HIV were at risk for cervical disease.

Meanwhile, rumors were circulating in the medical and public health community in New York City that there were many cases of invasive, rapidly progressing cervical cancer in HIV-infected women. Dr. Mary Ann Chiasson and a colleague at the New York City Department of Health decided to assemble in one room everyone in the city working on that issue. Fruchter and Marte attended as well as physicians from other New York City clinics. CDC people were invited so they, too, could learn what was happening. CDC had clout. It could get the word out throughout the country fast.

The meeting took place in April at the Health Department. The clinicians told the three CDC representatives that HIV-infected women at their clinics had a high rate of abnormal pap smears and might be at risk for a very high rate of cervical cancer. We should be doing pap smears on all these women and offering HIV counseling to women with abnormal pap smears in high-HIV prevalence places, they argued with urgency. The clinicians wanted people to sit up and immediately start *doing* something.

The CDC folks, expressing varying degrees of skepticism, said they needed to be convinced. Before they could come out with a definitive statement that HIV-infected women were at high risk for abnormal pap smears and cervical cancer and that, therefore, these women should have pap smears more frequently than once a year, the CDC needed much further data.

After the meeting, they wrote an article on the New York City data for the November issue of the CDC's influential *Morbidity and Mortality Weekly Report (MMWR)*.[1] The report did alert public health people and those running HIV clinics to the problem of cervical dysplasia in HIV-positive women. But CDC recommended that nothing change. HIV-infected women should keep on having yearly pap smears, the same as women who were not infected.

The *MMWR* report was written in the language of stern scientists adhering to a rigorous standard of scientific integrity ("methodological concerns about these four studies emphasize the need for additional assessment . . . ," "other possible risk factors," ". . . the community controls . . . may not be directly comparable . . . ," "limited sample sizes," "limitations of cytologic screening for diagnostic purposes," "complicated by complexities related to interpretation of . . . ").

All true. Also true: if you have reason to fear that valuable people are at special risk of cervical cancer, even without absolute proof of that danger, you err on the side of caution by increasing the frequency of screening. If the CDC had heeded the clinicians and recommended comprehensive gynecological care for every HIV-infected woman, and HIV counseling for every woman with an abnormal pap smear living in areas with high HIV rates, that would cost money. Lots of it. The money was saved.

· · ·

On a cool, sunny April day, Dr. Dooley Worth sat, furious, in a congressional hearing room on Capitol Hill in Washington, D.C., waiting with other female experts to testify before a House committee on a national drug control strategy. They were there to talk about what women need to free themselves from their addictions and why many treatments currently offered didn't work for women.

The House subcommittee had put all the women on one panel and scheduled that panel for last. The men on the first panels—physicians singing the praises of whatever drug treatment program they were running—spoke at length. Congressmen asked them questions about addicted women that they could not answer. Worth and the other women, silently waiting in the back, had the answers but were not allowed to speak then. It was driving them mad. So was the fact that as the men went on and on under endless questioning, congressman after congressman got up and left the hearing to go vote or sit on another committee.

By the time the women were called to testify, time had run out and so had most of the committee. The hearing was extended half an hour. As the women moved to the front of the now nearly empty room to take their seats at the witness table, committee chairman John Conyers of Michigan told them there was no time left for their presentations. Could they please summarize their statements briefly?

Angered, Worth read her entire statement as the chairman interrupted her, asking her to hurry. She listed all the barriers to effective drug treatment for women and then pointedly noted: "The needs of drug-dependent women are clearly defined. What we have to ask is: why are there only twenty-one comprehensive treatment programs for women throughout the country? Why are many privately funded, can take only small numbers of women and children, and are chronically short of adequate funding? What we have to ask is: why are we not funding what seems to work?"[2]

But only one congressman, the chairman, was present to hear her question.

ACT UP activists successfully pressured NIAID to admit them to the meetings of the physicians and scientists conducting ACTG studies. Women had been largely excluded from these trials, funded and managed by NIAID, even though they were often the only way to get HIV treatment. (By 1990, only 6.6 percent of trial participants were women.) Sitting in the meetings, the activists were angered to learn the conditions of one planned trial, 076.

ACTG 076 is a trial to test the efficacy of the drug AZT in preventing perinatal transmission of HIV. AZT would be administered to pregnant HIV-infected women beginning in the second trimester of pregnancy. (By the second trimester, fetal organs would have been formed, reducing the risk of drug-induced deformities.)

At the meetings, researchers spoke of the women merely as fetus-carriers, the listening activists felt. Though researchers claimed they would be assessing the effects of AZT on both the woman and the fetus, in fact attention was focused on the fetus. There were no plans to conduct frequent colposcopy exams of the women. No gynecological care would be provided for the women. There was no requirement that a gynecologist or internist be involved in the study to attend to the needs of the women; only obstetricians and pediatricians for the fetuses. AZT would be discontinued as soon as the woman was postdelivery. No medical treatment would be provided for the woman after the postdelivery period.

Examining the informed consent form to be signed by women in the study, the activists found it omitted mention of these facts:

- Female mice given AZT had an increased incidence of vaginal cancer in one study.
- No one knows the effects of AZT on the fetus in utero.
- Approximately 30 percent of the fetuses of HIV-infected women will become infected. Therefore, some 70 percent of the fetuses in the study would be administered a highly toxic drug in an attempt to prevent an infection they would not have gotten anyway.

The contradiction involved in this study was immediately evident to the activists: the original clinical trials supporting FDA approval of AZT as a treatment for AIDS had included only 3.5 percent women, partly out of concern that the drug might injure a theoretical fetus. What if the women in the study got pregnant during the trials and the AZT harmed the fetus? So the few women enrolled were required to document "appropriate" contraception or pledge sexual

abstinence during the trials. Routine tests were administered periodically to confirm that the women were not pregnant. The few women
who were enrolled were followed for the same complications associated with AZT use as the men; no assessment was made of AZT's
impact on gynecological problems.

Now the rules suddenly changed. Earlier, when the trials offered
a potential benefit to the HIV-infected woman in terms of her own illness and her own life, pregnant women were *barred* from those trials.
Now, when the trials offered a theoretical benefit, not to women
(researchers would not carefully monitor what the drug was doing to
the women) but to fetuses, pregnant women were actively *sought* for
the trials. Earlier, strict procedures were set up to ensure that no pregnant women were administered AZT. Now the women administered
AZT in 076 were *required* to be pregnant.

With the new interest in AZT's effects on fetuses, ACTG trial
sites were selected to target geographic locations with dense populations of women with HIV.

"Where were the same concerted efforts to seek out, enroll and
assess the effects of AZT on women in the original studies of this
drug?" ACT UP activists wrote.

If NIAID aimed to enroll 748 pregnant HIV-infected women for
this trial, why couldn't it seek out equally large numbers of women for
trials of drugs and prophylactic treatments that could potentially benefit the women themselves? they asked.[3]

ACT UP activist Linda Meredith commented: "The ACTG system sends women with HIV/AIDS a confusing and life-threatening
message: 'Don't get pregnant if you want access to clinical trials—but
we will only include you in a trial if you are pregnant so that we may
study the effects of treatments on your fetus.'"

At 7:30 A.M. on May 21, under drizzling skies in Bethesda, Maryland,
twelve hundred demonstrators—Linda Meredith among them—
streamed onto the campus of the National Institutes of Health (NIH),
three hundred acres of green hills and trees. A few were costumed as
"grim reapers," others as "scientists" in red-splattered lab coats. Most
wore black T-shirts and "blood"-smeared jackets. The demonstrators,
organized by ACT UP in one of its largest actions to date, had come

from New York, California, Ohio, Louisiana, Puerto Rico, Oregon, and Washington, D.C.

Activists marched from one colonial-style building to another among the institutes involved in AIDS research, chanting, "Ten years, $1 billion, one drug, big deal," and "We want a cure, this is war."

"National Institutes of Hypocrites" and "NIH: Nothing Is Happening" their posters proclaimed. At the entrance to each building, they found chained doors and a line of U.S. Park police on horseback.

While some demonstrators sang satirical ballads and others, in street theater, portrayed the characters Death, Life, NIH, and Drug Companies, still others strung red streamers through trees outside NIH buildings to symbolize governmental red tape. Some twisted themselves in the red tape and then spastically fell to the ground "dead." On an NIH lawn, a few activists set up a cemetery with several dozen cardboard tombstones: "We will not R.I.P."

Every twelve minutes, an air horn blared, marking the AIDS death of another person. At intervals, the thunder of hundreds of hands pounding on the back of protest signs added to the clamor of prancing police horses, songs, chants, and occasional screams. Pink and purple smoke bombs exploded. In interviews with reporters, demonstrators told tales of dead friends, dead children, dead sisters. They were storming NIH, they explained, to demand that all AIDS treatments be tested immediately and that all communities affected by AIDS—including women, children, people of color, and the poor— be represented in clinical trials.

When one protester leaped onto the roof of a building at 8:45 A.M., police in riot helmets and gloves began making arrests.

Shortly before 11:00 A.M., twenty-one demonstrators piled into a van they had rented and drove five miles up the road to a building housing the office of Dr. Daniel F. Hoth, director of NIAID's Division of AIDS. Hoth was responsible for the ACTG, including the 076 trial that appalled ACT UP feminists. While most of the activists walked to a back door, well-dressed Linda Meredith and Marion Banzhof walked in the front door. They had cased out the building twice before to determine where Hoth's office was and how to reach it quickly, and they had chatted with the woman at the security desk both times. This morning, security was beefed up. They were stopped at the desk. After answering a few questions, they said, "We're sorry.

We're late for an appointment," and got on the elevator. Two ACT UP men walked in pretending to be lost drivers needing directions. They engaged the security guard in conversation so she would be facing them and not the demonstrators waiting at the back door.

Exiting the elevator, Meredith and Banzhof walked to the back door to let in the others. When they had cased out the premises earlier, the door had been unlocked. Now it was locked. They passed five nervous minutes in the stairwell deciding whether or not to open the fire escape door, which would sound an alarm. They could hear the women waiting for them outside. They opened the door. As the demonstrators quietly walked up one flight and down the hall to Hoth's office, the alarm screamed.

Word quickly spread in the building that Hoth's office was under occupation. Within half an hour, the federal employees had been told to go home.

Two police officers entered Hoth's office and, while waiting for reinforcements, watched the occupiers. Hoth was not there. He was meeting in another building with Dr. Anthony S. Fauci, director of NIAID. They phoned him. He would not speak with them, they were told. The women then phoned the press. On Hoth's revolving erasable white board, they wrote facts on women and HIV. They had prepared summaries of the ways in which government-sponsored clinical trials on AIDS treatments ignored women, and they left about five hundred of these for Hoth to find when he returned: in drawers, on tabletops, in file folders.

They had come to Hoth's office to demand that NIAID form a Women's Committee that included HIV-infected women and women working with them and that would ensure women's access to the ACTG.

Police arrived and arrested twenty-one activists for loitering. All in all that day, police arrested eighty-two.[4]

Soon after attorney Terry McGovern began seeing exclusively HIV-infected clients in May 1990, a pattern became apparent to her: the poor, and particularly women, were having to fight hard, often vainly, to get federal disability benefits that came easily to more affluent white men. McGovern, a legal services attorney in New York City, had many gay male friends with AIDS or HIV. They had simply applied for disability benefits and gotten them. But her HIV-infected clients, mostly poor black women, had to go to hell and back to get theirs approved.

It had been in March 1989 that she had begun seeing increasing numbers of clients who were HIV-infected. The poverty law community, hobbling along on the slashed funds of the Reagan/Bush administrations, did not view HIV-infected women and IV drug users as a priority for their limited resources, and the AIDS service providers were focused on helping higher-income gay men.

Appalled at the suffering revealed to her by the women who came to her office, McGovern raised funds to set up an HIV project for poor people. In May 1990, she began seeing exclusively HIV-infected clients in emergencies: they were being evicted, or were losing their kids, or were getting no medical care at all. Many were coming because they had been denied disability benefits. They wanted a lawyer to defend them at the appeals hearings.

Social Security had two programs for people suffering HIV complications: Social Security Disability Insurance (SSDI) for those who have contributed to Social Security, and Supplemental Security Income (SSI), funded through federal income taxes, for the disabled poor who need not have paid into the Social Security system. To be judged "disabled," the Social Security Administration (SSA) requires that people have a severe impairment that prevents them from performing substantial work. The impairment must be one expected to last at least a year or to end in death. People with AIDS met those requirements, according to SSA. People with AIDS-related complex (ARC) were evaluated for disability on a case-by-case basis.

It generally takes SSA two to three months to process an SSI claim, but the agency can shorten that period for people with AIDS if the AIDS diagnosis is confirmed by a medical source. This is called presumptive disability. Benefits can continue up to three months during which time, Social Security will gather the medical evidence to confirm that the person is indeed eligible to continue receiving payments. Payments will then continue as long as the person is disabled.

As a member of ACT UP, McGovern heard that women were

challenging the CDC's AIDS definition, and she figured that the refusal of benefits to women and the poor was related to that definition.

ACT UP women had searched the medical literature and found at least sixty studies reporting symptoms in HIV-positive individuals that were not part of CDC's AIDS definition. CDC considered this anecdotal evidence but ensured that the information remain anecdotal by not funding studies that could demonstrate the link. It was the government's fault that there was only anecdotal evidence, ACT UP believed.

In the spring of 1990, McGovern began looking through the medical records of the clients in the five Legal Services offices in Manhattan. All the symptoms she had heard about at ACT UP meetings as afflicting women with HIV were in the clients' records. Yet the women were classified as "asymptomatic," without HIV symptoms.

"I think something is going on here," McGovern said to the attorney managing the Legal Services project on disability benefits. "All these people are being denied SSI."

Her colleague looked through all her own HIV cases. Clearly, there was a pattern: If you had CDC-defined AIDS, you got benefits. If you did not, you were denied them. It was a deadly situation for it meant that extremely sick women were being denied money for food and shelter. For medical care, too, because the disability benefits were often the women's only ticket to receiving Medicare or Medicaid.

There was an inequity in the system based on a discriminatory definition of AIDS, McGovern believed: the definition discriminated in favor of gay, non-IV-drug-using men.

McGovern contacted Risa Denenberg, a nurse practitioner working with HIV-positive clients at the Community Health Project, the AIDS outreach clinic in New York City where Carola Marte had seen so many abnormal pap smears. McGovern told Denenberg she was considering a lawsuit against Health and Human Services (HHS) Secretary Louis W. Sullivan, who headed Social Security, and asked her to come look through all the medical records she had.

News of the suit excited Denenberg. She and other health providers—most of them women—had been seeing the same symptoms over and over again in HIV-infected women, but these symptoms were not in the CDC definition. So they would watch as some of the women died, never having been diagnosed with AIDS. Something was wrong. Without government leadership, all she and other providers had been able to do was network with one another, at their own expense and on their own initiative.

HIV disease needed to be studied in women, Denenberg believed. CDC had done, and was still doing, expensive, long-term (MACS) studies on the natural history and prevalence of HIV in men. All their data was coming from those studies. If CDC didn't study the disease in different populations, then the only definition of AIDS that would ever exist in the United States would be one appropriate to white gay men.

But the disease was different in different bodies. Its major manifestation was suppression of the body's immune system. When the immune system is compromised, Denenberg knew, diseases a person previously suffered may come back. The disease had remained in the body kept under control by that immune system until, weakened, it was no longer able to do that. So the symptoms of people with AIDS partly depended on what they already had in their bodies. The symptoms also depended partly on the diseases and infections common in the communities in which the PWAs lived. The drug-abusing community is much more at risk of pulmonary infections, kidney problems, liver damage, abcesses, or endocarditis than non-drug-shooting gay men. Poor people are more vulnerable to bacterial pneumonia; gay men, to Kaposi's sarcoma. The patterns varied, too, in different parts of the world. PWAs in sub-Saharan Africa were more at risk of cryptococcus; those in the United States and Western Europe, to pneumocystis.

Women's bodies are different from men's. There are different organs. There is a hormonal cycle. Women have histories of different diseases. Those who suffered pelvic inflammatory disease (PID) before being infected with HIV might find the PID returning repeatedly after HIV, resistant to treatment. It made sense that the disease would not manifest in women in exactly the way it had in men.

But Social Security, ignoring all this, just fell back on the CDC definition. At the same time, Risa Denenberg knew gay men on Social Security who were doing so much better than the women she saw who could not get on disability. It wasn't that she wanted the disability taken away from the men; she wanted it extended to women.

Now, Denenberg marveled, along comes this incredible lawyer

working in a law firm for poor people. Terry McGovern saw her HIV-infected clients disabled and dying, never having gotten an AIDS diagnosis. Without any medical background, McGovern made the connection that physicians seemed ill-equipped to make. Women were visible to her as they evidently were not to many physicians. Poor people were visible to her. So she saw what was there to be seen.

Impressed, Denenberg volunteered her time to McGovern. Throughout the summer, the two went through all the medical records together. The symptoms they saw repeatedly in the records were chronic PID, refractory chronic candidiasis, vaginal candidiasis, cervical dysplasia that can lead to cervical cancer, chronic urinary tract infections, and recurrent genital warts. They repeatedly saw records of abnormal pap smears, some of which had not been followed up.

They also saw chronic bronchitis. That intrigued McGovern because it had been reported a couple of years earlier that between 1981 and 1988 in New York City, Newark, and other major cities, there had been a huge jump in the number of deaths of young women due to respiratory illnesses. She suspected those deaths were HIV-related, as had journalist Chris Norwood, who had uncovered them.

Reading through the charts, Denenberg found women who had had eight or nine gynecological surgeries and gradually lost all their female organs. There was the case of a thirty-one-year-old HIV-infected Latina who applied for disability in 1988. She was turned down at the initial and reconsideration stages. Judged able-bodied, her medical records included evidence of these HIV-related conditions and multiple hospitalizations:

1981: Two hospitalizations for PID; *1982:* hospitalization for laparotomy and partial right oopherectomy (removal of ovary); *1983:* hospitalization and treatment for abnormal pap smear, ovarian cancer treated with radiation and chemotherapy; hospitalization for PID; *1984:* treatment for pneumonia; hospitalization for laparoscopy and D&C; hospitalization for chronic PID and cervicitis; *1985:* hospitalization for pelvic pain due to chronic PID, and multiple adhesions to bowel, with procedures performed including laparoscopy, laparotomy, and hysterectomy for a tubo-ovarian abscess, and removal of left ovary and tube; *1986:* treatment for urinary tract infection and pyelonephritis; sonogram for chronic pelvic pain due to recurrent PID; treatment for pneumonia, left side; treatment for urinary tract infection, diarrhea and vaginitis; hospitalization for appendectomy, removal of remaining right ovary, ruptured cyst with dense pelvic adhesions, and renal stone treated with laser therapy; emergency room visit and treatment for complaints of mid-abdominal pain with vomiting of blood.[5]

Denied disability benefits and unable to afford housing without those benefits, this woman was sleeping on the floor of her parents' apartment.

Denenberg studied the charts of another woman, twenty-three, whose male companion had infected her sexually. She was unable to work due to increasingly painful outbreaks of PID, headaches, vomiting, shortness of breath, and dizziness. Her application for disability had been denied: the government presumed PID was not related to HIV. Unable to afford her own apartment, she was forced to live with a father who had molested her as a child, according to her social worker. Her two toddlers were in foster care. Every week, she took five buses to visit them, wanting to spend as much time as she could with them before her death. Partly because she had no adequate housing to offer them, she could not convince Family Court to return her children to her custody.

Health care was set up so that doctors were not recognizing the gynecological manifestations of HIV, Denenberg saw as she studied the charts and reflected on her own experience in the system. She recognized just what Pat Kelly was finding so maddening at Downstate in Brooklyn: women going to city HIV clinics for primary health care were not getting any gynecological care—though that was certainly primary for women—because of the systematic fragmentation and sexism of the medical system. If the women were not too embarrassed to mention a gynecological problem, they would be referred to the hospital's gyn clinic where personnel were not trained in HIV. There would be no communication between the two clinics over the woman's situation.

On the other hand, HIV-infected women who had not been identified as such were going to gyn clinics and emergency rooms for abdominal pain and getting much repetitious gyn care, with the physician never identifying their gynecological problems as HIV symptoms.

Women were either getting inappropriate gyn care and no HIV care or inappropriate, male-oriented HIV care and no gyn care.

Denenberg was appalled at the treatment many of McGovern's

clients were receiving. For example, the charts showed anemia going on and on, untreated. Often conditions were not followed up enough for a clear diagnosis to be made. So while she held the Social Security Administration responsible for its adoption of a discriminatory AIDS definition, she also felt that many terribly sick clients could not supply Social Security with the medical records to show what was wrong with them because, even though they had gone to the clinics repeatedly seeking help, nobody had done anything for them there. Some clients had been hospitalized four times with pneumonia in the early 1980s but because nobody had ever performed a procedure that could have diagnosed PCB (broncoscopy), this AIDS-defining condition had no chance of being identified.

The charts showed tremendous menstrual irregularities in HIV-positive women. Not only was this not being studied; no one was even raising the question, What's going on here? Were the irregularities due to weight loss? AZT? Heroin use? Or to the HIV virus itself?

After studying the charts, attorney McGovern interviewed the women, asking, "Are you having gynecological problems?" They would always say yes, refer to such problems as recurrent vaginal candidiasis or PID, and then add: "The doctors told me not to worry about it. They said it's completely unrelated."

It was clear to attorney McGovern that something was terribly wrong, though many people, including other poverty lawyers, told her they didn't see the problem. This sometimes made her feel crazy.

Hearing of the suit and believing that there was indeed a problem, several organizations said they wanted to join in on the challenge to HHS. So she signed on Cardozo Bet Tzedek Legal Services, the Center for Constitutional Rights, Lambda Legal Defense and Education Fund, and Brooklyn Legal Services, Corp. B as plaintiffs.

McGovern and her colleagues began meeting physicians treating HIV-positive women and gathering affidavits from them. The physicians agreed to testify in a suit against Health and Human Services. It would be the first compilation of anti-CDC evidence.

Bruce Sampson, drinking steadily in his small New Jersey town since he learned he had HIV, began beating his wife, Diane. In June she separated from him. Now she was a twenty-nine-year-old single parent with five young children under ten years of age.

Soon after testing positive, she had begun losing weight and feeling sick. She'd been run-down and tired before then, but after all, she'd just been through three pregnancies. She had attributed the exhaustion to that.

She got vaginal candidiasis, repeatedly. Vaginal warts. Terrible premenstrual syndrome. Some days she'd be needy, clinging to her family, her children: "Love me a lot!" Other days, she pushed them away: "Don't get close to me! Don't love me!" She felt dirty.

She had made arrangements for the children. An aunt a few years older than she and an uncle would raise them when she died. They would be cared for. Now, nothing mattered. She was tired. Tired of feeling, If I close my eyes, will I open them tomorrow? Tired of being scared. Just let it be done and over with, she thought. There was no sense fighting it.

Sometimes she'd take one of her children to the well-baby clinic for a vaccination and see that poster. It showed a mother in a perfect nursery holding a beautiful little girl in her lap. "She has her father's eyes," the caption read, "and her mother's AIDS."

When AIDS has already hit your house, Diane thought, that poster seems cruel.

Slowly, Diane came out of her lethargy. She had to make memories right now, she thought. She wanted her younger brothers and sisters to remember her in case, five years down the road, she wasn't there any more. She had to be the best sister she could be. She held the holiday celebrations at her house, seating her sisters, brothers, nieces, nephews, parents, aunts, and uncles all around her heavily laden table. She prepared a big Halloween party for the children of her expansive clan. Diane had to do everything she could right then, right there, in case tomorrow did not come.

Gradually, she realized: It didn't have to be over tomorrow. She could live for years with HIV.

After Bruce left, she sometimes felt enraged. Now she gave her rage full rein; he wasn't there to be hurt by it anymore.

"I hate him!" she screamed. "He had no right to do this to me! I didn't deserve this!"

Another woman's marriage falls apart, Diane thought, and people tell her, "Just forget about it. Put it in the past." That woman picks up the pieces and starts over. But the pieces she herself was left with—Diane didn't want them. She could never put HIV behind her.

She had to carry it with her, all through a shortened future. He's permanently scarred me, she raged.

Not that he did it deliberately. She realized that in calmer moments. We didn't know, she grieved. We just didn't know then.

Penny Abernathey's son James, now four years old, had a picture of his dad in his bedroom in Austin, Texas. When he was younger, his mother had told him his dad had gotten sick and died. Now James was older, his questions more specific.

"What did Daddy die of?" he asked.

"He died of a virus," Penny said.

"Tell me about the virus."

"Well, it lived in your daddy's blood."

"Do I have it in my blood?"

"No," Penny said. "But I have it in mine."

As James grew older, Penny incorporated more reality into her answers. The reality that someday his mother, too, like his dad, would die.

James had heard Penny say that her parents would be his guardians after her death. Hearing her speak of the virus to someone on the telephone, he would come and hug her and sometimes cry.

At work, Penny's supervisors, knowing her HIV status, continued to harass her. There was only one way she could figure out how to make them stop: tell everybody. An Austin television station planning a program on HIV in women gave her the chance. AIDS Services of Austin called Penny, one of its clients, and asked if she were willing to appear on the program. She was.

Once she went on television and said, "I'm HIV-positive," *everybody* in town knew. The people at work saw the program. So did the parents of children at her son's day care. Alarmed, the parents telephoned the day-care administrators. If that woman did not produce proof that her son was not HIV-infected, they said, they were yanking their kids out of day care.

Penny was ready. Before she'd entered the television studio, she'd been to her pediatrician and gotten documentation on James's negative HIV test results. She now made them available. Parents took their kids out of school anyway. But the day-care staff supported Penny, kept James, and bade farewell to those who left.

The television producers had counseled Penny: Tell us if you have any negative repercussions from this broadcast. We'll be happy to publicize it.

Penny went to work the next day and told her supervisors: "If I have any problems here, all I have to do is call up the media and they're going to be on you."

Their harassment of her stopped that day. However, her boss had told her that she would never be promoted because she would not be around for twenty-five years.

Penny watched the words come out of his mouth.

Dr. Sally Zierler held the unpublished results of the New England study in her hand. Women who, as children, had been sexually abused were twice as likely to be HIV-infected as women who had not. HIV occurred with a 40 percent frequency rate among sexual assault survivors.

The study Zierler had helped design also found:

- Forty percent of the 224 women in the study reported they had been raped or forced to have sex in their lifetime. (More than two-thirds of these had been abused for the first time in childhood or teenage years.)
- Compared with women who had not been assaulted, these women were more likely to be prescribed tranquilizers and to be heavy consumers of alcohol.
- They were three times more likely to work as prostitutes.
- Sexually transmitted diseases were more common among them.[6]

To Zierler, one implication of the study was that healing childhood sexual traumas was a public health priority.

Zierler and her colleagues felt the findings of their study, disturbing enough, understated the prevalence of sexual abuse. First, because women may be unwilling to talk about their sexual assault when they'd only seen the interviewer on one other occasion, hardly enough time to build trust. And second, because many women don't even remember their abusive experiences. This was not just a matter of conscious denial; it could also be a much deeper form of protection the child's mind provided her from an unendurable experience.

In recent years, a growing movement of adult survivors of childhood sexual abuse, feminist activists, and therapists had publicly named incest as a widespread phenomenon, helping to create an environment in which women felt safer in remembering. But there were still many people in their twenties, the age group questioned in the study, who might not yet have consciously remembered their sexual assault experiences, Zierler felt.[7]

Zierler wanted practicing physicians—pediatricians, internists, and obstetrician-gynecologists in particular—to know what the study had found. Clinicians, she felt, were appallingly limited in their understanding of the health consequences of sexual assault. Presented with an assault survivor, they typically would look for physical trauma to the vagina, and possibly evidence of sexually transmitted disease, and of pregnancy. Once in a while, an unusually sensitive physican might look for acute psychological damage. But by and large, clinicians were not attending to the long-term consequences of sexual assaults by making the appropriate referrals.

In their training, the physicians might themselves have participated in sexual assaults of women. Until medical students, under the influence of the feminist movement, had protested the practice, medical schools used anesthetized women in training students on how to do a gynecological exam. The anesthetized women had never been asked, and had never consented, to having a line of young men manually penetrate their vaginas. No one who participated, unprotesting, in such acts could have much sensitivity to sexual assaults of females.

In writing up the New England study, the major message was: Physicians need to recognize that sexual assault is so routine an experience, questions concerning it should be part of regular history taking. Physicians need to know how to ask these questions and what to do with the responses. They should be familiar with resources available in the community to sexual assault survivors and encourage their patients to seek counseling or other appropriate help. This was vital, not simply because of the implications for the HIV epidemic, but in terms of people's health generally. In recent years, many primary-care physicians, recognizing the health implications of drinking, had begun routinely including questions on it in taking medical histories. The same should be true of sexual assault.

Zierler submitted the paper to the *New England Journal of Medicine,* the most widely read and prestigious medical journal in the United States. Editors send papers submitted to the *Journal* out to experts to be reviewed and use these comments in deciding on publication. Two months later, the *Journal* rejected the Zierler paper. Only a one-paragraph comment from one reviewer was enclosed with the rejection letter.

So, Zierler thought in frustration, news on widespread sexual assaults on children's bodies and the health consequences of these assaults isn't worth the space in a clinician's journal.

Zierler telephoned the editor who handled her paper. She was concerned, she told him, that childhood sexual abuse was not considered an important agenda for the *Journal.* Judging from the minimal comment on it, the paper had not been thoughtfully reviewed, she noted. When the editor assured her that the *Journal* considered childhood sexual abuse a very important priority, Zierler asked, "If you think that this is very important, why has the *Journal* not published a single article on childhood sexual assault?"

He continued responding vaguely. Zierler told him she wanted to write something addressing publication bias, particularly involving women's issues, and wondered if she could use their conversation in her article.

"Absolutely not, you may not do that!" he said angrily.

Zierler sent the article next to the *Journal of the American Medical Association.* Within two weeks, she and her colleagues received a letter noting that "your topic is interesting" but rejecting the article. *JAMA* had apparently not even bothered to send the paper out for review.

Zierler had always known the *American Journal of Public Health,* focusing on preventive medicine, would be receptive to the paper. She sent it off to them and they promptly accepted it. Most clinicians do not read the journal. So now those physicians seeing survivors of sexual assault would most likely never hear of the study or its astonishing findings.[8]

Linda Meredith from ACT UP in Washington, D.C., sent Dr. Dan Hoth of NIAID a letter stating that in case he hadn't gotten the messages ACT UP had left for him all over his office, the activists would like to meet and talk with him. There was no response to the letter or to her repeated telephone calls. She sent another letter: We are giving you until the Sixth International AIDS Conference in San Francisco. If you don't meet with us, we will be back.

As the five thousand delegates to the AIDS conference assembled at its site in San Francisco, ACT UP activists, including Linda Meredith and Maxine Wolfe, handed them flyers that read "Put Women on the ACTG Agenda Now." Since April 1989, the number of newly diagnosed cases of AIDS among women had increased by 45 percent but women were only 6.6 percent of all ACTG participants, the flyer pointed out. "The ACTG agenda clearly reflects a priority of preventing HIV infection in children over treating HIV infection in women."

Inside the huge hall, as Dr. Daniel Hoth began his plenary address, the activists marched down the aisle with a huge banner and stood before him facing the audience all during his speech.

"NIAID: Form a Women's Committee," read the banner.

To Meredith, Hoth looked shaken. He declared that at some point in the next year, NIAID would present a conference on women and AIDS.

When Hoth finished, the activists chanted: "Women with AIDS cannot wait till later. We are not your incubators."

Activists were not the only angry women at the conference. Female physicians and scientists had begun three years earlier, at the international AIDS meeting in Washington, D.C. (where one result of male-dominated conference planning was hula dancers entertaining at a party for delegates), to object to the scant attention given women in the epidemic. In the three years since, the stubbornly maintained ignorance about the course of HIV infection in women remained.

At the San Francisco meeting, conference organizers invited one researcher to speak on HPV (human papillomavirus) in rectal lesions in men. They also invited Mardge Cohen, Rachel Fruchter, Carola Marte, and Pat Kelly to present their poster showing that HIV-infected women had an eight-fold greater risk of dysplasias (thought to be caused by HPV) than the community rate. Presenting a poster is less prestigious, and garners less attention, than giving a talk at a scientific conference. HPV in rectal lesions in men was considered worthy of an oral presentation to conference delegates assembled from around the world, but HPV in the cervix of women was somehow a less compelling topic.

Dr. Kathy Anastos of New York watched researchers present evidence that a depository in the body for the AIDS-defining infection cryptococcal meningitis is the prostate gland. Nobody mentioned that women don't have a prostate gland. Does this cryptococcus reside in women anywhere? Anastos asked herself. Is there a depository? Is there a difference if there is a cryptococcal infection in HIV-infected women and men?

That was an easy question to answer, Anastos thought, listening. Once again, you answer it by doing a long-term prospective study of infected women and looking at what happens. That was only one of the many unknowns about women. Anastos had learned of another in talking with Dr. Clara Jones, who took care of many HIV-infected people at Montefiore in the Bronx. Jones thought there was a nausea and vomiting syndrome in HIV-infected women that didn't seem to happen in men and that hadn't yet been defined.

And there was the vital question of male/female survival rates with AIDS. The studies all showed that there did seem to be a shorter survival time for women. Women were more likely to die the same month they were diagnosed than men. The average woman with AIDS survives 27.4 *weeks* after diagnosis, according to a study conducted by the University of Medicine and Dentistry in Newark, New Jersey, while the average affluent white man lives thirty-nine *months* after diagnosis.

It appeared that women die faster from AIDS than men but no one really knew. The question was: Is it because the majority of male cases are primarily white gay men while female cases are predominantly among IV drug users so that access to appropriate medical care is much more difficult for the women? Is it because women are diagnosed later than men? Or are there some real differences between men and women infected with the disease?

A study could be done with a male control group. It hadn't been done. Hadn't even been initiated, let alone completed. Maybe they needed a young lawyer like Terry McGovern to study a few groups of impoverished clients and work it out for them, the way she was helping to map HIV symptomology in her female clients.

While willful ignorance about the course of the disease in women persisted, once again the few papers on women that conference organizers did accept concerned women (bad Mamas) transmitting HIV to their fetuses; preventing infection in prostitutes; and locking up infected prostitutes. This went on and on, despite the objections women made to it year after year.

At the same time, researchers reported studies at the conference showing that heterosexual transmission was five to six times more efficient from a man to a woman than from a woman to a man (estimates that would grow even greater in future studies). Women were much more likely to be infected by a man than vice versa.

"Look, we've just heard you say that transmission from men to women is so much more efficient than from women to men," said a woman from a prostitutes' organization, standing up at the AIDS conference. "So why aren't you talking about locking up the johns?" Many female delegates erupted in cheers.

To get together a group of people—primarily researchers—to promote research on women and HIV and to work for better representation on those issues at the international AIDS conferences, Carola Marte and Mary Anne Chiasson called an impromptu, informal meeting. News of it spread by word of mouth. Close to one hundred people attended. They included some activists and a few men like Dr. Sten Vermund, who had been doggedly conducting and advocating research on HIV-infected women. When he had moved to NIAID in December 1988, he had proposed a women's study but couldn't get the money to do it. Clinicians like Carola Marte and activists considered him a strong ally.

They called their group the International Organization for Collaborative Research on Women and HIV Disease.

Following the meeting, Marte and Chiasson wrote, on behalf of the group, to the organizers of the next international AIDS conference, to be held in Florence, Italy, in 1991. They pointed out that the group had been convened as a result of a widely expressed concern over the lack of research data being reported on women, despite a rapidly increasing number of infected women and children globally. Noting the group's disappointment at the inclusion of few research reports on topics important to the care of infected women including gynecological diseases, they added: "We feel that it is important to correct the omissions of the 1990 meeting."

They requested a plenary session on research on HIV-infected women and an oral presentation and/or poster session on gynecological manifestations of HIV (as distinct from obstetrical issues).

They waited four months for a reply. Then their requests were denied. The organizers noted they were passing on their letter to organizers of an alternative conference focusing on political aspects of the AIDS epidemic.

This response was appalling. Marte wrote again: Maybe you don't understand. We're not asking for a political session. We're asking for a scientific session.

They didn't get it.

Women's efforts to place women on the agenda had once again failed.

JULY–NOVEMBER
1990

······································

A week after Linda Meredith's note to Dr. Dan Hoth, his office called ACT UP, inviting the women to meet with NIAID officials.

On July 27, seven women from ACT UP in New York and Washington, D.C., including Maxine Wolfe and Linda Meredith, met with Fauci, Hoth, and several assistants at NIH in Bethesda, Maryland. The women gave a presentation based on their study of the medical literature and interviews with physicians and nurses treating HIV-infected women and the women themselves. They began with the general position of women and moved on to a critique of NIAID drug trials.

In the discussion that ensued, Fauci disputed the women's contention that they were there because they had demonstrated at Hoth's office and at the San Francisco conference. He wanted to make it clear that they weren't there because they had acted tough, but because they had written a letter, because they were with ACT UP, a group he respected, and because they had made some important points that he wanted to pursue.

"Demonstrations don't get me," he told the women sternly. "If you come in and threaten, I can guarantee you 100 percent, if you threaten, you will get nothing, zero."

Did he want to speak with them about women and AIDS? the women asked him.

"Well, no," he replied, "because I want to tell you what the ground rules of how we interact [are], and if the ground rules aren't the right ground rules, we're never going to talk about women and AIDS. That's something you have to understand, because that transcends everything we're talking about. We won't talk about women with anything unless you understand that."

The women said they resented his manner and a tone that seemed to imply that if they didn't "act nice," like trained pets, they would get nothing.

He would do something about women and AIDS, he said. But he just wouldn't deal with them unless they acted in a "productive way." He had a very productive arrangement with the men of ACT UP in New York who could be adversarial but not confrontational, who sat down and talked civilly, he said. The women told him that he might well have an arrangement with some men in New York and might well have built up trust with them, but he had no agreement or trust with the women of ACT UP because NIAID had not done one thing for women.

They moved on to issues the women had raised in their presentation.

If, in fact, women's first signs of HIV infection were sometimes unlike those of men, if there were indeed various gynecological conditions like pelvic abscesses—he didn't know that this was so but it was certainly a possibility, he said—then that would be very important in developing preventive therapy for women. But to find out if this were true, maybe it wasn't necessary to design new studies. Maybe they could go back to data they had collected in previous studies, reanalyze it, and if they found any evidence that this might be the case, then perhaps they could design a pilot study. However, if they found no such evidence, investigating further would perhaps not be a good use of limited resources.

The fact that no information in the studies was gathered pointing to gynecological manifestations in women did not mean that they did not exist, the women responded. If the researchers weren't looking at women's pelvic organs, they wouldn't find anything. That did not mean it was not there.

And they were not looking. There was only one study protocol that called for doing pelvic exams on women, so, without a mandate from NIAID to collect relevant data on women, the researchers would not be looking for it, the women said.

That's a possibility, Fauci said.

". . . If there are centers in which they don't do pelvics," he added, "and there are women in those protocols, then I think the information that doesn't occur is important information."

The women brought up further information that was not "occurring." The researchers designing the ACTG 076 study to test whether AZT could prevent the transmission of HIV from infected women to their fetuses did not plan to collect information on the drug's effect on the women themselves.

". . . it is totally crazy to assess the effect of treatment on the fetus and have absolutely no regard at all of it on the woman," Fauci agreed. "We don't have any argument on that." If the protocol was inadvertently ignoring women, that had to be redressed, he said.

The women pointed out that *all* the protocols of trials involving pregnant women ignored the women. They asked him to ensure that after the women in the study did give birth, they were not just cut off from AZT and from all care. "If you follow through with the child, you also have to follow through with the woman."

They were absolutely right, he said.

Activists had earlier pointed out that in NIAID statistics the percentage of women enrolled in ACTG trials had been falsely elevated by combining into a single number all females: infants, girls, teenagers, and adult women. Fauci said they had gone back to check the statistics and that was indeed true.

They read him a list of demands. Dan Hoth, speaking in San Francisco, had mentioned a conference on women and AIDS to be held next year. That was too late. The situation was urgent. It should be moved up and viewed as an emergency conference.

We don't want a conference in which the government tells us what it knows about women and AIDS because we know the government knows nothing, the activists told Fauci.

HIV-infected women and the medical providers treating them should be assembled and asked what they were seeing and experiencing, they proposed. Let them talk to one another. If NIAID didn't want to bet its life on the accuracy of the information that emerged, it could just do what scientists routinely do: say "may." Such and such "may be true." Putting that information out quickly would at least alert women in ways that might save their lives.

NIAID agreed to form a steering committee for the conference incorporating these front-line providers and the women they served. This steering committee could meet in September to draw up the agenda.

The men agreed to move up the conference from February 1991 to December of 1990.

Women will constitute the fastest growing proportion of new cases of AIDS, the National Academy of Science knew. In preparation for its third report on AIDS, *AIDS: The Second Decade,* it asked a group of high-level experts to write papers for a chapter on women. The experts included Drs. Anke Ehrhardt, Mindy Fullilove, Dooley Worth, Wendy Chavkin, and Judith Cohen.

When asked to write on female intravenous drug users and partners of drug users, Worth told the Academy committee that very little research had been done on women in either category so little information was available. Much of what was available was coming out of service programs that had never been set up as research projects.

"It's not that we don't know what the problems are," she told them. "We've worked with them. We do know. We can write about what the women's needs are and how AIDS is affecting them. But we may have to back some of that up with secondary data."

They might have to use data about intravenous drug users, but not specifically female users.

The women worked hard on their papers. At their first meeting with the Academy committee, Worth felt they were treated like graduate students. Their position was that since they were each experts in their fields, they could identify the issues for the Academy and discuss them. But it became clear during the meeting that the Academy did not want a discussion of the issues but rather an overview of what could be documented in a way that met its standards. Throughout that discussion and those at future meetings, it seemed to Worth that they were obsessively demanding documentation for every other sentence.

The women sent their papers in. No word came back for months. Then their papers were returned to them. The National Academy of Science decided that there was insufficient research on women to justify a whole chapter devoted to them. So it dispersed some of the material on women throughout the book, leaving its sole chapter on women a chapter on prostitutes.

Why? Because there was plenty of documentation—hard data, polished data—on prostitutes. There have been zillions of studies on prostitutes because that's where men in power wanted to look—where men's safety might possibly be threatened by virus-infestation of the women whose bodies they bought.

"So now they're using their bias—what they focused on, women as 'vectors of disease'—to say that we can't talk about the other women because there's no information on them," Worth noted bitterly.

Since there had never been enough research on women, then, of course, most writing on women was "speculative."

Worth had written on the vast majority of the women in the United States who, at that point in the epidemic, were dying of AIDS: intravenous drug users and the female partners of users. When Worth got her chapter back, she found they had cut out almost all of what she had written about the women. The final thick book, published in 1990, contained only three pages on these women—the majority of women dying of AIDS in the United States. Three pages! *All* her recommendations for aiding these women had been cut out.

The National Academy of Science had a lot of influence and the five women experts had hoped it would use that influence in taking a stand.

"They could say, 'We are missing this and we are missing that and this should be done,'" Ehrhardt explained.

But no. The National Academy of Science was content to represent women with a chapter on prostitutes and pages of tables with statistics, women as numbers buried in another chapter.

Outraged, the five women met and decided to speak out.

"I have to go to battle with the Academy about this," Worth said. "I just don't give a shit anymore about what happens to me." She laughed bitterly. "This is just unacceptable."

For Worth, the issue was that something was coming out that did not represent women. Once again, the information was skewed. Even though Judith Cohen's information on women in prostitution was excellent, the mere fact that the only chapter on women was one on prostitutes perpetuated the view of women as disease vectors no matter what was said in that chapter. The final book didn't even mention lesbians. In her junked chapter, Worth had had a whole section on lesbian IV drug users.

Ehrhardt, Worth, Cohen, Fullilove, and Chavkin wrote to the Academy protesting its failure to highlight the issues actually affecting women. There was nothing they could do about it, the Academy replied, after a long delay. Ehrhardt heard informally that their protest was being written off as "irrational," and an "overreaction."

When the book came out in late 1990, the women agreed, they would go public with their criticisms. They fired them off in a letter to the prestigious journal *Science*. Protesting the Academy's treatment of women in the book, the letter, published January 25, 1991, noted:

> Minimal space is allocated to the host of critical questions that have been raised for American women by the HIV epidemic. When we protested to NAS about this dearth of information on women, it said that hard data resulting from large-scale quantitative gender-specific research were unavailable and that the available data focusing on women and AIDS were "too soft" for inclusion in the report.
>
> We believe that the judgment of NAS not to use existing data because they are "too soft" is a grave error. First, such an approach suggests that we lack the tools to provide a careful analysis of preliminary data. This is not so. . . . Second, such an approach denies policymakers and planners a presentation of the existing material. Public health officials are often forced to make decisions on the basis of incomplete data, and this instance is no exception. The use of incomplete data for policy decisions is greatly facilitated by careful, exhaustive review. It is this careful, exhaustive review of the incomplete data the Academy might have provided on this complex issue. Because of the threat AIDS poses to the women and children of our society, errors of omission, such as those described here, are not simply matters of neglect: they are matters of life and death.[1]

In a reply to the women's protest letter, the Academy's AIDS research committee stated that it was the policy of the National

Research Council to refrain from publishing scientific materials when peer review "indicates that the materials do not provide adequate scientific evidence to support their conclusions." The committee shared the women's concern that much remains to done, it noted, adding, "Much of the needed research has not even begun . . . "

On a hot August day in Brooklyn, a group of women, mostly young, some African-American, some Latina, some white, some HIV-infected, some not, sat in the office of an AIDS education organization, Lifeforce, discussing whether governmental policy on AIDS was active or merely passive genocide.

"There was a small article in the *Times* yesterday reporting a comment by President Bush," said one HIV-positive white woman in her forties. "He said he felt real sorry for all those folks with AIDS but he didn't know that the way to get at the problem was to spend a lot of money. Now is that active or inactive genocide? I assume that rather than spend the money, they feel we are 100 percent expendable. In general, who does AIDS affect? Gay men. Drug users. Women of color, mostly. If you lose a few that come out of other communities—that's what it costs. In general, it would be wiping out whole classes of people that they don't want to mess with, especially if it costs money. In that sense, it's active genocide."

"We can talk about President Bush," a young black woman responded, "but let's bring it even closer to home—the state representatives who are right here in our little neighborhood and go back and forth to Albany. We went, as representatives of an AIDS coalition, to visit these guys. Their attitude was that this was a disease that affected people who weren't voters, so why bother? That they were dealing with a dispensable population that was sick and dying and wouldn't be around long enough to vote anyway. These are the people who are in power positions to determine what services we do and don't get, the monies we do and don't get and whether we live or die."

Genocide by neglect? No, she said. Active genocide.

Ada Setal takes eight-year-old Faith out of school at eleven-thirty and arrives with her at the Downstate Medical Center renal clinic at noon.

Immaculately groomed, Ada wears a blue polka-dot suit, white pearl necklace and earrings, her hair in a bun.

A hospital employee introduces Ada to a journalist writing about women and AIDS. Ada agrees to tell the journalist about the organization she cofounded, ACTUAL, and about her own experiences as a caregiver.

Faith colors in the waiting room. When she looks up to grin at and talk with the journalist ("Are you going to help me with my homework?"), dozens of colorful barrettes swing at the ends of her ringlets. Her eyes are bright, trusting.

Ada talks to the journalist and hours go by. Faith is not called. Faith gives the journalist sum after sum to do. "It's okay if you don't get this one because it's hard. What's twenty-seven and—" She thinks. "Three?"

Ada speaks of how difficult it is for caregivers having such long waits—three, four, five hours—to see a doctor. Some kids are restless and can't sit still. The caregivers are worn out. They're up all hours of the night when the kids need them. They start out tired. Then, after those hours waiting, they may have to get the children on a bus and get back home.

Ada tells the journalist how necessary it is to be patient; how life will either make you or break you; how, if you're not willing to be made, it will break you in many pieces. You *must* be patient.

It's four-thirty-five. Faith is finally called. Ada marches up to the reception window angrily telling the woman there that waits of this length are unacceptable. The journalist realizes that Ada had actually been lecturing herself on patience but had found herself unconvincing.

Now, a solid, imposing figure, Ada Setal walks with dignity down the corridor off which the examining rooms lie, declaring to no one in particular in a loud voice how outrageous this situation is. Heads turn. Faith skips ahead of her, then skips back to the waiting room, holds her hand out to the journalist and leads her down the corridor.

A doctor in a white coat comes to Ada in the corridor and, speaking deferentially, tries to mollify her. Fails. Her face is stone stern. She had stopped him hours earlier outside and told him of the unacceptable wait and he had brushed her off, too busy to talk. She reminds him of this now and he apologizes.

The resident, a young woman in medical training, calls Ada, who is still agitated, into the examining room. The journalist walks in, too, with Faith. The resident is annoyed. Who's this? she asks Ada. Ada, pulling the roll of paper down over the examining table to prepare for Faith's exam, tells her firmly: "Don't you worry about her. She's my friend and support person and she's going to be here." She allows no discussion of the point.

The resident studies Faith's chart a long time.

"Have you ever been here before?" she asks.

Ada, in exhaustion: "I come here nearly every week."

"Is she HIV-positive?"

"Yes." (Faith, in fact, has full-blown AIDS.)

How did the child get it, the resident wants to know. Ada tells her. Tells her she's Faith's grandmother.

The resident, still looking over the chart, notes that Faith has missed several of the weekly visits and strongly implies that Ada is negligent for not having brought Faith in.

Ada, exasperated at this resident she's never seen before, replies that it is not necessary for her to bring Faith every week when she is doing fine, that she, Ada, knows very well when something is amiss and will make an appointment when that happens.

The older doctor comes in, agreeing with Ada that there's no reason for her to come every week.

The resident continues looking over the chart. Faith plays clapping games with the journalist. She sing-songs children's rhymes, rhymes she's learned on the sidewalks or in the schoolyard. The journalist smiles, the palms of her hands held out as Faith rhythmically claps and slaps and chants, half-listening to the child as she tunes in to the encounter between Ada and the physicians. Suddenly her full attention snaps to the child when she hears:

"And I asked my mother," clap, slap, "to come out and play," clap, slap, "but she couldn't come," clap, slap, "'cause she was dead," clap, slap, and on and on, more claps and slaps, never missing a beat, and when she finishes, the journalist hugs her and asks, "Did you make that one up yourself, Faith?"

Faith grins and giggles and buries her face in the journalist's chest.

The doctor is still trying to mollify Ada: "I just want you to know we're on your team. We want quality care for Faith."

A lab worker comes in and asks the resident if she wants any lab work done on this patient as the lab will close in five minutes. In all the hours Ada and Faith spent in the waiting room, no urine or blood samples were taken for tests. They will have to return to the clinic the next day to have that done.

Ada suddenly remembers her van. It's in the parking lot and she's afraid the lot closes at five.

"Can you drive?" she asks the journalist, frantic. Panicked, she searches for the parking ticket and hands it over. The journalist runs out, Faith leading her, skipping, to the parking lot several blocks away. They get the van. Ada runs into the lot.

"I've got Faith's file!" she shouts, waving it in her hand. "They just left me there with the file."

The three stand in the parking lot laughing.

"Get in the van," Ada tells the journalist after asking her where she's staying. "I'm taking you to Fifteenth Street."

On the drive, Ada tells the journalist of something that's breaking her heart: her twenty-five-year-old son Anthony was caught in the Riker's Island riot August 15 and badly beaten. She tells the tale at length. Then silence.

"Mr. Rabbit—wasn't he great?" Ada suddenly asks the journalist, grinning. "He said, 'Oh, Brother Fox, please don't put me in that briar patch! Oh, do anything! Do anything with me but *please* don't put me in that briar patch! Oh, God, I don't want you to put me in that briar patch!' That's just where he wanted to be because he was home."

Ada laughs, her eyes gleaming.

"That fox got sucked in!" she laughs.

She plays the fox: "Oh, my God, he's afraid of the briar patch! Oh, that's just where I'm going to put him 'cause he's scared to death of the briar patch. I'll throw him right in the briar patch."

Now Ada is the little rabbit, shouting: "Oh, thank you, Mr. Fox! I'm home! I'm home!"

Faith, listening to the story in the back seat, squeals with laughter. Ada and the journalist laugh heartily as Ada's eyes gleam.

"So my life is: 'Throw me in the briar patch! Heap it on me! I'm home! Bring it from the west, from the south, from the north, from the east. Bring it and heap it on me! I'm home. I know where I'm at.'"

She speaks in a strong, powerful voice.

"I will survive. That's my story. I will survive. Mr. Rabbit says: 'Hey, I'm home! You gave me a favor! You brought me to be scratched up so I'm home!'"

Her laugh is high, screechy. Suddenly the laughter is gone, her voice quiet, deep: "So that's my life."

A condom manufacturer has donated a van to Dr. Joyce Wallace, the Greenwich Village physician who, early in the 1980s, had conducted small studies of HIV in prostitutes. The van serves as a mobile HIV testing site. From her office in Manhattan, Wallace is continuing these studies. Several evenings a week, one or two of Wallace's employees— Janice and Pam tonight—go out in the van with the driver, Joe, to sites in New York City where women work the streets. The employees offer each woman ten dollars to be tested for HIV and answer questions for the study and another twenty dollars when she comes to the office to pick up her test results.

This is a hot August night. They are taking a journalist out with them.

After crossing the Brooklyn Bridge, the van stops on a desolate street. A young black woman climbs into the van, and softly answers the questions. (Born in 1968. Yes, she always uses condoms with johns. No, she has no health insurance. Yes, she uses crack. She has a five-year-old child and another seven months old.) She's been on the streets two months, she says, and begins weeping.

"I want to go home," she says over and over. "I don't want to be on the streets."

They keep asking, "Why can't you go home?" She never answers, just repeats, "I want to go home. I don't want to be on the streets." After some minutes, she asks, "How do I find out about getting into a program?" They give her a pamphlet, "Getting Off Drugs," and a referral to a drug rehabilitation program. That program takes people with and without insurance, they tell her. Reaching for the equipment on a tiny table in front of her, Janice pricks the woman's finger and takes a blood sample. Test over, she gets out of the van.

Quiet. Everyone turns to the window. The young woman is sitting alone on the brownstone steps of an apartment house reading the pamphlet they had given her on AIDS prevention for "working girls," prostitutes.

Joe drives to another part of the city and parks near a group of women standing on the sidewalk. The workers test woman after woman. Joe turns off the motor during the long stays at each location and the air-conditioning goes off. It is hot. Pam and Janice are tired. They had already put in a day's work when they set out on this evening shift. Pam has a standard explanation to give the women on how the test works—one that compares the virus and the antibody to the army and the navy—but as the van gets hot and Pam more exhausted, the explanation gets increasingly confused.

A group of women are waiting outside the van to be tested. The ten dollars is the attraction. One woman looks dazed, glassy-eyed. She wears black leather shorts and an improvised halter—a black belt around her small breasts. Holding a compact mirror before her face, she puts eye makeup on and then lipstick. When she climbs into the van and sits on the back seat beside Janice, Pam smiles and remarks on her unusual use of the belt. The woman, Rehala, stiffens, taking offense.

"No, I was just admiring your creativity," Pam assures her, and Rehala relaxes her defense. She answers all Janice's questions. Yes, she always uses condoms with johns.

"Even sometimes the guys that don't want to wear condoms, at the end, they didn't even know they had the condom on. I had it on my tongue. I learned to—you know what I'm saying? 'Cause I actually got scared."

As Janice prepares to take a blood sample from her finger, Rehala mentions that they'd already done a test on her in May. She'd never come into the office to get the results.

Pam looks up those test results on sheafs of paper.

"You tested positive," she tells her.

Rehala begins sobbing. There is a sudden dead silence in the van surrounding her sobs.

"I'm scared."

Her right leg shakes.

The women awaiting their turn outside are looking in at Rehala sobbing through the van's large side window that is covered, but incompletely, by curtains.

Anguished words—"AIDS," "time bomb"—erupt from her lips. Pam and Janice rush to tell her urgently that she does *not* have AIDS. She just has the antibodies to the virus. It's not the same thing. She can't absorb what they're telling her. She half-rises, making a move to leave the van.

"Let me explain some things to you before you get out," Pam says firmly. "What did we just talk about? About not saying that you have AIDS. Now don't shut down on me," she says, looking at the woman's anguished face.

Rehala continues weeping.

"You must have come into contact with the virus but you can live for years and years . . . if you take your medication. Don't shut down now. This is not an end. It's the beginning of taking care of yourself."

There is laughter outside the van. Inside, dead solemnity.

"Nobody is telling you you have AIDS. What we're telling you is you are going to have to pay an exceptional amount of attention to yourself now. We're going to give you a lot of information. We're going to give you a letter that you're going to take to the clinic."

The doctor who runs this testing program is going to open up a drop-in center for women like herself so if she doesn't have a place to live, she'll be able to come there and get some social work help, medical care, she tells Rehala.

"So don't shut down on me because you got a lot of options," Pam says earnestly, sliding over the fact that that drop-in center, while planned for, does not at this moment exist.

"Are you using drugs right now?"

"Heroin."

"Are you going to get off heroin?"

Long silence.

"It's very important, you know, to keep yourself healthy," Pam says. "We're also going to give you our telephone number. So we can help you as much as possible. All you have to do is call us and we'll do what we can to get you in where you need to go. Understand? But you can't shut down on me. You have to talk to us."

But Rehala does not speak. There are only Pam's lulling, desperate words. Trying to comfort, she grabs any words that come to her.

Then silence. The sound of a car pulling up on the corner.

"This is the letter I was talking about," Pam says, handing Rehala an envelope. "You're going to be tested as to whether you need to take the medicine or not. . . . You're going to be alive and healthy for a long, long time. But it's all about taking care of Rehala now. You're going to do this, aren't you?"

Silence.

Then Pam's continuous low hum of details, telling Rehala where to go to try to get into a detox program, where the HIV clinic is. ". . . Monday through Friday, 7:30 A.M. On the second floor of the building. You're going to be there. Tomorrow. Aren't you? With your letter in hand."

Rehala sobs in anguish: "My brother just died from AIDS two months ago. My mother wouldn't even talk to him! She didn't even want to know him! She won't hug me no more. She won't touch me as it is now."

Sobbing.

"Sometimes I just want her to hug me, you know. I want her to hug me!"

More anguished words choked in sobs.

In the face of Rehala's grief, awesome as an erupting volcano, Pam now throws forth the words of a distanced professional like charms to protect her from the fiery lava: "How can you deal with her? What do you think you can do about that?" Rehala doesn't even bother to brush the words aside. They fall of their own weight.

Her sobs carry more choked words. How her mother will reject her when she learns she is HIV-infected. In a tiny, fragile, broken voice: "How can I tell her?"

"You don't need to tell her," Pam says firmly. "The only people you have to talk to about this are the people in the hospital who are going to help you."

Now, more pieces of her life, offered in anguished phrases: There is a lover, an older policeman. At his approaching retirement, they had planned to live in a small town in the South near his family that, to her amazement, had warmly welcomed her. Now that vision of her future has blown to bits.

"How do you expect him to live with a walking time bomb?" Rehala cries.

She's in the pain of drug withdrawal. She got out of jail just an hour ago and is only out here on the street because she's dope sick and needs a fix, she tells them.

It's hitting her in waves, what this news means. Now another wave thunders over her: "If I got it, he got it."

She sobs a long time. Then: "I can't believe I'm sitting here thinking I can tell him he gave it to me. He didn't! Oh, God!"

Trying to comfort, Pam tells her she can now start taking good care of herself and get into a drug treatment program.

Rehala, her voice cracked, completely real, tells them she is in an out-patient detox program. Three days ago, she tells them, when she was not soliciting, but was simply walking down the street, she was arrested for prostitution and kept, until an hour ago, in jail where she couldn't get her daily methadone dose.

"I was tired," Rehala tells them. "You know when you get tired? When I was in the street, I was tired. It was just the pain of detox that I go through. I can't stand—like, diarrhea, knots in my stomach, the way they detox me. I was going to NA [Narcotics Anonymous] meetings. I was doing so good. I stayed away from these people." She throws a contemptuous glance out the window at the pimps and prostitutes in the street outside.

"I was just coming out of a store and I went around the corner"—her voice rises in despair and her next words are cries—"and the cops just told me to get in the van! I said, 'I'm not doing anything!'"

Despair.

"I'm like out there [in jail] three days! You know what it is to keep on methadone?" She sobs. "Do you think they care? They put the handcuffs on me and just said, 'Yeah, yeah.'"

She tells the women that a john who said he had AIDS had raped nine women working that block. She was the seventh, she said.

"He put a gun to my head and said, 'Now you suffer.' It was in the papers. I got a bullet wound in my thigh. Believe me, it was no joke. He left one girl paralyzed."

Her policeman used to come to the hospital when she was recovering from the attack.

"He used to kiss my feet," she sobs, "and tell me, 'You're going to be all right,' and everything. You know?"

Pam is reasonable: "I think if you talk to him about this—"

"I can't. I don't see what in the hell he sees in me anyway! I always tell him that. I don't know—something—I don't understand."

Her voice is low, miserable.

Rehala tells the women, in words, some bitter, most anguished, a few inaudible, that she had been desperate to get off drugs and had finally gotten into a methadone program.

"A week later, I was walking on the street, they [the police] picked me up. They locked me up for welfare fraud. I never been on welfare in my life! I said, 'I needed a Medicaid card. I wanted to go on the methadone program so I don't have to go out on the street . . .

"So what I did—I was living out on the street—I tried to kill myself."

She doesn't tell how. But in the course of this arrest and attempted suicide, a local television news camera crew, hidden, filmed one of the cops roughing her up, dragging her. A reporter from that television station later interviewed her and broadcast the story. In the interview, Rehala said she wanted to get off drugs, she was tired, she needed help getting into a drug treatment program.

"I told twenty million people that I'm tired. You should have seen how many people called in. [Drug treatment] programs that people couldn't get in, that had waiting lists for a month, was ready to take me in. I started to feel good. I'd be walking down the street and people would say, 'You the girl that was on TV?'

"And those sons of bitches locked me up for welfare fraud and I've never been on welfare! I just disappeared. I could not believe how the system is so stupid here. I want help! I told them! I showed them my arms—shooting drugs. I JUST WANT A MEDICAID CARD SO I DON'T HAVE TO BE OUT ON THE STREET!! You know what I'm saying? Help me! And then they lock me up for welfare fraud. I couldn't believe it."

They talk for a long time.

Then Rehala pulls herself together and climbs out of the van, trying to act as if nothing had just happened.

Everyone in the van is hot, exhausted, left flat and breathless in the wake of the volcanic eruption.

Silence.

Pam, anguished, says she can't do this anymore, can't keep giving people their "positive" results.

"I go home and I think about it and then it bothers me. Maybe it bothers me more because I know my sister's down there on the street and I—I'm thinking that one day I'm going to have to deal with that."

"You know," Janice says, "it's getting worse. When we first started going out, nobody *ever* came out with positive results."

Sirens scream in the night around them.

"Now, isn't it every week?"

There is a book of daily meditations for people living with AIDS. Perry Tilleraas wrote it: *The Color of Light*. If Rehala had had a copy, she could have read the entry for November 30 that begins with a quote from the Upanishads: "That which is the finest essence—this whole world has that as its soul. That is Reality. That is Atman. That art thou."

"I am the soul of the world," the meditation begins. "I am that which is the finest essence."

Those are words we need to hear again and again, Tilleraas wrote, for knowing who and what we are restores us to sanity.

A few weeks later, in another part of New York City, five years after the last violent days of her own life on the street, Katrina Haslip was free. Paroled from Bedford Hills Correctional Facility September 10, she felt overwhelmed at the prospect of job-hunting. She'd never had a legitimate job before, never written a résumé. But she was exhilarated, too, at her freedom and sobriety. After five years in prison, she enjoyed every small thing: A walk in the park. A friendly conversation. In a tragic way, she thought, the HIV virus had saved her life. It had pushed her to live with awareness, rather than with drugs.

She moved into a residence in Brooklyn for women coming out of the court system. She walked in the door, met the other residents, and immediately asked if anyone were worried about living with her as an HIV-positive person.

"Can we talk about it now?" she asked them. "Because I don't want anyone to feel like I'm putting them at risk."

They talked and the women accepted her warmly.

She landed two part-time jobs. HIV outreach and educational work with women of color in Brooklyn for Lifeforce, an organization still in development. A baby ACE, Katrina thought affectionately. Recognizing ACE's maturity, by comparison, gave her a new pride in the prison organization.

The second job was to consult for the Brooklyn AIDS Task Force. In its eleven-week project at a family health clinic on Coney Island, she was to provide AIDS information to the community, dispel myths, help break the stigmatization of people with AIDS.

She worked with Ada Setal, an older woman she met at Lifeforce and came to admire. First the two women showed videos, set up a literature table at the clinic, and gave out free condoms. People would take the condoms but leave the literature. Ada suggested pulling people in with refreshments. So they set up food on the table, along with the pamphlets, and as people stood and ate, they could get into conversations with them about their worries over AIDS. Katrina found people—from children to the elderly—hungry for information. She felt she was doing badly needed work.

As she worked, she saw with elation that her skills actually were *her* skills. They were not, as she had feared, abilities that could only blossom inside prison walls.

In the midst of her elation, worry. An HIV-infected friend told her she had recently gone to a New York City hospital emergency room with PCP and high temperatures. She had waited almost nine hours for someone to attend to her and had finally left the emergency room, returning home untreated. Katrina was appalled. Was that what lay before her? The medical care system worried her more than her disease. She thought she could handle her own physical deterioration. But waiting long hours in an emergency room, deathly sick and ignored? No. That terrified her.

She had medical insurance at a third job she took on at an AIDS task force, but couldn't use it for any HIV-related conditions. She was afraid that not only would she be thrown off the medical plan for having an undisclosed "prior condition," but that everyone in the office would be thrown off as well. That is exactly what had happened to the task force earlier when an HIV-infected employee's claim had been invalidated. Katrina didn't want to be responsible for everyone's loss of medical insurance. She was on programs that gave her assistance in paying for such treatments as AZT. But she had to pay for all other medical care herself. Soon, the bills would begin to accumulate.

The primitive consciousness about AIDS that prevailed in the outside world shocked Haslip. In her prison community, she had gone through an agonizing internal struggle to become open about her HIV status. Speaking the truth about her life, unashamed, had been a triumph in her development, one that had strengthened her. Now, in the "real world," she felt pressured to regress. Those few family members who knew of her infection were urging her to keep her status hidden.

"I'm willing to support you," one brother had told her, "but you can't be blabbing about this to people."

Haslip didn't want to be guarded because it meant suppressing who she was. She didn't give a damn how the community responded to her. In fact, she welcomed their negative attitudes because that was the opening people gave her for breaking the HIV stigma. But she knew her openness could expose her family to abuse.

Then, astonished, she saw the abuse her Brooklyn community heaped on an HIV-infected child. Parents, wanting the child barred from his elementary school, were picketing that school. The school offered the parents an informational workshop on HIV run by the Department of Health. They refused it. They wanted the child out, period.

Katrina couldn't believe it: here on the outside, people were still dealing with unfounded fears about casual contact! It was unreal.

Inside the prison, ACE encouraged women to challenge it every time they heard others being stigmatized. Refusing to let cruelty go unchallenged was a deliberate part of building a community where people cared about the next human being. If, in an argument, someone yelled, "Oh, shut up, you old AIDS-ridden bitch!" other inmates would confront her: "Well, at least she knows what she has. Do you know what you have?" Or, "Does it make a difference? Then why did you say that?"

But on the outside, the cruelty went on unchecked. And it was— literally—too close to home: in Flatbush, down the street from Katrina. It made her feel vulnerable. It made her rethink the implications of her openness for her family. Their employment. Their ability to keep insurance coverage. Their positions in their own communities.

Yet she wanted to defy the stigmatization, even against those odds. This was *her* drama and she should be able to play it out the way she wanted to, she believed. She was ready to break barriers, as great women like Sonia Perez had before her when it had been even harder to do than it was now.

But Katrina tried to meet her family halfway. Sometimes—on the job, for instance—she was open. Sometimes, when she felt disclosure might harm her family, she hid her status. She hated how hiding felt.

One day, walking down Eighth Avenue at dusk, a stranger walked close to her and she felt frightened. She thought in astonishment that in her days as Lady T, she had been willing to come up against strange men day after day, exposing herself to abuse and violence. She had been drugged then and could do it. Now she was sober and it frightened her.

She was a different person. She sensed it. So did her old friends in Niagara Falls. She felt that she was now the person who, for many years, had been dying to come out.

On a crisp September day in yet another part of New York City, Washington Heights, Dr. Anke Ehrhardt turned the last page on the grant application she would submit to NIMH that week, well pleased. Finally, they would get some real data on women. The design of this study on how HIV infection affected women was excellent. She and Zena Stein had fought the battle two years earlier to admit women into the Center's natural history study, but they had not thought to include gynecological measures for the women. This study would fill in that essential gap.

It would enroll four hundred HIV-positive women from three inner-city hospital clinics in New York and a control group of one hundred women from the same neighborhoods but HIV-negative.

The project would generate one of the first systematic studies of HIV's impact on the mental and physical health of women along the HIV disease continuum. Data from the study would help in developing strategies specifically geared to women for medical care, HIV-prevention activities, and community outreach to infected women.

Most innovatively, the study would examine HIV's impact on gynecological conditions such as vaginal candidiasis and cervical dysplasia, and on the menstrual cycle. Physicians treating HIV-infected women had been commenting that the women's periods often stopped. But there had been no systematic study of the phenomenon. Such menstrual dysfunction could result from a variety of factors including viral infection of the reproductive organs or weight loss.

Menstrual dysfunction was very likely a marker of endocrine dysfunction. The endocrine system interacts with the immune system but no one knew its role in the deterioration of that system. Of the handful of studies done on the endocrine system in HIV disease, *none* had focused on women. When researchers examined the endocrine system in one study on thirty-seven men and three women, they just removed the women from the group and measured the men's testosterone! They completely ignored the women's endocrine system.[2]

There were now also no published data describing the psychological impact of HIV infection on inner-city women. To increase understanding of the context of HIV infection, Dr. Dooley Worth, the medical anthropologist, would oversee interviews with some women in the study. These would illuminate the context in which sex and drug use took place. Worth would analyze the interview transcripts, coding them for sexual and physical abuse, initiation into and pattern of drug use and sexual behavior. The women would also be asked about their relationships and experiences as mothers. From listening to women at length, the researchers would learn the obstacles to changing high-risk behavior among inner-city women.

Ehrhardt would send the proposal in. It would be reviewed by a panel of scientific peers and, if approved, given a priority score. At thrice-yearly meetings, the NIMH Council decides, given the budget, its cutoff priority score. If the cutoff point was 180 and a grant came in at 220, it would not be funded. If it came in with a priority score of 160, it would be.

This was an excellent study. Ehrhardt, who had earlier received the largest multimillion-dollar grant ever awarded by NIMH, had no doubt it would be approved and funded.

Charlotte and Steven Schafer, the couple who had met at Columbia University, moved back to Vermont where Steven had grown up. They bought land and built a house. As a result of AIDS, Steven was now paraplegic and wheelchair-bound. They had no money problems. The investment bank Steven had worked for had an excellent health and disability plan. Charlotte's parents supported her.

The first six months were hard for her, staying home, cooking and cleaning—chores she despised with all her heart. Steven had done both when he had been well in New York.

But after a while, it was okay. She was content to care for Steven. He was not going to live long and Charlotte loved him. He had had a screwy life. She was thankful that at the end of it, she was there to see that he was not made to work for every bit of attention and caring he got.

They were living with a heavy secret and it isolated them. No one around them knew Steven had AIDS. In rural Vermont, he felt, telling was too big a risk to take. He was afraid they were going to burn their house down. He was always saying that.

Charlotte found the secrecy lonely. And stifling. She had to keep paying attention to what she said.

"What is it that Steven has?" people would ask her.

"A neurological retroviral infection," she'd tell them. "That's all I know about it."

There might well be people around them who would be helpful and caring, she thought. If they had any brains, they already knew what was going on and were probably hurt by the secrecy. But as long as there was a chance that people would treat Steven cruelly, she could not risk the truth.

As she cared for Steven, the deeply buried awareness that she herself had HIV disease occasionally broke through to consciousness. And it worried her. The first gynecologists she had gone to, in both New York and Vermont, had known nothing about HIV in women.

Then, when she asked, Steven's doctor referred her to a gynecologist who knew something. This man had several other HIV-positive patients and knew much more than the previous physicians had. But most of his knowledge was about HIV's repercussions in childbearing.

Charlotte did not ask him one question about childbearing. He volunteered the information: that she could have children; that the chances of bearing an HIV-infected baby were such and such; that the pregnancy and delivery could be managed without difficulty.

Sitting there, Charlotte felt irritated. What did babies have to do with *her,* Charlotte Schafer? Here was this man behind a desk assuming that, faced with a dying husband and a fatal illness in herself, the only thing she could possibly be thinking of was having babies! How presumptuous! Babies were the last thing on her mind. She would have none. When she was intent on finding out what this disease might do to *her,* it was jarring, disorienting, to have all the answers come back with a baby in them.

Yet the same scenario played out each time she went to a gynecologist.

Charlotte was now confronting the lack of information on HIV in women that feminist activists like Maxine Wolfe and Linda Meredith had been railing about for the past several years and that feminist medical care providers like Pat Kelly and Carola Marte, on their own time, had been trying to help remedy. Caring for Steven, Charlotte saw that physicians knew a great deal about the illness in him and very little about it in her. Though physicians could tell Steven what might happen to him and what signs he should look out for so a preventive treatment could be started promptly, they could not tell her how the disease progressed in women.

Her gynecologist assured her the disease followed essentially the same course in both men and women. Though certainly women were as susceptible as men to such AIDS-related conditions as PCP, Charlotte thought, quite rightly, that her gynecologist's answer was bullshit. As long as researchers didn't *do* the studies on women, didn't actually *do* pelvic exams on women and see what was happening, they couldn't possible know.

Now, when Charlotte Schafer needed information to keep herself alive and well, there was this vacuum of knowledge into which gynecologists tossed irrelevant statistics about theoretical babies.

Charlotte worried whether, when she fell ill, appropriate medical care would be available to her. In the midst of her worry, she wondered bitterly whether worry and upset impair a woman's immune system. In fact, the HIV Center's proposed study on HIV and women that Anke Ehrhardt was just sending off to NIMH would assess the "effects of hopefulness, hardiness, sense of personal control, and other factors which may contribute to health or the progression of illness."

One way Charlotte dealt with Steven's illness was knowing as much as she could about it. Knowing things was a way of gaining control. Not a great way, she thought, but at least *some* way. It was frustrating, oppressive, not to have that coping mechanism for dealing with her own disease.

One day Charlotte read an article in *People* magazine on the Pediatric AIDS Foundation, an organization cofounded by Elizabeth Glaser, wife of the television actor Paul Michael Glaser. Glaser's children were infected with HIV, and Elizabeth was, too. Elizabeth was as affected by the disease as her children, Charlotte thought, but the article's whole focus was on the children.

As she had seen in her encounters with gynecologists, children preempted women in importance, even when the children did not and never would exist. When children did exist, women were not even in the running for attention and concern.

Charlotte found it hard to protest the focus on children as the truly "innocent victims." No one was suggesting the children should not be cared about and for, she thought, but if you said, "Care about women, too," well, there was always the feeling that that didn't matter as much. According to the media, Charlotte felt, there was a battle for dollars, attention, and energy among those with AIDS, and if women dared to lay claim to any resources for themselves, they were selfishly denying them to the children.

It was tough being one of the "guilty victims." The issue of blame was always an undercurrent in encounters with physicians. Of all the doctors they had dealt with, only one had treated AIDS as a disease, nothing more. All the others made judgmental comments.

The harsh judgments drifted into them both like polluted air; they needed constant vigilance to keep them out. Stephen felt some guilt about his past and discomfort over his bisexuality. As he lay dying, he struggled with issues that got to the core of his self-respect and identity. Harsh judgments from outside made his struggle harder and made it difficult for him to do what Charlotte wanted him to do: be peaceful and live knowing that he was loved and cared for.

In the background, playing softly, her own illness. Death did not terrify Charlotte. What did was the fact that she would be alone, that there would be nobody there to care for her the way she was caring for Steven.

⋯ ⋯ ⋯

They weren't going to fund the study of women, the fastest growing subgroup of people with AIDS in the United States. NIMH had turned down the HIV Center's grant. Anke Ehrhardt couldn't believe it. Dr. Patricia Warne, a colleague who had also worked on preparing the proposal, was stunned. Before submitting the proposal, they had sent it around to critical scientists, including study design and statistical experts, who had judged it superb.

The study would have provided a wealth of data quickly. They had the perfect setup for the study at Harlem and Presbyterian hospitals. Such an opportunity lost!

When Ehrhardt and Warne got the "pink sheet," the reviewers' critical comments on the study, their astonishment turned to outrage. The women's study proposal was given a priority score nowhere close to funding level. It was an incredible insult.

Reviewers had not even *read* the proposal on the women's study carefully. The study was not a longitudinal study as the reviewers indicated on the pink sheet, but a cross-sectional one. It was to run for three years, not five.

The HIV Center's argument that women had been neglected in AIDS research, clinical care, and prevention strategies was convincing, the reviewers acknowledged. But they were not persuaded that HIV had a different impact on men and women in a number of the areas (like parenting) to be studied, or that the "relatively expensive" study would add new information.

Was this for real? The reviewers were actually maintaining that men and women have similar mental, social, and sexual experiences!

If women and men had similar parenting experiences, that would mean, then, that bearing children and rearing them was roughly the same experience for men and women, including for the many men who did not even live in the same building, or city, their children did. If women and men had similar sexual experiences, then, experientially speaking, to be raped is roughly equivalent to raping.

The lack of social support networks and community and medical services will be related to demoralization, depression, and anxiety in both men and women, the reviewers wrote. (It was true, Warne noted, that social support is important for both men and women, but often the men *have* it and the women don't!)

The reviewers questioned whether the proposed study of women would provide any new information when there already were women involved in the HIV Center's Follow-up Project.[3]

Good point. Except, of course, Warne noted, that the follow-up study had seventy-five women in it, not four hundred; that the women in the follow-up study were all drug users and those in the women's study were both drug users and partners of drug users; and that no gynecological exams were performed in the follow-up study and no information gathered on what was going on in the women's pelvic organs while the proposed study included pelvic exams and at last would have provided information on how HIV affected gynecological health.

Physicians treating HIV-infected women had indeed been seeing effects and speaking of them when they could get away from their clinics to conferences. Grass-roots female health professionals—Carola Marte, Pat Kelly, Mardge Cohen, and Rachel Fruchter—had done ground-breaking work on one of those effects: the connection between cervical dysplasia and HIV infection. With the proposed women's study, that work would have been followed up. Researchers would have described the prevalence, type, and severity and the history of gynecological complications including not only cervical dysplasia, but HPV infection, other STDs, and menstrual irregularity associated with different stages of disease.

But there was no need to do another study. That would be a waste of good money. They already had seventy-five gynecologically unexamined women. That was plenty.

One of the conceptual and design flaws in the study, the NIMH reviewers observed, was that the researchers appeared to place too much faith in what poor women of color said happened to them. The women could be prone to "selective retrospective recall."[4]

They further noted that "since counseling is not a popular treatment method in poorly educated minority groups," counseling might not be an appropriate way to handle women who had just learned their HIV status.

Yet there was no evidence that counseling was ineffective in "poorly educated minority groups," Ehrhardt and Warne knew.

They found the reviewers assessment of inner-city minority women shocking: ". . . the proposal includes the study of the effect of HIV on gynecological health, with the assumption that gynecological abnormalities will be of concern to these women and if so, should be identified. Much of the study is directed toward collecting information related to gynecologic disease and HIV infection, along with gathering information on sexual desire, arousal, and satisfaction. Although this information may be useful, its relevance to this sample is not obvious. Inner-city women who are trying to care for children and manage the other risks in their lives may not care about the topic."

It was stunning. When they got their fury over the racist and misogynistic comments in the pink sheet under control, Drs. Ehrhardt and Warne composed a restrained response: "It is unwarranted to assume that women of color do not care about their health; are not bothered by STDs, gynecological cancers, or vaginal infections; and do not seek sexual satisfaction."

Marie Tulman, the HIV-positive grandmother, hated it when her AZT treatment induced neuropathy. A tingling, a numbness, then painful muscle spasms would start in her feet and move up through her whole body. When that happened, she could not walk. Couldn't lie down, either. It was too painful in that position. Once she'd had to stand the whole night, ironing, ironing, and looking for more to iron.

The doctor never told her, "You are no longer just HIV-positive. You're now into AIDS." But she knew it. There were certain things you just don't get until you moved right along into AIDS, she thought. She was getting them.

Since joining Lifeforce and training with other women to be AIDS educators in Brooklyn, she had learned a great deal about the disease. Her growing knowledge increased her irritation at her young doctor. Sometimes she got so mad at him, she gave herself a headache. She would describe her symptoms and he would lean back in his chair and tell her her T-cell count was too high for her to have such symptoms. He left his assumption unstated: what a woman experiencing the disease had to say about it was not valid; only what doctors wrote about it was.

One day, she exploded at him: "I know no one has bothered to even study the virus in women or what happens to women with these drugs like AZT. You don't know! You're telling me that this can't happen to me because it didn't happen to white men! Take your book and stick it up your ass!"

Another day he responded to her account of her symptoms: "That's not HIV-related." She shot back: "Let me tell you one damn thing: Dead is dead. I don't give a damn what it's coming from at this point."

Terry McGovern, the poverty lawyer, had told Maxine Wolfe of ACT UP she would sue Health and Human Services (HHS) over denial of disability benefits to women with HIV. Wolfe wanted ACT UP's Women Action Committee to mount a concurrent demonstration in front of HHS in Washington, D.C. So they quickly arranged that McGovern would file suit October 1 and ACT UP would demonstrate the following day. The activists invited HIV-positive women to join the demo. It would be the first women's speak-out on their problems as PWAs.

McGovern's lawsuit contended that HHS maintained a discriminatory definition of disability that kept women from getting benefits by not considering manifestations of disabling HIV-infection common to women.

It sought a regulation providing presumptive disability benefits to all claimants with proof of HIV and medical evidence that the claimant was disabled or unable to work and the creation of an appropriately inclusive listing of disabling HIV-related impairments.

In front of the massive building housing HHS on Independence Avenue October 2, two hundred demonstrators picketed in a circle, holding tombstone-shaped signs, each proclaiming a different symptom of AIDS found in women. "Women with AIDS," the signs read, "Dead, But Not Disabled." Katrina Haslip, Marie Tulman, Terry McGovern, Maxine Wolfe were among those chanting, "Land of the free, home of the brave, is putting women in the grave," and "How many women have to die before you say they qualify?"

As had become a common tactic, every ten minutes a horn sounded marking another AIDS death and the demonstrators fell to the ground. After each such "die-in," an HIV-positive woman stepped into the center of the circle and described her symptoms and Social Security's rejection of her claim for disability benefits.

Phyllis Sharpe, a thirty-nine-year-old mother of six and a plaintiff in the suit against HHS, stepped into the center. She was speaking, not to the crowd, but to the imposing building behind it, a mammoth structure surrounded on three sides by a concrete plaza in which a U.S. flag waved. She felt great talking back to this building that was obliging her to live with hunger.

She had applied for disability benefits in April 1989, she said, and was later told her application was lost. She reapplied in January 1990 and was awaiting a decision. She had hated to give up her job—it was such a good one. But with her shortness of breath, pain, fatigue, and persistent vaginal yeast and urinary tract infections, she could no longer perform the heavy physical labor of laying train tracks for the Transit Authority in New York City. She had never suffered these recurring ailments before her HIV infection, she said.

Without the disability benefits, she said, it was hard to eat balanced meals. She ran out of money at the end of almost every month. She would eat whatever was left in the house. If it was just rice, rice. If it was a can of green beans, she would eat that. But many times, she said, she went without. If there was any food, she gave it to her three youngest children.

Marie Tulman could not stand and speak in the center of the circle. She had taken the long bus ride to Washington although her neuropathy was acting up. Walking around with the other demonstrators, she suddenly stopped. She could not move. Her legs felt blocked. It was the neuropathy. Some demonstrators, both women and men, saw what was happening, lifted Marie up and carried her to a corner. She had forgotten to bring the potassium tablets she needed. Someone ran quickly to buy bananas for her.

Sitting in the corner while one demonstrator massaged her pained legs, she thought of what she so urgently wanted to talk about: what dying women go through trying to get benefits.

Tulman herself was in limbo. From May until that October, she had not heard a damn thing from SSI except that she needed a new set of records because her application was now more than six months old.

Katrina Haslip stepped into the circle's center. Two months earlier, she had been in prison. This was the first demonstration she had ever participated in or even attended.

Now, in public and before reporters, she declared she was HIV-

infected. Men did not have to stand up in public and detail their bodily ailments in order to fight for disability benefits, she said in anger.
She said she was worried about what help she would be entitled to
from HHS should her disease progress, should there be symptoms like
abnormal pap smears.

The only way women were meeting the government AIDS definition was on autopsy, she said.

"Women don't *get* AIDS," she told them, repeating an activist
slogan. "We just *die* from it."

Terry McGovern had been to many AIDS demonstrations but
this one felt different. This one wasn't about federal dollars for drug
testing as some of those organized by gay men had been. This was
about gravely ill women having a place to lie down, a roof to shelter
them, in the last months of their lives. Here were women trying to
prove to the government that they were dying.

This was the first time she had seen women do a public speak-
out. She was happy to see the women's words hitting the air. Watching
Katrina Haslip, she felt inspired. Katrina was so alive, such a fighter.

HIV-positive women around the country, reading in newspapers of
the suit against HHS, began telephoning Terry McGovern: "I've been
having this gynecological stuff for six years," they'd tell her. "My doctor doesn't believe me. Nobody believes me." The lawsuit, McGovern
saw, was legitimizing the experiences that women had been reporting
for years.

In November, Risa Denenberg, the nurse practitioner who had
gone over the medical records of McGovern's HIV-infected clients in
preparation for the suit, set up a gynecological service within the HIV
clinic at Bronx Lebanon Hospital where she had recently begun work.
Physicians assume women with pelvic inflammatory disease have been
having intercourse but Denenberg was seeing HIV-positive women
with severe PID who told her they were not sexually active. She
believed them. Giving up sexual activity was a common response of
both women and men to news of their infection. So the infections she
was seeing had to be reactivations of old infections. In other words,
they were opportunistic infections.

She knew this was an important and basically unreported finding. She was able to recognize this phenomenon because of a scientific advantage she had over many male providers: she believed what women told her.

There was a dramatic switch in 1989 to a greater percentage of HIV transmission through heterosexual intercourse and to a greater percentage of infected women. This switch was reported in a number of places.

"When I first came on board in 1987," Evelyn Figarowa of the Woodfield Family Services in Bridgeport, Connecticut, said, "we didn't have one woman in the [HIV buddy] program. It was interesting to see our first woman [in 1989]. And then it was like, all of a sudden, all the new referrals that we got were all women. It seemed for a while there that most of the referrals came from women."

From July 1990 to June 30, 1991, there were fifty-eight PWAs in the buddy program—thirty-nine men and nineteen women. The program had no women at all in 1988; in such a short time to suddenly have a three-to-two ratio of men to women Figarowa found extraordinary.

In the Brown University AIDS program, where an estimated 95 percent of all the HIV-infected women with AIDS in Rhode Island were seen, before June 1989 almost all the HIV transmission—81 percent—was attributed to sharing of needles by IV drug users.

"Around June of 1989," Dr. Charles Carpenter of that program reported, "we began seeing a lot more heterosexual transmission. During the next nine months, the ratio of heterosexual transmission to IV drug use transmission was roughly fifty-fifty. During the nine-month period starting in March 1, 1990, the bulk of the transmission has been by the heterosexual route: roughly two-thirds. That's been a very striking change in the recent past. It's been statewide. Throughout this period, the ethnic backgrounds of the patients have remained roughly the same: 15 percent black, 15 percent Hispanic, and 70 percent Caucasian."

So, in a short period of time, the dominant mode of transmission in women in Rhode Island switched from IV drug use to heterosexual transmission.

In the women infected through sexual contact, the median number of sexual partners the women had had throughout their lives was small, Carpenter reported. Only three. Though a standard AIDS prevention message to women is "Reduce risk by lowering the number of sexual partners," some American women are learning what had long been the case for African women: with even one or two lifetime partners, you can get AIDS.

In New Jersey, Dr. Patricia Kloster, chief of the only women's HIV clinic in New Jersey, reported that in the mid-1980s, the HIV-infected women she saw at University Hospital in Newark were about 80 percent IV drug users. The remaining 20 percent of patients had been infected through heterosexual intercourse or by unknown means. But by 1989, 48 percent of the women had been infected through sex.

Dr. Carmen Zorilla, who has been working with HIV patients in Puerto Rico since 1986, reported that in 1987, 28 percent of the women with AIDS acquired it through sexual contact. By 1990, this had increased to 43 percent.

"We can observe a clear pattern of increasing prominence of cases attributed to sexual transmission," she said. "Without sophisticated mathematical analysis, we can predict that within the next two years, heterosexual transmission will be the principal cause of AIDS in women in Puerto Rico. Most of our patients—82 percent—acquired the infection through the sexual route."

Dr. Janet Mitchell, chief of perinatology at Harlem Hospital Center in New York, and colleagues looked at former IV drug users at a methadone program in New York City, a third of whose clients were women. These seven hundred women had a higher rate of HIV infection—61 percent—than the men in the clinic—on the order of 56 percent. This, she pointed out, was probably because the women were doubly exposed to HIV—through shared needles and sexual contact.

"So you don't know how they got it," she said. "You don't know which came first—the chicken or the egg. . . "[5]

The CDC's method of classifying the way in which a person became infected with HIV could be hiding even more cases of heterosexual transmission in women. The transmission categories are set up hierarchically. That means that the first risk behavior a person admits to is the one her case is classified in. So a woman who admits to IV drug use and has HIV would be counted as having acquired the disease through dirty needles. But most often that woman is also sexually active and may actually have been infected through sexual intercourse.

Women with AIDS are twice as likely as men with AIDS to be reported without an established risk factor, Dr. Ruth Berkelman, chief of the CDC's surveillance branch, reported. (According to Dr. Judith Cohen, director of the Association for Women's AIDS Research and Education [AWARE] in San Francisco, this is partly because some women die so soon after they are diagnosed that there is no time to schedule an interview with them to determine what their risk factor may have been.)

Many of these cases in which the risk factor had not been pinpointed may actually be due to heterosexual transmission, the CDC's Berkelman noted. She reported that between 1988 and 1989, there was a 33 percent increase in AIDS cases attributed to heterosexual transmission in the United States.

"AIDS cases attributed to heterosexual transmission are rising among both men and women, but more cases are occurring among women than men," she stated.[6]

The dramatic change in the AIDS epidemic was also happening in the predominantly white, middle-class suburbs of Long Island, New York. In fact, Long Island has more people with AIDS than any other American suburban region. A full 28 percent of the clients served by the Long Island Association for AIDS Care (LIAAC) are women.

In the next few years, many women living in suburbs who feel perfectly safe, who have no idea they are at risk, will get AIDS, LIAAC director Gail Barouh predicted. By 1994, she calculated, 42 to 45 percent of LIAAC's cases would be women.

Because the AIDS message had focused on categories of *people* at risk rather than on *behaviors,* women who did not belong to those categories—*they* were monogamous and nondrug-addicted—felt unjustifiably safe. But maybe their husband, identifying himself as a heterosexual, sometimes had sex with men.

Jeri Woodhouse, assistant to Manhattan Borough president Ruth Messinger on special projects including AIDS, worried about this.

People working with street youths in the city talked with her about the men who drive in from the suburbs, pay the street youth—boys and girls—for sex, and then drive home to the suburbs where their wives have no idea that their husbands have a secret sex life.

It's hard for women who've been married for a long time to know how to discuss this openly with their husbands, Woodhouse said. Suburban women tell her, "If I want to bring up that issue, he assumes I'm accusing him of cheating on me so I can't speak to him about it." Or, "I married him thirty years ago. How do I now say, 'Let's use condoms?' when we've not used them all these years?" Or the women fear their husbands will get angry and turn it around on them: "If you're thinking of this, you must be fooling around."

Among white, single women on Long Island, Gail Barouh now saw blanket denial that there was any problem, a chanting of charms that made them feel safe: "He doesn't look gay." "He hasn't gone out with a lot of different people; he was in steady relationships." "He looks safe so we don't need condoms." "He's into bodybuilding so he wouldn't be using drugs." "We used condoms at the beginning but we've been going out six months now so we don't do that anymore."

In the support groups LIAAC ran were women whose sisters had died of AIDS. Yet they themselves were sleeping with men without condom protection.

Thus a number of experts believe the current scale of the problem among married women in the suburbs may be somewhat underestimated to the extent that HIV infection in women is not being identified or counted.

"These [HIV-infected] women are going to their gynecologists," Figarowa of Woodfield Family Services in Connecticut says. "They're getting frequent infections, and it's attributed to anything else [other than HIV]. The doctor would never ask—and the wife would never have any idea. Unless they're tested or their husband comes down with the illness."

She could as well have been speaking of Patricia Daugherty in rural Maine.

In Brooklyn, Marie-Lucie Brutus of WARN believed the false sense of safety middle-class white women felt about AIDS was due not only to the CDC's use of risk groups rather than risk behaviors but to the politics of knowledge. Poor women of color will be the ones mostly counted in official statistics on AIDS, she said, because they go to the places where counting is done: hospital clinics and social agencies.

"But the ones who do not go to the places where you can count—you don't know about them."

It was true that women in poor communities were being hard hit by the AIDS epidemic, she emphasized.

"Food, shelter, clothes to cover us in winter—those are primary needs and these women don't have it! Let alone education. If they don't have it, of course they are going to be the group that will be most likely to be infected with a virus that is transmitted sexually. Because the drugs are already there. The alcohol is already there. The misfunction of the families is already there. All the social ills that are a breeding ground for any problem are already there."

But because white middle-class women tend not to go to agencies where the counting is done, we don't know where the disease may be spreading, undetected, Brutus pointed out.

"That's why I keep telling people not to be complacent," Brutus said.

Within the next three to five years, Barouh predicted, AIDS would be as much a woman's problem as a man's problem. At least on Long Island. What was happening on Long Island would happen in other areas, she feared. In many ways, Long Island was a suburban trend-setter.

Barouh could sum up Long Island's response to the AIDS crisis in two words: denial and apathy. Politicians were quiet about AIDS. County executives did not speak on it publicly or consider it in their long-range planning. Long Island had done little to deal with its current AIDS problem or to prepare for the more massive AIDS epidemic that was coming.

Barouh was worried because many of the prevention strategies for women had not worked. Obviously. She and her colleagues at LIAAC thought training HIV-infected women to educate women in the community on AIDS prevention would be effective. But that was difficult because the HIV-infected women felt they needed to hide to protect themselves. Like Katrina Haslip, they had to consider the consequences of their openness to their families. Would their children be thrown out of school and the whole family out of their housing? Would they lose their jobs? It was a big risk.

Early in the year, when a woman who lived in Huntington, Long Island, revealed that she worked for an AIDS organization, a swastika was painted on her fence, Woodhouse reported.

"The women who are infected in the suburbs tend to believe that they are isolated cases, alone and stigmatized, so they are not going to tell anybody around them about it."

The women most directly affected by AIDS in the suburbs weren't talking.

When the numbers of women infected got real bad, then something would be done, she felt. But government agencies were keeping the numbers low through a narrow definition of AIDS. Those artificial numbers were going to explode. Soon more and more people would know people with AIDS. It would be harder to keep the problem under wraps. Then maybe something would be done. When it was a colossal disaster.

Just three months after her release from Bedford Hills maximum security prison, Katrina Haslip sat with a small group of activists from ACT UP, including Maxine Wolfe, around a table in a conference room at CDC headquarters in Atlanta, Georgia. Continuing ACT UP's strategy of confronting the federal officials handling the epidemic, they were there to convince CDC officials to include in the AIDS surveillance definition the symptoms unique to women.

When CDC arrived at its earlier definitions of AIDS, it had been content to gather together the clinicians treating white gay men and, later, children with AIDS, and ask them what they were seeing in their patients. Those conditions went into the definition. But now, when it came to defining the conditions women were experiencing, suddenly they needed studies, hard scientific proof. Suddenly it was impossible to simply gather together the clinicians who were treating women with AIDS—like Mardge Cohen, Janet Mitchell at Harlem Hospital, Carola Marte—and ask them what they were seeing.

Sitting down at the conference table with the government officials, the activists laid out their reasons for changing the CDC's surveillance definition of AIDS to include the symptoms unique to women.

One of the most important was to alert doctors, especially gynecologists, to the possibility that symptoms commonly found in American women could, in some cases, in fact be early warnings suggesting the presence of HIV/AIDS. If CDC alerted physicians, they could pay attention to PID and HPV that didn't improve with treatment as it normally would. By the time doctors recognize AIDS in a woman, she has PCP and is ready to die. But women were coming in with signs of AIDS long before then—signs physicians did not recognize because CDC had not alerted them.

Since many clinicians don't read medical journals, they look to the CDC for information on AIDS. If every doctor in the country received a letter from CDC stating, "We're changing the CDC definition and these are the conditions appearing in women with AIDS," physicians would see that letter. Every major newspaper in the country would carry the news.

As Patricia Daugherty in Maine and Evelyn Figarowa in Connecticut had learned, physicians were less likely to ask white women—particularly white, middle-class women—questions that might lead to an AIDS diagnosis.

There are other ways to achieve the goals of alerting physicians to possible HIV infection besides changing the surveillance definition, the CDC officials argued. Moreover, women who are HIV-negative also get some of the symptoms seen in women who are HIV-positive. Conditions such as PID, vaginal candidiasis, and certain cervical dysplasia were common among American women, they asserted. Women with these common conditions might be frightened that they were HIV-infected when they were not.

(Maxine Wolfe's translation of this argument was: "We don't want to scare nice women.") CDC already included in its definitions caveats to distinguish a common condition from that condition appearing in someone who is immunosuppressed, activists pointed out. Why did CDC only have a failure of imagination—an inability to create similar caveats—when it came to women?[7]

One ACT UP activist told the CDC officials that when she read "HIV asymptomatic," she knew that meant *most* HIV-infected women because "symptomatic" means a symptom on the CDC's deficient list.

Furthermore, it was vital to acknowledge conditions appearing exclusively in women in order to begin developing preventive measures and treatments for them. When PCP was recognized as an AIDS infection, clinicians began devising treatments for it, they noted. Then PCP stopped killing people to the extent that it had before.

During the meeting, CDC officials presented their arguments for not expanding the surveillance definition. To their minds, revising the definition would make it more difficult, though not impossible, to track the AIDS epidemic. The definition was useful as an epidemiological tool for tracking the epidemic because it captured the most severe manifestations of HIV infection. Officials were trying to estimate two things:

1. The number of people severely affected
2. Where the epidemic was going. Was it going up in the heterosexual population? Was it plateauing in homosexual men?

When the CDC changed the definition in 1987, they pointed out, it did a better job of capturing women, IV drug users, and people of color, but it decreased the CDC's ability to track the trends and do projections.

Dr. Gary Noble, CDC Deputy Director (HIV), presented another reason for not changing the definition:

". . . We would be laughed out of the country for inflating the epidemic and the curve and simply trying to bring more money into AIDS research," he said.

That flabbergasted the activists. If women's ills were a source of amusement, that was hardly new, they pointed out later in the meeting after they had had time to recover. The medical system had a history of abusing women and had never treated women's bodies with respect. What women experience is constantly trivialized. This was a point the women's health movement made and endlessly documented.[8]

There was, moreover, no danger that, with additional conditions listed in the definition, physicians would rush to diagnose ordinary cases of PID as AIDS, the activists argued.[9]

"Most doctors dismiss almost every complaint women have," one added. "They just do. 'You're fatigued. Every woman gets that.' We're still living in 'hysteriaville' in terms of the image of women by most doctors. So I don't think that by putting any of that stuff in, you are suddenly getting a rash of cases that are not AIDS."

Instead, she said, she thought they would be giving health workers caring for HIV-positive women some indicators of AIDS before the point at which the women got sepsis and died the next day. Again, CDC alluded to a problem of including "less severe diseases," i.e., vaginal candidiasis, in the definition.

"Everybody goes back to that because in a way, you think it lets you off the hook and you don't have to talk about the other things," one activist noted. "I can't tell you how many women I know in New York City who have hysterectomies because they are HIV-positive and they had PID and they don't know what the cause of it is. They say it's not gonorrhea. It's not chlamydia. They say, 'Could it be tuberculosis? What is it?' But eventually, snip, snip. Okay, now the woman has a hysterectomy. Now what's going on? They are not alerting people earlier on to think that this PID maybe has to be treated differently, instead of going, "Oh, she's HIV-positive." And if I read another chart that says, 'HIV-positive, asymptomatic, refractory PID,' and know the client is in the hospital, there is something wrong. And that problem comes from here. If that woman is in the hospital, HIV-positive, with an IV in her arm, and they are talking about, 'Well, what should we do?'—well, how come nobody thought earlier? We're not coming up with treatments. We're not coming up with prophylaxis."

This was exactly what Charlotte Schafer, in Vermont, feared. Her doctors would know so little of HIV's progression in women, they would not give her the treatment that could spare her unnecessary suffering and prolong her life.

The officials at the meeting finally mounted the high horse of Science and reiterated a common argument: that no one has *proven* a causal relationship between HIV and cervical dysplasias; that there is insufficient data; that the CDC feels a need to be correct.

"Why only for women do you need total causal proof?" one activist asked.

To the assertion of one CDC official that this was "not all a men/women issue," that the conditions in drug users were also not so well represented in the definition, one weary activist replied: "I do know that women have a specific set of organs that do not appear anywhere in that case definition and that somehow every time that gets raised, issues of scientific validity come up, issues of needing more evidence come up, issues of not fucking with the definition come up. 'We'll do anything. We'll give them more care. We'll give them this. We'll give them that,' but it's the one thing that's untouchable."

To look at illnesses such as vaginal candidiasis that were not cap-tured by the AIDS case definition, the CDC had set up a Spectrum of Disease study, Dr. Ruth Berkelman, chief of surveillance, told the activists.

The activists were well aware of the study. Once again, like most of the others, it was studying white men. From a source inside CDC, they knew that only 7 percent of the four thousand people enrolled to date (280), were women, a fact the CDC acknowledged when con-fronted with it.

ACT UP dismissed the statistical problems involved in changing the AIDS definition. It was vital that AIDS be correctly diagnosed and caught in women. It was not so vital that the CDC's future projec-tions be exactly correct, they argued. If, years down the line, they found that their projections were not accurate, they could simply state that fact.

The activists argued that women couldn't afford to wait for years while the CDC conducted studies to absolutely *prove* a causal relation-ship between the conditions appearing in women and HIV infection.

"Nobody waited for years to do those studies for gay men," Wolfe said. "Nobody did it for children. They sat down people who worked with children and they said, 'What's going on?' They didn't review the literature. If you sat down doctors who see lots of HIV-positive women, they will tell you what those women are getting and you can change the definition. . . . Right now, it needs to be included. Nobody else had to wait. This is very, very typical. White men do not have to wait to be included. Everyone else needs proof beyond a shadow of a doubt."

The problem even extended to the clinical trials NIAID con-ducted—the ACTGs, they continued. NIAID did not require that a gynecologist be on the staff at the forty-seven sites where ACTG stud-ies were based. In every woman who was ever in a clinical trial, researchers had been looking for male markers.

"And that goes back to the CDC definition," one activist pressed on. "Lots of drug trials say 'CDC-defined AIDS.' . . . When they set up a research team, it means that they will not put a gynecologist on."

So they could be giving a woman a drug that was making her gynecological problems worse and they wouldn't know it because nowhere was there anything published that suggested they ought to monitor what was going on in women's organs.

Gary Noble questioned the logic of putting HPV in the AIDS definition if it did not significantly alter the person's life expectancy.

"Well, Kaposi's sarcoma is in there!" the activists shot back. "Come on!"

"Well, we've been thinking we should take KS out . . . ," Berkelman noted.

Several times during the meeting, Haslip was on the verge of tears, overwhelmed by the officials' attitude. One of those moments came when a CDC physician asked how vaginal candidiasis could be life-threatening. Haslip had seen a progression in her friends from vaginal candidiasis to vaginal warts to abnormal pap smears to cervical cancer and on into death and she feared that she was somewhere along that progression herself. She was suffering from recurrent, persistent candidiasis. Her gynecologist wanted to biopsy what appeared to be developing vaginal warts. How many more women had to fully go through the whole progression before the medical and public health establishment started to do something about it? No one was listening, she told the CDC people in frustration.

"I don't understand why you don't get it," Katrina said.

"Can someone tell me why you care about oral candidiasis [thrush] in men, and vaginal candidiasis is not important?" another activist asked.

Gary Noble responded with a question: "It is more severe in HIV-infected men, right?"

"Oral thrush?" an activist replied. "Well, you haven't studied vaginal thrush in HIV-positive women, so I don't know how you can make that statement."[10]

The activists laid it out: when CDC told them they couldn't change the surveillance definition until data came in from studies proving a causal relationship between the symptoms in women and HIV; when CDC then told them it had only managed to enroll 7 percent women in its Spectrum of Disease study; when their CDC source told them, and the officials acknowledged, CDC couldn't enroll more women until it received additional funds; then what CDC was saying was that nothing would change. That was unacceptable, the activists said.

The definition had been changed in 1985 and 1987 and they were open to changing it again, CDC said. They didn't know when. It depended on the evidence.

One ACT UP activist, herself a health professional, said she had participated in the design of the Spectrum of Disease study in Atlanta. "We were told that we should not try to capture data on vaginal candidiasis because too many women get it."

"Who told you that?" Berkelman asked.

"People working on the ad hoc committee to design that data base. And when I asked, 'Could you pull that data up?' about two months ago, I was told they could not, that it was not collected and entered, that they would have to go through the questions by hand to look under 'Other infections,' that it might appear under [that] in the Atlanta data."

Berkelman would have to look into that, she said.

This meeting between CDC and ACT UP illustrates the crazy-making politics of knowledge operating to exclude women:

- What we have is an AIDS definition that excludes the symptoms appearing exclusively in women.
- This definition cannot be changed to include women's symptoms until (adhering to a High Scientific Standard created exclusively for women) data exist *proving* a causal relationship between these symptoms and HIV infection.
- Studies cannot provide the data demonstrating that causal relationship because:

    a. Women have been largely excluded from the studies. (This fact has been partially obscured by swelling the woman count through the inclusion of female infants and children.)

    b. On the few women who do manage to be enrolled in studies, no pelvic exams are done because male medicine has thrown women's pelvic organs out of medicine. So HIV-related conditions appearing in those organs are not seen or noted.

    c. The study sites are not located in areas where the highest proportion of HIV-infected women live so it becomes difficult to enroll women in the studies.

As if in a Funhouse of Scientific Knowledge, mirrors reflect grotesque images off each other: CDC, in its AIDS definition, reflects back the NIAID studies that omitted women; NIAID reflects back images from the medical system that tossed women's pelvic organs out; Health and Human Services (HHS) reflects back the CDC definition of AIDS in an image of dying, but not disabled, women.

Small-town gynecologists in Vermont and Maine and big-city internists in New York provide care for women based on a knowledge as distorted as reflections in funhouse mirrors. No wonder the women receiving that care sometimes feel they're crazy. Patricia Daugherty's pain in her pelvis shows in the mirror as a pain in her head, reflecting Medicine's view that she has pelvic pain in her head because she doesn't like being a woman. Reflecting back at empty-armed Charlotte Schafer is an image of herself holding a baby, what any woman, fatally ill or not, *must* be wanting. Women who get angry and challenge funhouse knowledge, like Dooley Worth and Judith Cohen, look in the mirror and see their anger reflecting back as "irrationality." Marie Tulman, Katrina Haslip, Terry McGovern's clients, including Phyllis Sharpe, stand side by side, look straight into an entire mirrored wall, and see reflected back at them nothing. Nothing at all. What they feel, what they experience—none of it is reflected in the funhouse mirror.

Six days after the meeting between CDC officials and ACT UP activists, CDC representatives visited AWARE, the project in San Francisco that had been following women with HIV since 1983, one of the first in the country to do so. They questioned AWARE investigators, including Dr. Judith Cohen, for three hours and left.

On November 28, the CDC telephoned and informed Cohen and the rest of the AWARE staff that their study on women was no longer a priority with CDC and it was cutting off its modest funding as of December 1.

That meant funds to cover the fieldwork, including the salary of the nurse practitioner, would disappear in two days. CDC left only enough funding for the analysis of existing data.

It was very unusual for an ongoing project that was producing valuable data to be cut off in the middle, Cohen knew. Why was CDC doing this?

She'd been given only one answer: their study on women was no longer a priority.

···

The day the AWARE project lost its funding in San Francisco, 350 ACT UP activists from around the country were on their way to Atlanta to prepare for a demonstration at CDC headquarters December 3. Their earlier demonstrations at NIH and HHS had challenged the barring of women from clinical trials and the denial of disability benefits to women with HIV/AIDS. This one would challenge the CDC's AIDS definition, the basis for the denial of those benefits. Combined, the demonstrations threatened to break some mirrors in the Funhouse of Scientific Knowledge.

The activists had already mailed letters to the thousand-odd CDC employees informing them of the upcoming demonstration and explaining their reasons for it, a major one being that the CDC's artificially low disease surveillance statistics, based on an incomplete definition of AIDS, resulted in inadequate funding for AIDS research, education, treatment, and prevention. Since ACT UP's dealings with CDC (detailed in the letter) had not resulted in a change in the definition, they were coming to demonstrate. The target of the demonstration was CDC policymakers, not employees, the letter emphasized. Employees could show their support by joining them or by calling ACT UP Atlanta to find out how they could help.

The day of the demonstration, torrential storms poured more rain on Atlanta than Maxine Wolfe had seen in her whole life. Some clad in slickers, others holding umbrellas over their heads, the activists marched in the rain for five hours—from their hotel to CDC headquarters. Medical professionals who were ACT UP members or sympathizers marched with them, ready to assist if any of the many HIV-infected among them fell ill.

Jane Auerbach, a tall white recovering drug addict who herself escaped the virus, was there because many of her friends had not.

"All my running partners—the ones I did drugs with—they're all positive," she told a journalist. "It could have happened to me. A lot of my friends have died. It's close to home and scary."

By "acting up" in ACT UP, she saw herself as defying what she considered the government's unstated policy: to keep inner-city people on drugs, on methadone, so they can't raise their voices in protest.

To Auerbach, the demonstration was exhilarating. They were in the rain, many of them sick, but all fighting together.

At CDC, several activists chained themselves to the building.

While most activists demonstrated outside in the rain, fifty stormed the building. They occupied the office of Dr. Gary Noble, one of the officials activists had met with two weeks earlier. Several chained themselves to his desk.

Once in the office, three teams, each composed of three members, took their positions. The first team went to the fax machine and began sending out a letter it had prepared in advance, typed on CDC stationery, to the media and various organizations, informing them of the demonstration and reasons for it.

The second team, composed of computer whizzes, was to figure out how to get into the government computer system. But they didn't need to. As soon as they were seated at the computers, a female CDC employee asked one of them, "Do you know how to get into the code?"

"No."

"Well, let me do it for you."

ACT UP had found people inside who were with them.

The phone team telephoned the media. They were occupying Dr. Gary Noble's office, they'd say, and explained why. They wanted CDC to document the full scope of the AIDS epidemic by expanding their definition of AIDS; change their surveillance reports so information is collected and published according to the routes of transmission (what someone might *do* to contract HIV), rather than continuing to use the misleading "risk group" label; abandon their policy of advising HIV-infected women to delay pregnancy, establish one of giving women accurate information on which to base their own decisions about pregnancy, and so forth.

The police arrived and began the first of their ninety-odd arrests. At one point, while the police were absent from the office, escorting activists into a van, two of those left erased the message on Dr. Noble's telephone answering machine and recorded another: "Hello. You have reached Gary Noble's office. Unfortunately, Dr. Noble is not here. However, ACT UP *is*. This is why we are here." They gave their rap.

Outside, the police were dressed in yellow slickers and—apparently because PWAs were among the demonstrators—surgical gloves, white and superfluous. Raindrops clustered on the clear plastic visors of their helmets.[11]

As the arrests went on, Terry McGovern, the poverty lawyer from New York who was suing Health and Human Services (HHS), was among the rain-drenched demonstrators. She, too, was outraged at the gross undercounting of people with AIDS.

It's almost, she said, like an invented game board has been placed on this epidemic: If you are in the box, you have AIDS. If you are outside the box, you don't. When you are in the box, you get benefits and are able to care for yourself and live longer. If you are outside the box, you have to spend the last few years of your life trekking around to hearings and fighting to convince government workers that you are actually dying.

It is always women who are outside the box.

After the meeting with Dr. Anthony Fauci, director of NIAID, the Women's Action Committee of ACT UP assembled a list of sixty candidates for speakers and for the steering committee of the National Conference on Women and HIV Infection. They gave the list of peer educators, physicians, nurses, PWAs, and researchers to NIAID.

The whole point of the conference, as ACT UP saw it, was to assemble the medical care providers actually treating infected women—the people who knew what the clinical manifestations of HIV in women were—and the women themselves, ask them what they were seeing and experiencing, and let them talk to one another so that they could work on solutions and so that patterns among HIV-infected women could be identified. This conference would do for women what had been done for men early in the epidemic.

Activist Linda Meredith was appointed to the steering committee. For two days in September, the committee hammered out a conference agenda. But within weeks, NIAID redefined the agenda and included speakers at its own discretion, Meredith asserted in a letter to Fauci. In a telephone conversation with Caitlan Ryan, the NIAID employee charged with coordinating the conference, Meredith was told that someone like attorney Terry McGovern could not be invited to speak on legal issues because she was suing the federal government. Speakers were primarily selected based on their seniority within the community, ethnic background, and "reluctance to 'Fed bash,'" Meredith wrote Fauci.

As the official agenda began to be formulated, ACT UP found, it was clear that the majority of plenary speakers were not going to be women working in the epidemic but instead government employees putting out their line.[12]

Meredith resigned from the steering committee November 5 when ACT UP concluded that it did not want its name connected to what it saw as a manipulation.

DECEMBER 1990

Thirteen days before Christmas 1990, women poured into Washington, D.C., from around the country for the National Conference on Women and HIV Infection that would open the next morning in the Sheraton Washington Hotel. Activists, many in jeans, T-shirts, and sneakers, arrived in buses and would sleep in spare rooms and on living room floors of D.C. hosts. Some carried sleeping bags, posters, banners. Women with AIDS from states including Florida, Georgia, New York, and California arrived. Professionals—physicians, researchers, social workers—flew in, wearing suits and carrying briefcases. They checked into the hotel.

Many of the women buzzed with exhilaration (*finally* some attention was being paid to women in the HIV epidemic) and anger that this attention was coming so late.

Mardge Cohen arrived from Chicago, and Carola Marte from New York, both annoyed that after their study pointed to the increased rate of cervical dysplasia in HIV-infected women, CDC was still recommending nothing more than yearly cervical checkups for the women.

Judith Cohen and Connie Wofsy flew in from San Francisco, having just learned that CDC was abruptly cutting the funding for their study on women.

Anke Ehrhardt, Zena Stein, and Pat Warne put in their day's work at the HIV Center in Manhattan and then headed for the airport, smarting from the recent news that their grant for a woman's study had been turned down with an insultingly low priority score.

Vickie Mays flew to the capital from Los Angeles, frustrated that still there was no study for women comparable in scope to the MACS study on men. The funds just weren't there for the women.[1]

From New York came Kathy Anastos; Risa Denenberg, the nurse practitioner who had pored over the medical records of Terry McGovern's clients, helping the poverty lawyer file suit against HHS on the women's behalf; Maxine Wolfe, veteran of many ACT UP demonstrations, and fresh from meetings with CDC and, earlier, NIAID officials; Denise Ribble, the nurse/activist who had confronted Robert Gould on his misleading *Cosmopolitan* article; T.J. Rivera, in a purple brimmed hat, now paroled from Bedford Hills and working on HIV education; Katrina Haslip, eager to confront after the frustrating meeting at the CDC in Atlanta.

Linda Meredith, the southern lesbian activist who had resigned from the conference steering committee, lived in D.C. If the feds turned this conference into a dog-and-pony show, trotting out federal officials to lecture on HIV infection in women when they hadn't troubled to study it, she wasn't going to sit still for it.

Women acutely aware of all the obstacles to drug treatment for women were there: Gloria Weissman from NIDA; Hortensia Amaro from Boston; Dooley Worth from New York.

Marie-Lucie Brutus, with her stillness and dignity, arrived from the bustling WARN office in Brooklyn.

Sally Zierler, frustrated by her inability to get a study published in a medical journal showing a relationship between childhood sexual abuse and subsequent HIV infection in women, had come to Washington from Providence, Rhode Island.

Leslie Wolfe, who, in the Center for Women Policy Studies (CWPS) in D.C., had been working on legislation mandating research on and services to HIV-infected women, was setting up the CWPS table in the exhibition area. She was there to get support for the women and AIDS bill that the Center had written and that Representative Constance Morella (Maryland) had introduced. She piled petitions supporting that bill on the table. Later, in the hotel lobby, she met with a small group of women, several of whom, including Anke Ehrhardt and Vickie Mays, were plenary speakers. At Wolfe's suggestion, the women all readily agreed to urge support for the legislation as they spoke in the conference plenaries and workshops over the next two days.

After the meeting, in the nearly deserted exhibition area, the women saw Caitlan Ryan, the NIAID employee facilitating the conference, who seemed exhausted and worried. She said that after ACT UP's pull-out from the conference steering committee, she was worried that the activists would demonstrate. She had beefed up security for the conference and had been asking various conference participants to respond to any demonstration with calls to let the speakers speak, she told the women. The speakers didn't see why there was any problem with women demonstrating. Why try to control it?

As women drift noisily into the enormous twelve-hundred-seat ballroom Thursday morning, Katrina Haslip, red ribbons tied around her African-style dreadlocks, hands out ACT UP information sheets headed "What NIAID Won't Tell You About Women in Clinical Trials."

Speakers on the first panel are two government officials—Dr. Jim Curran, director of the CDC's Division of HIV/AIDS, and Dr. Ruth Berkelman, chief of CDC's surveillance branch, and one maverick epidemiologist the steering committee had managed to get on: fifty-two-year-old Dr. Judith Cohen, director of AWARE in San Francisco.

As the buzz of hundreds of people conversing in groups of twos and threes in the aisles trails off and people settle in their seats, Dr. Jim Curran, director of the CDC's Division of HIV/AIDS, moves from his seat at the speakers' table on stage to the podium. He is in trouble the moment he stands before the hostile audience.

There were too few ob/gyns involved in the HIV epidemic, he is saying at the podium when a woman's voice rings out from the audience, interrupting him: "You won't change the definition!"

Unnerved, Curran continues: "We need to have a better understanding of the impact of HIV infection on gynecologic conditions, including those that have long been underestimated in our society and misunderstood as public health problems, like PID, cervical dysplasia, and cancer—"

A shout erupts from below him: "Put them in the definition already!"

Eyes glued to his text, Curran continues: "—and contraceptive efficacy and safety in HIV-infected people."

Katrina Haslip, holding a sign reading CURRAN, DO YOUR JOB, rises from her seat along with about thirty-five other ACT UP women. Clapping rhythmically, they move to the front of the hall.

"Anyone who thinks the CDC is not doing its job, join us!" one shouts to the audience angrily.

"We want action!" they chant. "Change the definition!"

Muscles throughout the cavernous ballroom tense with the chanting; some stand up in the aisles to see better; alertness sharpens since what is going to happen at the plenary is no longer predictable; the government has its agenda for the conference, but here is a group that has another.

The women fan out, standing beneath the stage from which Jim Curran continues to lecture. They face the audience. Long, thin strands of red crepe paper snake among them to represent the red tape women are tied up in. Some hold signs: CDC ASSASSINS, CUNNILINGUS COUNTS, WOMEN DIE FASTER! CHANGE THE DEFINITION!

"If you have questions for him about the definition of AIDS the CDC has, ask him!" an activist urges the audience.

Several women shout that they want to hear Curran.

"What does he have to say that we don't already know?" the activist, enraged, shouts, the strain on her vocal chords audible, causing a tensing of neck muscles in the audience. "Ask him about the definition! Stand up! Make him accountable!"

Many women in the audience rise from their seats and walk forward to join the ACT UP demonstration.

Curran plows on reading his prepared text, though, in the heat of angry chants and shouts below him, it sounds jarringly artificial.

"The second research question: Are current therapies for HIV that have been studied primarily in men adequate for women? What are the special problems that women face in the family? Often women face these problems alone when they are infected with HIV. Yet we describe them merely as vectors to their children and perhaps as unwed mothers."

"*We* don't!" a woman shouts from the back of the auditorium, a thousand people away from Curran. "*You* do!"

The decision on whether or not a woman should have a baby is that woman's choice and not the choice of policymakers, Curran maintains, ignoring the demonstrators' challenges. Much more information is needed about contraception and gynecologic needs, he adds. As Curran clings desperately to his text, angry women interrupt him, shouting, challenging, confronting. One woman holds up a sign just beneath him: THIS MAN IS LYING.

Trying to ignore the pandemonium, he maintains that they all had common challenges of dealing with social stigmas based on gender, race and ethnicity, sexual orientation, and HIV and AIDS.

"Based on your risk groups!" a woman from the audience screams, as applause and shouts welcome her assertion that CDC has helped create that stigma.

Curran still clutches his prepared speech: ". . . We must focus for two days on women—"

"We've been working ten years on women!" booms a voice from deep in the enormous hall. "Where have *you* been?!"

Sitting in the turbulent audience, Anke Ehrhardt notices that bodyguards or security men have quietly walked up on stage, their eyes alertly scanning the hostile audience below them.

The eyes of many other women in the front of the ballroom are focused not on the stage but on the balcony above and to its right. A man, apparently on the security force, is quietly walking around taking photographs of the demonstrators below him and the women shouting at Curran. As others in the audience notice clusters of women looking above, they, too, turn their heads, see the photographer, and whisper among each other. One woman stands on her seat and stares at the photographer, focusing the attention of a yet greater portion of the audience on the lone man on the balcony. A young woman with a camera comes forward and begins taking photographs of the photographer. Standing in the right-hand aisle, a conference organizer, seeing the growing attention to, and anger at, surveillance of the protesters, speaks hurriedly into a walkie-talkie. Within minutes, the photographer disappears.

Curran's opening address has turned into a call-and-response between him and his listeners—women infected with HIV or working with those who were.

"So I hope to be able to continue to join with you in the next two days—"

Response: "You never *started* to join with us!"

"—and in the end remember that stigma and the futility and suffering of AIDS knows no gender, no sexual orientation—"

Response: "How come you haven't studied cunnilingus then?"

"—no race/ethnicity. It knows no social class."

He lurches to a halt, and sits at the speakers' table on stage, as the activists chant: "Change the definition! Change the definition!"

"Dr. Curran, I don't think you're done yet!" a woman shouts. She wanted to know, she says, why CDC, in the face of evidence of a relationship between HIV and cervical cancer, has not put cervical cancer in the case definition. She knows HIV-infected women who have died of cervical cancer.

"I want to know why you don't put PID in the definition when women who are HIV-positive are getting hysterectomies instead of treatment. I want to know why you don't put vaginal thrush as a part of the definition when you include oral thrush."

Her voice weakens as the microphone she is speaking into is shut off from a central control.

"Turn the mikes on!" women shout, and then chant for a full minute, "Answer the question!"

The AIDS surveillance definition includes diseases that define the end-stage of HIV infection and carry with it a substantially poorer prognosis, Curran at last replies.

"Doesn't cervical cancer carry a substantial prognosis of death?" she counters.

"And that are clearly shown to be *caused by* HIV infection," he adds.

"Herpes?!" she shouts, referring to a condition found in men and already in the case definition. Was he going to claim that *that* had been clearly shown to be *caused by* HIV? "Come on! Get over it!"

Katrina Haslip walks to a mike (now turned back on) in the aisle, waiting to question Curran. She is angry. It feels good to be interfering with the presentations of government officials who were making decisions about her and other PWAs without their input.

A woman shouts to Curran that she may die of her cervical infection, which she believes is related to her HIV infection.

Curran asserts that the papers given the CDC by ACT UP on cervical cancer were studies that had been supported by CDC.

He was crediting CDC for studies it had never supported, Carola Marte thinks, from her seat in the ballroom. He is wrong on all counts. Since that study had come out under her name as one of the clinicians reporting, she wants to clarify that her group's research was *not* funded by the CDC, that they did not know of any funding by CDC for dysplasia. She joins the line at the mike.

Cervical cancer was not in the surveillance definition, Curran was explaining, because there was inadequate scientific data to show that it was *caused* by HIV.

"Because you don't *do* the research!" one woman interrupts in frustration. "Because the data doesn't exist, you're going to let women die!"

"We are committed at CDC to undertaking more studies—" he tells the belligerent women.

"How many more women have to die!"

Katrina Haslip's electronically lifted voice rises over the shouts as she stands at the mike: "You know women are dying of cervical cancer, PID, and all these other illnesses—that they're reflections of HIV infection in women. Why doesn't the CDC concentrate on more studies looking at the natural history of HIV infection in women? And why haven't they taken more of a leadership role in—"

The throb of a rhythmic clapping drowns the rest of her question.

"I agree with that," Dr. Curran tells Katrina Haslip. "I think that a very high priority is additional studies of HIV infection in women, particularly related to gynecologic disorders and problems and cervical cancer. So I think you're absolutely right. I think CDC and NIH both see this as a very high priority. We're going to fund more studies."

How hollow those remarks are to all the women in the room whose studies on women have been underfunded or turned down and cut off from funding altogether.

Signaling an end to Curran's presentation, moderator Eunice Diaz of the University of California School of Medicine in Cerritos, a member of the National AIDS Commission, turns to the demonstrators: "I would like personally to thank all of you who have come forward in an expression of anger and frustration, putting your reputations on the line."

The audience applauds the activists as they return to their seats.

Dr. Ruth Berkelman of the CDC comes to the podium. An internist and pediatrician who has worked at public hospitals and community-based health centers and has taken care of many HIV-infected women, Berkelman provides basic statistics on the epidemic in women. She notes that CDC has recently implemented a Spectrum of Disease project to describe all illnesses and conditions for which HIV-infected persons are seen and to describe their level of immune function.

A furious Linda Meredith soon challenges Berkelman, calling from a mike, "How *dare* you report the Spectrum of Disease Study's data about women!"

Meredith points out that, as so often before, women have been largely left out of that study—only 7 percent of its participants are women. It can hardly be cited as evidence that the CDC is now paying attention to women.

As she speaks, two activists unfurl a large banner from the balcony above her. The banner crowns the speakers' heads: CHANGE THE DEFINITION!

The third speaker, epidemiologist Judith Cohen, is soon a favorite with the audience as she delivers a speech frequently interrupted by applause, whooping, and laughter.

"My experience—I didn't get this gray hair for nothing—" she says, peering over her glasses, "is that those who direct the research, programs, and the policy often don't know what's happening in the real world."

The women cheer her.

Cohen speaks pointedly of ways in which the number of HIV-infected women could be underreported and undercounted in the epidemic, including through the hierarchical classification system; how, following the 1987 change in CDC's case definition of AIDS, cases of AIDS in women suddenly increased by 38.5 percent.

If you ask biased questions or you look in only some places, you get biased information, Cohen tells the women. She refers to a recent article on testing for drug use in women who came in for prenatal care and delivered in Florida. There was no difference in the proportion of illicit drug use among women in different racial or income groups.

"But the number of cases of illicit drug use reported to authorities at birth was ten times higher for blacks and for poor women than for others," Cohen says.

A woman, her voice hoarse from the morning's shouting, yells from the back of the mammoth ballroom: "We love you!"

A surprised Cohen lifts her eyes from her text on the podium: "Thank you. I love you, too."

Applause and whoops celebrate the exchange.

After addressing issues as an epidemiologist—the scapegoating of women in prostitution in the AIDS epidemic; the need, as yet unmet in many studies, for clinical assessments that include women's body parts and signs and symptoms; the need for larger, more representative cohort data, and for pooled and cooperative efforts—she adds:

"Speaking as a woman, I think it's time to get down and get real. We need to work on these tasks now. We need to assess and plan and develop—even on the incomplete information [on women] that's already available and not use it as an excuse to do nothing."

Holding up the National Academy of Science book on AIDS, she tells the tale of how the chapter on women got cut out. The audience boos.

She had begun by quoting comedienne Lily Tomlin: "Reality is the major source of stress, for those who are in touch with it." She goes on: "Let's remember that our reality is that there's a long history of not much research on women. You want a prevention example? Some of you know about the Mr. Fit trial. A huge heart disease prevention trial—on men. You want a clinical trial? How about the study of aspirin as prevention for heart disease? . . . It looked at male M.D.s because they were, quote, 'easy to follow.' How about all the nurses? They were in the same offices. The one I love the most—the close-to-twenty-year study of 'normal aging.' In men. Who gets old in this culture? Not us, if we keep on the way we're going."

Amid laughter and applause as a defiant Cohen returns to her seat on stage, a woman shouts, "I hope you took some notes, Curran!"

According to the federal officials' conference schedule, questioning of the three speakers and the discussion period is to begin now, though the women jump-started the discussion within minutes of the conference opening. Now a woman asks CDC official Berkelman why women were not being counted as PWAs. She herself had been HIV-positive since 1984, had had cervical problems in those years, including cervical cancer, but never had PCP—a condition that many men with AIDS had and that CDC classified as AIDS-defining.

Many women get cervical cancer, Berkelman replies. Women shout angrily at her reply.

"Yes, they do, but my [cervical problems] continue," the woman insists. "I keep having paps and they keep coming back positive, more cone biopsies and tests. I've been through pure hell with the medical system trying to take care of the problem. They *do* take care of it but it comes right back. It does not go away. I've had the cone biopsy. I've had the colposcopy. I've had all of these things done. It continues to come back. I know as an HIV-infected woman that when you have these cervical problems, they keep recurring. I've had no other symptoms, other than that I've been HIV-positive since 1984 and have been diagnosed with cervical cancer."

"I'm an HIV-positive woman," one twenty-eight-year-old white woman from Boston says, standing at the microphone in the aisle. "I have persistent vaginal thrush. I've been hospitalized for PID. And I've been denied Social Security twice. There was a comment made to me, 'What good would it do women to know that they had AIDS?' What good it would do me is that—I know I'm sick. I know there's no cure. I know I'm dying." Her voice rises and vibrates with emotion: "Allow me the dignity to not die in poverty!" Thunderous applause breaks out around the young woman, through which she demands: "Allow all my sisters in this room that dignity, too!"

While the Public Health Service officials had tightly controlled the program, arranging it so that federal officials would talk at women, the women have turned the formal program into a speak-out on their reality.

It was a kind of coming-out experience, Cohen thought, not just for the women with HIV but for women like herself—epidemiologists, physicians, researchers—who were saying things they were, as professionals, definitely discouraged from saying.

Many professionals seemed to have reached the point Dooley Worth had when the National Academy of Science cut the chapter on women out of its AIDS book: an "I-just-don't-give-a-shit-anymore-what-happens-to-me; this-is-unacceptable" point.

"It was scary," Cohen later told a journalist of her speaking out, "but it hurt a lot less than keeping my mouth shut all those years."

From the back of the room, a woman asks Cohen to tell the history of the funding of the San Francisco study on women.

"Very briefly," she says as the women laugh in response, "I'm sorry to say that right now, we are in negotiations with the Centers for Disease Control because two weeks ago, in the third year of a five-year cooperative agreement, they decided that what we were doing, and following in women in high-risk communities—looking at risk behavior and syphilis and HIV infection—was no longer a priority and they have terminated our field operations."

The women, enraged, chant, "SHAME! SHAME! SHAME!"

"I'd like to make a quick clarification on funding," says a small, slender woman at the mike. "I'm Carola Marte of New York City. I'm one of the clinicians who took part in the recent *MMWR* publication of the CDC on cervical dysplasia. I'd just like to clarify that that study was *not* funded by CDC. It was done by what we considered a group of grass-roots professional women who were concerned, because we were working in the clinics, about the amount of cervical dysplasia we were seeing."

Contradicting the CDC's recommendation of yearly paps, she adds that her center and all others dealing with HIV-infected women are recommending full pelvic exams with pap smears every *six months* because they are concerned about the data published so far.

A white woman from Kansas City, Missouri, stands at the mike and announces that she is HIV-infected and works in health care. "I had to call the CDC myself and the Health Department in our area to report myself as an HIV-infected person because no one was interested in reporting me," she says. "That's why the numbers [of women] are underreported, I'm sure. I would love to be a part of any epidemiological studies. I would love to be followed to see what kind of health problems women have. But no one is interested in following me."

A large, imposing African-American woman stands at the mike and tells the audience she believes physicians had withheld her HIV diagnosis from her when she was hospitalized with osteomyelitis in 1987: "And in 1990, because my surgeon was worried about himself getting infected when he had to perform my hysterectomy because of repeated bouts of PID and really bad cervical cancer, he . . . told me, 'I think I got all the cancer, but you tested positive for the AIDS virus and from AIDS, you die.'

"Then he came back the next day and his only advice to me was: 'In six weeks, when you heal from your hysterectomy, should you decide to have sex, make sure your partner wears a condom.' I assure you, just having my insides ripped out, sex was the furthest thing from my mind."

Her voice rises in power, till it sends chills down the collective back of the audience: "I decided that my mission in life is to put a face on AIDS. I will not distort my voice! I will not cover my face! And I refuse to live in the shadows! I'll stand on any corner anywhere, telling people: 'My name is Wendi Alexis Modesti and I have AIDS!'

"I know that my job is to go out to my sisters and to my community and to explain and educate so that what happened to me won't happen to them."

In the break, hundreds move slowly through the halls in the crush of bodies. In long lines at the coffee tables, women speak in anger, disgust. A male reporter from the *Boston Globe* interviews Carola Marte in the hall. Stunned by the morning's events, he tells her he'd been covering AIDS for years, yet had been completely unprepared for the high level of anger that had obviously built up in women.

Back in the ballroom, as the late-morning panel gets under way, Dr. Anke Ehrhardt continues the women's speak-out. Addressing prevention, she points out:

"To tell women to use condoms reflects a lack of knowledge about anatomy, gender role, and power differences between men and women. I thought this morning: We really cannot win. In terms of [AIDS] case definition, we get treated like men without penises. And in terms of prevention and condom use, we get treated like women with penises."

The women laugh.

Lesbians, she notes, were excluded from HIV research, clinical care, and prevention efforts.

"Our rationale is that transmission from woman to woman is

rare." She pauses, then adds dryly: "Since we are doing no research on this issue, we will hardly find out how rare it really is."

Again, the audience laughs and applauds.

Over the previous two years, she says, she and Zena Stein had tried, with passion, frustration, and little success, to raise consciousness on the need for an HIV prevention method women can control—a chemical barrier that, in cream or jelly form, blocks viral infection—and to stimulate research on such methods.

"So far, we have learned from scientists that the development of such a virucide is certainly imaginable. And think for a moment of all the technical advances we have in this country. We go to the moon. We go to Venus. But we do not have the priority to develop such a method."

Existing spermicides needed to be tested for their virucidal qualities. Tests had been conducted on only one—nonoxynol-9—and when found unsuitable as an HIV prevention, research on virucides was abandoned.

"We gave up *one* spermicide because *one* study showed it had a couple of side effects! There are lots of other spermicides [to test] or we have to develop new ones and test them."

Keeping to the strategy Leslie Wolfe had proposed the night before, Ehrhardt urges the women to support the Women's Health Equity Act that would allocate $10 million for women's HIV research and $10 million for prevention and community outreach. Fact sheets on the legislation were available at the Center for Women Policy Studies table outside the ballroom.[2]

"We can do it!" she says. "Let's do it now."

Another speaker, Rashidah Lorraine Hassan, an African-American woman majestic in flowing Muslim dress, walks to the podium, her posture making it clear she is well beyond self-assurance. That she and her people are of infinite value is an immovable rock of knowledge within her. Cofounder and executive director of Blacks Educating Blacks About Sexual Health Issues (BEBASHI) in Philadelphia, a former member of the Black Panther Party, Hassan says she is hearing from the women that morning "the need to be validated by the male-oriented structures to do what we actually can do ourselves. I don't want to talk anymore about allowing them to allow us to research on ourselves. I don't want to talk anymore about allowing them to allow us to develop clinical models of treatment and care. And I don't want to talk anymore about what *other* women can do for women of color. We can do it for ourselves. We don't have to have permission from anyone to do it.

"I was just a nurse in a neighborhood surrounded with black people dying with AIDS who didn't know they were supposed to get it. I didn't ask permission to organize BEBASHI. . . ."

Coming somewhat to CDC's defense, she points out it isn't the only agency responsible for public health. Nobody had talked that morning about HERSA (Health Resources and Services Administration), which is responsible for the funding of health care.

Women didn't need any agency's permission to act, she says. Anticipating that the women would respond that they needed government money to conduct research, she says brutally, "Well, they're not giving it to you. So get over it."

Her audience loves her blunt manner and greets her words with applause, laughter, whistling.

If women waited for the money to come, she told them, nothing would ever happen. The civil rights movement didn't start after appropriations had been made, she points out. People met in churches and used community resources, as she had in launching BEBASHI.

"If nothing else, my past history has taught me clearly that if you want something very badly, the only way to get it is to take it. Nobody ever invited us to power, ever negotiated, interfaced, or dialogued about it. Those who had it took and kept it as long as they could keep the strength to hold it. We are the seed of this creation. They can't do it without us.[3] So therefore, we already have the power. We need only to assume it. I think we have five more minutes to do it."

In the discussion period following the speeches, a middle-aged woman, her voice agonized, speaks into the microphone. She works with imprisoned women, she says, and has just started a program in one of the local city jails.

"We don't have any type of testing. The information I'm allowed to bring in is screened very closely. Some of the women in this program have already discussed that they're HIV-infected. One has a baby at home. One is exhibiting some serious clinical signs of PID, ongoing. The doctor that works in the jail is retired and I don't think he's ever seen PID anyway.

"I don't know what to do. I'm terribly frustrated. The agency I work for felt that I didn't need to come [here] so this is my Christmas present. My husband paid my way [to this conference] because my agency wouldn't. I need help. I need help and information on what I can do and who I need to see to get things like this taken care of."

Her voice is desperate, agonized.

"I mean, I'm just really here for help."

Ehrhardt, referring to the ACE program at Bedford Hills, tells her that Katrina Haslip from that program is here at the conference and suggests the woman speak with her.

Next on the conference agenda are workshop sessions.

In the afternoon, HIV-infected women hold a speak-out before about 150 warmly supportive women in the hotel's large Delaware Suite. One woman stretches out on the floor behind the last row of chairs, her body tired, face attentive.

Katherine Ritter, a young white woman from New York City who was diagnosed with HIV in 1986, speaks of how hard it was to come by her diagnosis:

"I had had a kidney infection for over a year. They'd been pumping me with sulfur. I had suggested to my doctor, well, maybe we should test me for HIV. 'No, you really don't need it. We'll beat this with another medication.'"

She finally got a diagnosis by going on her own to the Board of Health. Once she knew, she took measures to protect her health and stay alive as long as she could, she said. The delayed diagnosis deprived her of a chance to begin safeguarding her health earlier. Once diagnosed, Ritter had trouble getting into clinical drug trials:

"I was considered unreliable just because I was a woman, because of a hormone difference, and also because of that great theory that if you bleed, you can breed, and heaven protect the unborn—or even the unthought-of—fetus.

"I was sterilized and had papers to prove it. Yet I still had great difficulty. I have girlfriends that are lesbian. I mean, there is no chance that they are going to get pregnant. Just like with myself. They also have had problems with the bleed/breed theory, and getting into studies and trials. They are just shut off."

When Ritter sits, Terry Stout nervously takes her place at the microphone. She is young, blond, slim. In May 1988, she was diagnosed with HIV after her husband, long ill, was found to have AIDS. She was five months pregnant at the time of her diagnosis. Her husband died soon after. Her son, now twenty-eight months old, has AIDS. She cares for him without any help. Her family lives in Michigan, she in Florida.

"I have fears that someday I may not be able to care for my son. It is not so much that I am giving in to the HIV, but I have chronic arthritis in my back. My son is totally physically handicapped and he requires a great deal of lifting. I'm afraid one day I might wake up and I won't be able to care for him.

" . . .My in-laws are in Florida and I've lost their support. There is nobody there but me. We have all lost a mental health grant down in south Florida that has been my main strength, along with my spiritual awakening. I'm doing everything I can every day, twenty-four hours a day, to care for my son, and I come second. . . ."

Betty Jean Pejko, diagnosed with AIDS in March 1988, stands next at the microphone, telling the women she had been excited to learn her city, Chicago, had low-income housing for disabled people.

"I went right away and applied for that program and they were about to accept me until they read on my application that I have a child.

"Then I was informed that I couldn't go into disabled housing because we are blended in with the senior citizens and they don't need noise from children. But they assured me that I could apply for the other program. It has an average waiting list of fifteen to twenty years. Well, I have to be an optimist: I signed up."

The women laugh.

A twenty-year-old African-American woman from Atlanta comes to the microphone, speaking bitterly of how it had felt that morning to listen to Drs. Curran and Berkelman discount women's symptoms.

"Right now, I have so much pain and frustration inside of me," she tells the women.

There was no reason why such symptoms as hers—"I have fifteen-day periods every month and I'm told it's normal"—should not be documented and thoroughly studied, she says.

"But we, as women, are not important. I am told I am fourth on the ladder because I'm a black woman. I'm even lower down because

I'm still considered an adolescent. I'm twenty years old and was diagnosed on my eighteenth birthday. It frustrates me because I don't know if I will live to see twenty-one. . . .

"It frustrates me when I see on television so many millions of dollars have gone to this country, to that country, and we have people who are ill and dying right here in the United States. When is our President and all these bigwig officials who make these six-figure salaries going to realize that we have women, children, men who are dying in this country and who are not getting care because the bigwigs don't care?

" . . . I used to do interviews and ask that I not have my face shown because I didn't want people to harass me or discriminate against me. Even with my face not shown, I suffered discrimination from a hospital in Atlanta, Georgia, that refused me care when I had a high fever. I went to another hospital the next day and was told that if I had not come in, I would have died.

"I want to say this straight to the CDC: we are not numbers on a page. . . . I'm so burned up I can't even really tell you just how angry I am."

As the young woman moves to her seat, her mother, whose family turned from her when they learned her child was infected with HIV, takes her place at the microphone, radiating dignity.

"My child was seventeen years old, very smart, honor student, real good in school," she tells the upturned faces of the women in the large room. "She was on all types of committees—just great. Every time I walked in her school, they made me feel so proud because my kid was really good. . . ."

One day, apparently after her daughter had applied to join the army, an army official telephoned and, saying he needed to speak with her alone, made an appointment with·her.

"AIDS was the last thing on my mind," the woman continues. "When he told me, I turned and looked at him and I smiled. I said, 'Man, don't play with me. This is my kid you are talking about.' Because I was blind like so many others. I thought that this was a disease that only homosexuals get. . . .

"I had begged God for my children. Twenty-five years ago, I had toxemia. I lost my first child. I was told to have another child would kill me. But I begged Him. I said, 'Lord, if you give me just one, I'll be the best mother possible.' Well, he not only gave me one more—he gave me three, of whom I am very proud . . . "

Speaking of Social Security's denial of disability benefits to women, she continues: "It frustrates me to go to the Social Security Board, to these different little meetings with her and watch a judge tell my child, 'Well, you know you look well. You can work.' He has not followed her home. He does not know how it feels to watch your child in pain every night and you can do nothing about it. He does not know how it feels to hear that child stand up and pace that floor. He does not know how it feels to lie there and cry till your heart pains because there is nothing that you can do."

As participants, moved by the women's speak-out, applaud, the afternoon session ends.

That night after dinner, in a meeting open to any conference participants, activists plan their activities for the next day. They read a resolution prepared by the Center for Women Policy Studies—a long list of whereases ("Whereas as many as 65 percent of HIV positive women get sick and die from HIV-related infections that do not fit the CDC definition of AIDS . . . ") and a shorter list of "Be it resolved"s, announcing the conference's support for passage of woman-focused AIDS legislation.

"I feel more in a 'fuck you' than a 'be it resolved' mood," a weary and disgusted Linda Meredith comments.

They decide on a simple Unity Statement with three demands that had been the focus of ACT UP demonstrations over the past several years and that most women at the conference could readily agree to: a CDC AIDS definition that reflects immunosuppression as it affects women; a Social Security Administration policy to cover the disabilities of women; clinical trials designed by NIAID to study and treat the conditions of women.

While a CDC handout at the conference justifies the exclusion of women's conditions from the AIDS surveillance definition ("There is no scientific evidence that conclusively links HIV infection to life-threatening illnesses specific only to women"), the women redefine the issue that needed to be addressed at the conference: what the male-dominated government was doing to ensure that data on women did not come into existence. The unethical exclusion of women from studies cannot be used as an excuse to continue ignoring women, the women assert. They are naming and challenging the politics of knowledge.

The activists agree to ask each conference participant to sign a copy of the Unity Statement, stand in solidarity with a group of HIV-infected women who will read it aloud together at one of the mikes, and then walk to the front of the ballroom to personally hand their signed statements to either Dr. Anthony Fauci, head of NIAID, or Dr. Daniel Hoth, director of NIAID's Division of AIDS.

Several activists volunteer to write up the statement and photocopy it.

By 8:00 A.M., activists holding piles of the Unity Statement are stationed at every entrance to the ballroom, handing a statement to each person entering.

The speakers for this plenary session are Drs. Fauci and Hoth, and a physician treating HIV-infected women, Dr. Howard Minkoff, director of Maternal-Fetal Medicine at SUNY in Brooklyn, the same institution in which Dr. Rachel Fruchter and Pat Kelly work.

"Is PID changed by HIV?" Minkoff is asking from the stage. ". . . I hate to use the same words that have emanated so often from this podium, but the data is quite preliminary."

The numbers in the data at his institution are very small, he says, and confirmatory and further study is needed.

Following his speech, Sally Zierler, standing at a microphone in an aisle, asks him: "One of the implications [of your talk] is that the endocrine system must be involved in regard to HIV infection. I wonder what studies have been done to look particularly at estrogen receptors or other endocrine functions that are affected by HIV."

"I get tired of using the word 'preliminary' but for your question, I don't have to use the word 'preliminary data,'" Minkoff responds. "There is no data whatsoever. No one has been looking at that, to my knowledge."

A counselor for the New York City Department of Health involved in anonymous testing for HIV says it troubles her at this conference "when I continue to hear that there are no studies, or that the studies or information is small. The people in government should be prepared . . . not to tell us all what we know or get to find out from one another . . . *but what is going to be done?*"

An ACT UP woman in dungarees walking down the aisle sees Dr. Anke Ehrhardt in an aisle seat, leans down and pats her blond head affectionately before continuing on, one gesture of the bonding going on among female professionals, activists, and PWAs.

"My new friend," Ehrhardt says, smiling, to the colleague beside her.

Dr. Daniel Hoth is up next. He is supposed to give a twenty-minute speech on clinical trials for women with HIV. Since women had been basically barred from the trials, Linda Meredith, looking at the title of his speech, thinks, "Jeez, I wonder what he's going to do with the other nineteen and a half minutes."

Now he stands at the podium.

"This morning I am here to talk to you about women and HIV therapeutics but quite frankly, I can say very little about the treatment of women and HIV infection because we simply don't have much information," he says nervously. "There just aren't sufficient numbers of women in therapeutic clinical trials. It's as simple as that. I stand before you simply stating: we haven't done enough. The reasons are complex. It certainly wasn't intentional. I won't waste your time with details.

"What's important is what's next. What is the future? And that is that the NIAID will do everything that it can to get the answers to questions women and their doctors need to know to select the best treatment. That means more women on clinical trials. That means more study of diseases affecting women specifically. That means eligibility criteria for most trials that admit women as they exist in the real world. That means being as concerned about women as the fetus. . . .

"Well, I could go on and on but enough for now. . . . *Since I can't say much specific here about women and HIV therapeutics*, I'd like to tell you . . . "

Listening, Meredith is flabbergasted. Hoth, assigned to talk on clinical trials for women, goes on to give a twenty-minute lecture on how AZT works in men's bodies. She would have been embarrassed to do what he was doing but he obviously didn't care. She is surprised at the blatancy with which government researchers addressing the plenaries do not take the conference seriously. With a master's degree in immunology, she has worked in medical research for years and given papers at many scientific conferences. Hoth and his colleagues, she thinks, would never address a scientific conference that concerned anything other than women at the level they are doing it here. It is insulting.

Hoth winds up by noting that there is, at present, no evidence of any difference in safety and efficacy for antiretroviral therapies for men and women. He acknowledges that that had, however, never been systematically evaluated, that adequate numbers of women simply hadn't been enrolled in these trials to evaluate their effect.

"But my take-home message is that if we don't *look* at this question, we'll never know. And we *will* do so. We *will* look at that question."

"When?" women shout from the audience.

To increase the enrollment of women in ACTG trials, ensure the inclusion of gyn exams in the trials, and increase knowledge about the safety and efficacy of treatments in women, the ACTG had recently established a Women's Health Committee, he announces, confirming what activists had been told earlier.

(That big banner spread before him at the San Francisco conference six months earlier, NIAID: FORM A WOMEN'S COMMITTEE, seems to have been effective.)

In the discussion period, a group of HIV-infected women gather around a microphone in the aisle and together chant the Unity Statement. Hundreds of women rise in support as the women read it, then walk to the stage to hand their signed statements to a startled Hoth and Fauci. (Displaying openness, Fauci sat down at an impromptu, lengthy meeting that afternoon and listened to and answered the questions of a group of HIV-positive women.)

Dr. Janet Mitchell, chief of perinatalogy at Harlem Hospital Center and an outspoken African-American critic of the medical care provided poor people of color, and Dr. Ruth L. Kirschstein, acting chief of the newly created Office of Research on Women's Health at NIH, are among those on the next panel.

The Office of Research on Women's Health had been created only two months earlier in response to outrage over the paucity of research on ailments affecting women, in stunning contrast to generous funding of research on ailments as they affect men. The Office of Research on Women's Health is staffed by a total of two persons. That includes Kirschstein, the chief. It exists in temporary quarters. It has had no money whatsoever appropriated for its work.

In her address, Kirschstein notes that a starting appropriation for the Office of Research on Women's Health of $2 million had been in the NIH Appropriations Bill as it was passed in the Senate.

"That did not survive in the final appropriation," she observes, hastening to add: "I've had discussions with the acting head of NIH and I'm *sure* he's going to provide us with some money and I know the department plans to ask for considerably more than that for the fiscal year 1992."

The funding level to that Office of Research on Women's Health was key, Janet Mitchell points out when she takes the floor. Without adequate funding, the Office was little more than window dressing.

Minorities, she tells Kirschstein, "know about window dressing. We know about all the special programs that get set up with no appropriate funding. . . . If you are not funded, you are not going to be able to do a thing. And they're going to scapegoat you because [they'll say] 'we set up this office for women. . . .'"

In the discussion following the next plenary panel, a community researcher, noting all the inadequacies of university-based research delineated throughout the conference, asks Dr. Mitchell if any efforts have been made to reach out to ob/gyns and other community-based physicans who could be gathering data on HIV-infected women.

"The majority of women who are presenting to physicians have no idea that they are HIV-infected," she continues. "Since the women weren't identified as HIV-infected, physicians couldn't collect appropriate information on what was showing up in them."

She had been enormously frustrated in her efforts to get ob/gyns in her own hospital to help identify HIV-infected women by asking questions and referring for testing, Mitchell says.

"So all the candidiasis, all the abnormal paps, all the trichomoniasis, all the things you're talking about—I don't really know what the prevalence is because I can't get my physicians to understand the importance of telling the women at Harlem they are at risk simply because they live in a high-prevalence area."

It isn't that ob/gyns are too dense to understand the situation; it is more that they just don't want to have to deal with HIV-infected women, Mitchell explains. They maintain their ignorance of HIV in order to keep themselves removed from the epidemic.

A community physician from Berkeley, California, jumps into

the discussion. From the beginning of the epidemic, she says, community-based physicians have been conducting largely unfunded community-based research. In the last year NIH allocated a community program for AIDS research, and she and others now get limited funding to do the community-based research they had all previously been doing as volunteers.

But the funding has been so inadequate that they can't put all their patients on an observation data base (ODB) where they can follow them and get natural history data. Instead, she says, individual sites have to decide whether, for example to put their IV drug users or their women on the ODB because there isn't enough funding for both.

The ACTGs provided a fair amount of information, but certainly not enough relating to women, minorities, and IV drug users.

"Yet when supplemental applications went in this year from ACTG sites to add sites that would serve women and minorities—sites like mine in California were denied. Most of us believe that the reason they were denied was that women with HIV infection are thought to be only in New York and New Jersey. Yet there are many women on the West Coast and throughout the United States who are HIV-infected."

"What Dr. Mitchell is saying about ob/gyns I just have to echo," she adds. "It takes me at least ten to fifteen calls every time one of my women patients needs an abortion or a colposcopy."

The refusals were always clouded by funding issues, she says, such as assertions that they don't take Medicaid patients.

"But the bottom line is, 'I don't want to take care of HIV. That's somebody else's problem.'"

Dooley Worth crystallizes the major question facing the women gathered together in Washington at this conference and, indeed, the question facing women throughout the nation. Speaking at an afternoon workshop on culturally specific strategies for HIV education and prevention, she unexpectedly speaks not about black, white, Latino, or Asian-American culture but about the culture of power in the United States: the domination by men of the social, economic, and political resources.

"Behavioral change, which is what AIDS prevention is about, is really a change in power relations between men and women," she asserts. "This can't be promoted successfully if we don't . . . act on what I would call the structural determinants [of behavior] which are: poverty, poor housing, a lack of educational opportunities, acculturation problems, lack of health care."

Outdated ideas of disease and how diseases spread created barriers to women's participation in AIDS prevention, she continues. Such outdated ideas also created the notion "that somehow AIDS is the result of bad personal behavior such as intravenous drug use."

In that concept was embedded another: "that the government cannot address the roots of such bad behavior, such as intravenous drug use. There's an assumption that it cannot do anything about solving poverty, racism, or sexism."

That viewpoint "assumes that individuals, even impoverished minority women, have adequate resources to lead healthy lives, to engage in personal AIDS risk reduction. . . . It ignores the evidence that vast changes in the ability to deal with other infectious diseases have been the result of improvements in the standard of living, not through magic bullets."

Not only did women need to look at the link of AIDS to power differentials and sexual behavior: "I think it's time for all of us to decide what we're going to *do* about it. We *know* what's going on. How can we collectively do something about this culture of power and how it affects women?"

AFTERWORD

The story of women and AIDS continues, although settings, characters, and numbers will change. Some new studies on women have been announced; their significance remains to be determined following a woman-centered analysis of their designs and budgets. In 1991, the CDC did announce plans to expand the AIDS definition, but as of May 1992 the planned change still did not include gynecological manifestations.[1] In New York State, women had to fight back an attempt by the AIDS Institute to redirect the Women and AIDS Project away from women and onto adolescents. They succeeded. But then the Institute stopped funding the Project altogether. The Women and AIDS Project held its last formal meeting in March 1992.

So it goes on.

And we *know* what is going on, as Dooley Worth said. The question she posed at the Washington conference in 1990 remains for us to answer: What are we going to *do* about it?

From the beginning of the AIDS pandemic, there have been women who, despite the risk and cost to themselves, have questioned, organized, and fought. The women you have just read of in this book represent only a small number of them. There are many more throughout the country and the world who, on a daily basis, are working to save lives.

We need to join with them: looking at AIDS policy, treatment, and research and becoming a chorus of voices on our own behalf; confronting city, state, and federal governments; exposing the politics of scientific knowledge; working to scrap a medical care nonsystem that so demeans our lives it provides medical care as if it were just another widget to be marketed and sold; advocating a health service respectful of women and people of color; voting out of office politicians who ignore our challenge to the male hogging of resources and our calls for an equitable distribution of state and federal funds; challenging the economic exploitation of women—limited career opportunities and low, unequal wages—that, by keeping women dependent on men for survival, sets us up for sexual exploitation.

We need to name sexual exploitation of women as a public health issue—it is key to the worldwide spread of the AIDS pandemic—and as a human rights violation. We can politically challenge it in all its manifestations: incest, rape, prostitution, sexual harassment, pornography.[2]

The story of women and AIDS, becoming more horrifying with each passing year, will be with us for the rest of our lives. AIDS is a young pandemic. Its major effects are yet to be felt.[3]

To get through it, we need to follow the moral leadership provided by the women of Bedford Hills Correctional Facility: Challenge the HIV/AIDS stigma and the cruelty that accompanies it. Build community. Educate and support one another in preventing the spread of HIV. Care lovingly for those among us who are struck with the disease.

We can thwart the patriarchal tactic of divide and conquer and refuse to be tranquilized by assertions that AIDS has to do only with *some* women, *other* women, *those* women. All women, no matter our race or our economic status, are at risk, and we are bound to the fate of one another. Like the women of Bedford Hills, we are in this together.

We can change the plot in the story of women and AIDS by joining with those women, in resistance to our subordination, who know that the Upanishads are right on this: Rehala, the young woman who learned of her HIV infection in a van on a desolate New York City street, is of infinite worth. She is the soul of the world. As Katrina Haslip and Patricia Daugherty are. As Helen Cover was. As we are. We are not dark shapes in dark shadows. Silent. Invisible. So unworthy we can allow ourselves only tiny little breaths. No. We are the soul of the world. We are that which is the finest essence. We can act together to command the respect and justice that is no more than our due and by our actions make visible at last the invisible epidemic.

Most important, each and every one of us can add our own names to a new kind of quilt—a quilt of resistance to oppression and affirmation of our worth.

RESOURCES

AIDS Coalition to Unleash Power (ACT UP)
Women's Action Committee
496-A Hudson Street, #G4
New York, NY 10014
212-989-1114
Activist group.

Association for Women's AIDS Research/Education (AWARE)
San Francisco General Hospital
955 Potrero
Building 80, Ward 84
San Francisco, CA 94110
415-476-4091

Centers for Disease Control (CDC)
Hotline: 1-800-342-AIDS

National AIDS Information Clearinghouse
P.O. Box 6003
Rockville, MD 20850
800-458-5231
Maintains listing of AIDS service organizations and educational materials. Resources, free publications, information on clinical trials.

National AIDS Network
2033 M Street, NW
Suite 800
Washington, DC 20036
202-293-2437
Refers volunteers to organizations providing help to people with AIDS.

National Association of People with AIDS
P.O. Box 18345
Washington, DC 20036
800-673-8538

National Minority AIDS Council
300 I Street, NE
Washington, DC 20002
Provides referrals and assistance to minorities.

National Resource Center on Women and AIDS
Center for Women Policy Studies
2000 P Street, N.W.
Suite 508
Washington, DC 20036
202-872-1770
Publishes *The Guide to Resources on Women and AIDS,* an excellent
resource.

National Women's Health Network
1325 G Street, N.W.
Washington, DC 20005
202-347-1140
Distributes a vital report offering policy recommendations on women
in the HIV/AIDS epidemic: "New York City Task Force on Women and
AIDS Policy Document."

The Positive Woman, Inc.
P.O. Box 34372
Washington, DC 20043
202-898-0372
A nonprofit volunteer organization dedicated to improving the quality
of life for HIV-infected women. Produces a bimonthly newsletter, *The Positive Woman: A Newsletter by, for and about the HIV Positive Woman.*

University of Massachusetts/Boston and the Multicultural AIDS Coalition
566 Columbus Avenue
Boston, MA 02118
Publishes *Searching for Women: Literature Review of Women, HIV and AIDS in the United States*. Price, including postage: $11.50.

Women's AIDS Network—San Francisco AIDS Foundation
333 Valencia Street, Fourth Floor
San Francisco, CA 94103
415-863-AIDS

Women and AIDS Resource Network (WARN)
55 Johnson Street
General Building
Suite 303
Brooklyn, NY 11202
718-596-6007

See the following sections of *Women, AIDS and Activism* by the ACT UP/NY Women and AIDS Book Group (Boston: South End Press, 1990) for these excellent and extensive resource listings: "Resources," by Bea Hanson; "Bibliography" (well annotated), by Polly Thistlethwaite; "AIDS Videos by, for, and about Women," by Catherine Saalfield. The Glossary by Brigite Weil is also extremely useful.

ACKNOWLEDGMENTS

The force propelling the birth of many valuable books, videos, and guerrilla actions, Sandra Elkin played a role for me in the creation of *The Invisible Epidemic* that she has played for uncounted others and that goes completely beyond the function of a literary agent: on a nearly daily basis, conceptualizing, questioning, probing, shaping, challenging, cheering on. In a thousand generous ways, she made this book happen. Sandra Elkin is a mover and shaker, a brilliant, passionate, and powerful woman. She gets bored when I try to thank her so I'll say only: My friendship with her is a shining jewel in my life.

During the often difficult labor of writing this book, African dance was a source for me of joy and awe. I thank the gifted dance and drum teachers in the Boston area for the years they've devoted to developing their art and for the generosity of their teaching, sharing with me and others the rich cultures of Africa and of the African diaspora. I am grateful to: Eno Washington (whose spirit always becomes visible when he dances), Ife Bolden, Stone Montgomery, Ibrahima Camara, Fatou Carol Sylla, Nuru Dafina, DeAma Battle, Akila Stanley, Noel Staples, Ramzieh Hassan (with her magnificent African-Arabic style), Assane Konte, Fatou Ndiaye, Abdoulah Diakite, Mauricio Marques, Edir Passos, Cornell Coley, Sadio Diatta Rosche, and Mohamaed Kalifa Camara.

With her expert editing, strong support, and *savoir-faire,* Janet Goldstein steered this book through all the complicated passages to publication. I am grateful, for the third time, to be the beneficiary of such skill, commitment, and caring.

I am most grateful to those I interviewed, who generously shared their experience, expertise, and time with me. They often made me feel that the book was a collaborative project. They wanted it to exist and played a major role in making sure that it indeed does.

The affirmations Elizabeth Corea wrote for a meditation tape we made together enriched and supported me as I worked on this book. Six-year-old Sarah Elizabeth Renninger, who, like her mother, Elizabeth, is creative, hungry to learn, and eager to dance, has brought me joy.

Tom Marlin telephonically led me through many a computer crisis, saving the day as he has done for years. He is family to me, with a special and treasured place in my life.

A special thanks to Rosemary and Jim Maconochie for the innumerable times they've rushed to the rescue during household emergencies. I'm sure my neighbors thank them, too; any attention to my lawn has come from them, not me. They've been my personal 911. I've really felt their support on this and other levels.

Friends helped me, not only in various ways with the book itself but also by talking things over with me, by being solid friends. I treasure in my life: Denisce DiIanni, Lia Coulouris, Monika Weis-Imroll, Jo Lynch, Jan Raymond and Patricia Hynes (my subconscious's image of ideal adult women), Cynthia Fertman, Fred Setterberg, Asnath Masipa and my sister Masepeke Mapule of the Republic of South Africa, Mary Mangan, Ly Cheik, Fran Boronski, Rhyena Halpern, Renate Klein, Gundula Kayser, Teresa Alabernia, John Alibrandi, Ana dos Reis, and Kathy Barry.

I thank Ferdoos, Akram, and Burhan Atallah, whose extraordinary hospitality, education, and protection under difficult circumstances I will always count among the gifts of my life. I also thank Al and Diane Pesso for their important work.

I was the beneficiary of skillful, efficient, and generous help in the scheduling of interviews, transcription of interview tapes, and location of research materials. I thank: Kimberly Grant, Shereen Goodman, Rosemary Maconochie, Tee Provost, and Erna Kelly. A special thanks to Erna Kelly, who, throughout this project, was always ready to transcribe quickly and on short notice in all my declared emergencies, and who helped me buy and set up office machinery. She always aided me beyond the call of duty.

Many people kindly helped me in a variety of ways during the eighteen months I wrote this book. Some read sections of the manuscripts and gave me valuable comments. Others connected me with HIV-positive women, often taking a great deal of effort in doing so. Some sent me materials on women and AIDS. Others aided me during machinery breakdowns, and kept household chaos at bay. I'm deeply grateful to: Anke Ehrhardt, Linda

Lofredo, Carola Marte, Waffa El-Sadr, Nina Ridgewick, Mason Klink, Pat Kelly, Lynnette Dumble, Rita Arditti, Shannon Joslin, Patricia Foster, Robert Martin, Diane Fedele, Greg Zammuto, Ed Hardy, Charles Armstrong, Toby Simon, Lois VanLaningham, Patricia Warne, and Peternelle van Arsdale.

I am also grateful to Marie and Ed Corea; Katy Corea; Ginny, Gigi, Mike, and Dan Caple; Jim Jr. and Jenna Marie Maconochie; Ed, Charlene, Ted, Andy, Bryde, and Nicholas Corea; Teresa, Jay, and Lila Barbuto.

I thank Andrea Dworkin for writing *Mercy,* a novel in which "the bait"—the woman—talks back with a power, a fierce intelligence, a stunning beauty that must be unparalleled in world literature.

As I researched this book, I often thought with gratitude of nineteenth-century feminists who struggled to open universities and law and medical schools to women. Our foremothers consciously saw themselves working for the women of the twentieth century so that we would not suffer as they had. It was because of their struggle that today there are some women in law (like Terry McGovern) and in medicine (like Helen Rodriquez) with the skills to challenge the politics of male knowledge and, frankly, enough exposure to this knowledge and to academia to be unfettered by any awe of it. If it were not for the struggle on our behalf of these earlier feminists, we would lack many of the tools we now have to save our lives in the face of the AIDS pandemic.

I want to acknowledge the role Helen Cover played for me as I wrote this book. She lived and, in her late twenties, died in a world diseased with sexual and racial injustice. Helen Cover never became the person she had the potential to be. That the richness that was Helen was numbed out, painted over in a layer of dirty, dull yellow, and then tossed aside as if of no value— that is a crime.

In investigating Helen's story, the more I learned of her, piece by piece, through person by person, the more I felt the enormity of her loss to us. I could see her—fatally ill, in pain, cold, homeless, friendless—leaning down to draw a picture on the street because she had within her that drive to create art. I have grieved and raged for who she might have, but never did, become. I often felt I was writing this book for her.

NOTES

··

In addition to the sources listed in the notes, this book is based largely on interviews, usually multiple, that took place between August 1990 and January 1992 with the following persons: Vicki Alexander; Hortensia Amaro; Kathy Anastos; Byllye Avery; Jane Auerbach; Kathy Barry; Gloria Boyd; Kathy Boudin; Marie-Lucie Brutus; Mary Beth Caschetta; Wendy Chafkin; Maryanne Chiasson; Judy Clark; Judith Cohen; Mardge Cohen; DiAna DiAna; Alexis Danzig; Risa Denenberg; Anke Ehrhardt; Sandra Elkin; Waffa El-Sadr; Anna Forbes; Mindy Fullilove; Rachel Fruchter; Diane Hartell; Katrina Haslip; Eileen Hogan; Charlotte Davis Kasl; Pat Kelly; Alisa Lebow; Annamarie Lewis; Sondra Lieberman; Linda Lofredo; Elaine Lord; John Lynch; Carola Marte; Vickie Mays; Lynne MacArthur; Terry McGovern; Lucy McKinney; Linda Meredith; J. Kevin Mulroy; Lesley Noble; June Osbourne; Nampet Panichpant; Katy Porter; Scott Porter; Janice G. Raymond; Marilyn (T.J.) Rivera; Helen Rodriquez-Trias; Renée Scott; Kathy Selzer; Ada Setal; Phyllis Sharpe; Tamar Sohol; Edith Springer; Marie St. Cyr; Zena Stein; Ida Susser; Katy Taylor; Mario Tomasetti; Marie Tulman; Sten Vermund; Silvia Vitali; Joyce Wallace; Rodrick Wallace; Patricia Warne; Gloria Weissman; Marcia Weissman; Marie Wilson; Leslie Wolfe; Maxine Wolfe; Jeri Woodhouse; Dooley Worth; Sally Zierler.

I also interviewed many HIV-positive women, not all of whom I could write about. Throughout the text, I refer to Penny Abernathey by her maiden name to avoid confusion that might arise in the reader if I changed to her married names: first Knox, then Vehrs.

For nine of the HIV-positive women I did include, I created the pseudonyms: Patricia Daugherty; Charlotte Schafer, Diane Sampson; Rosemary Star; June Winkler; Rehala; Donna; Joanna; Mary. For some of the relatives and friends of these women, I created the pseudonyms: Steven Schafer; Bruce Sampson; Margaret; Sally; Carol; John; Al; and Miss Lily. Pseudonyms for workers in Dr. Joyce Wallace's employ are Janice, Pam, and Joe.

1981–1982

1. The aspirin/heart study was NIH-funded (Hilts, 1990).

Since most studies on heart disease have been carried out on men, ignorance about heart disease in women reigns. One result: Two recent studies showed that physicians treat women with heart disease less aggressively than men, even though in the women, the disease tended to be further advanced. Women were half as likely to undergo cardiac catheterization and much less likely to have bypass surgery or a procedure to unclog blocked arteries.

A recent review of seven major studies on high blood pressure found that treatments that work for men may be ineffective or even harmful for white (though not black) women. These conclusions are tentative because there is little information on treating hypertension in women.

Even though women apparently suffer clinical depression much more often than men, research on antidepressants was initially done only with men. There is now evidence that the effects of some antidepressants vary during the menstrual cycle. This means that a dosage can be too high for a woman at some times and too low at others.

Ailments that especially affect elderly women, including osteoporosis, receive unequal research attention (*New York Times,* Sept. 9, 1991).

In a report published in July 1991, the Council on Ethical and Judicial Affairs of the American Medical Association concluded that women were far less likely than men to receive a kidney transplant or a diagnostic test for lung cancer.

Commenting on this report, a *New York Times* editorial stated: "Stereotypical attitudes and prejudice by doctors may well be one reason. The council cites evidence that 'physicians are more likely to attribute women's health complaints to emotional rather than physical causes.' And doctors may consider men's role in society 'greater than women's'" (*New York Times,* July 26, 1991).

2. For feminist critiques that document the risky drugs and unnecessary operations provided women in the U.S. medical system, see: BWHBC, 1992; Cohen and Estner, 1983; Corea, 1985a; Scully, 1980; Seaman and Seaman, 1977; Hynes, 1991; Gross, July 14, 1991; Hilts, Sept. 10, 1991.

3. The conception and phrase "politics of otherness" is that of Sandra Elkin, a New York City–based media expert who produced the AIDS education video *AIDS Is About Secrets.*

4. Norwood, 1988.

5. Wallace stressed that results in this largely self-selected group did not prove that prostitution in the United States was necessarily a significant risk factor for the immune-deficiency syndrome. Subsequent studies found it not to be, though in many countries it decidedly is. (Wallace et al., April 17, 1982, and Wallace et al., Jan. 18, 1983.)

6. Kinsella, 1989.

7. The CDC has at least three different systems for referring to AIDS/HIV. None of these systems includes even one gynecological symptom (ACT UP, 1991).
    a. A classification system for HIV disease. People who have tested positive for HIV are divided into groups beginning with "HIV, asymptomatic" and progressing on to a listing of conditions. Because this classification does not include any gynecological symptoms as manifestations of HIV disease, this means, as ACT UP points out, that an HIV-positive woman would be considered asymptomatic even if she had a number of gynecological conditions (such as severe PID resistant to treatment) known to be associated with HIV.
    b. An international classification system. AIDS is defined in this system according to CDC's surveillance definitions. The person reporting each case codes "associated conditions" under the following categories:
        With HIV
        Due to HIV
        With an AIDS-like disease
        Due to an AIDS-like disease
        With AIDS
        Due to AIDS
    c. A surveillance definition. Used for reporting the extent of the epidemic in the United States. This definition has a more limited set of conditions than those in the other two systems. It includes AIDS cases diagnosed "presumptively," meaning that the persons so diagnosed show certain AIDS conditions but laboratory tests have not been performed confirming them. It also includes people with no laboratory evidence of HIV, but with HIV diseases or conditions and in whom causes other than HIV have been ruled out. The figures emerging from this definition are the ones used for determining the extent of the AIDS epidemic and on which budget requests for fighting the epidemic are based.

1983–1984

....

1. In May 1983, researchers from the Pasteur Institute in France claimed to have isolated the AIDS virus, setting off a long, bitter dispute with U.S. scientists over who discovered the cause of AIDS first. The virus was eventually named the human immunodeficiency virus (HIV).

For details on the Franco-American dispute over who first discovered what came to be called HIV, see: Hilts, May 7, 1991; Hilts, Sept. 16, 1991; Kinsella, 1989.

2. Meyer-Bahlburg et al., 1991:9–10, 20–21.

3. Kinsella, 1989, is the source for the media reporting on "casual contact" as a transmission mode for AIDS. This book's "time line of the plague" has been particularly helpful in providing a year-by-year context for the events concerning women during the epidemic.

4. "Gladys Thompson" is a composite, created to represent the women like this whom Anastos met and reacted to in this way.

5. Three weeks later, a relative of the woman's said he had convinced her to turn herself in to authorities in exchange for his release from jail. He was facing charges of larceny and forgery. He made his role public when he complained that court authorities had reneged on a promise to drop the charges against him. They had promised to let him off if he helped them, he alleged, because they were anxious to get the woman in custody where she would not infect anyone through her prostitution (Hamm, March 21, 1984).

Court officials denied they had promised to drop criminal charges but did acknowledge that the man had been released on a promise to appear in court in the hope that he would contact the missing woman and convince her to turn herself in.

Other sources discussing the woman in prostitution in New Haven include Hamm, Feb. 15, 1984; Barbuto, Jan. 24, 1984; Hladky, 1984; Guilfoy, 1984.

6. Sources for information about the Bedford Hills Correctional Facility are interviews with inmates and with the superintendent, Elaine Lord, and Linda Lofredo. Also, Clark and Boudin, 1990:92.

7. Flam and Stein, 1986.

1985

....

1. Kinsella, 1989.

2. On the availability of HIV test in New York City: Norwood, 1988

3. Guinan and Hardy, 1987.

4. Berkelman made the comment in a meeting with women's health activists at CDC headquarters in Atlanta in 1990. The activists, as described in Chapter 9, were challenging the CDC AIDS surveillance definition that left out women-specific conditions.

Berkelman continued her observation: "The surveillance system is dependent on the medical care system. If the medical care system isn't working, if people aren't being HIV tested and aren't being diagnosed, that's a problem."

Of course, if the CDC doesn't alert physicians to, for example, the fact that recurrent vaginal candidiasis resistant to treatment may be a tip-off to suspected HIV-infection, it will be more difficult for physicians to come to an appropriate diagnosis.

5. In 1990, Dr. Isaac Weisfuse's blind test of 2,238 consecutive inmate admissions in New York City jails found a 25.6 percent HIV positivity rate among women. The rate was 43 percent among those women admitting to IV drug use. (New York City Department of Health, 1990. Information sheet entitled "Living Well with HIV Requires Changes and Choices.")

6. Amaro's perceptions on the framing of women's health issues: interview with Amaro; Amaro, 1990 and Amaro's speech at Women and AIDS breakfast meeting, Oct. 4, 1989, at the HIV Center in New York City.

7. Cauley, Demkovich, and Ryan, 1990.

8. For some details on these cases, see Chapter 5.

9. Kolder, Gallagher, and Parsons, May 7, 1987.

10. Gardiner-Caldwell SynerMed, 1991, p. 4.

11. On federal documents in 1990 stating physicians should not prescribe pentamidine for pregnant, HIV-infected women and on exclusion of women of child-bearing potential from ACTG trials: presentation by Dr. Howard Minkoff at Women and HIV Conference, December 1990 in Washington, D.C.

12. On ACTGs and their committee structure: ACT UP, May 1991.

13. On denial of Medicaid funding for abortions: New York City Task Force on Women & AIDS, Policy Document, 1992. Sixty-four percent of New York City abortion clinics denied appointments to HIV-infected women: Katherine Franke, Abstract, V International Conference on AIDS, June 4–6, 1989, p. 855, cited in ACT UP/NY Women & AIDS Book Group, 1990.

14. Researchers had found decreased levels of helper T cells during pregnancy and decreased lymphocyte function. See Minkoff, 1987.

On the scarcity of information on HIV's effect on health of women in pregnancy: Risa Denenberg in ACT UP/NY Women and AIDS Book Group, 1990; Howard L. Minkoff, 1987. General sources for section on HIV and pregnancy: Working Group on HIV Testing of Pregnant Women and Newborns, 1990; Mitchell, 1988.

15. Ellerbrock and Rogers, 1990.

1986

....

1. Corea, 1985a.

2. Jeanne Maguire of Harvard School of Public Health compared implicit policy to body language at a workshop during the conference "Women and AIDS: Keeping Women in Focus" in Boston in April 1991.

3. Held Sept. 26, 1985, this was the first public hearing of its kind inside a prison. It was cosponsored by three New York State agencies: the Department of Correctional Services, the Governor's Commission on Domestic Violence, and the Division for Women. Ronnie Eldridge, then director of the Division for Women, suggested the hearing during a meeting with the Inmate Liaison Committee at Bedford Hills. As Superintendent Elaine Lord recalls it, there was a discussion about why women were in the prison, what brought them there, why the women had such long sentences. Some members of the Liaison Committee had fifteen-year minimum sentences for killing their husbands. They spoke of the years of battering and sexual abuse they had been subjected to by their mates and of their futile attempts to get protection and help from state agencies such as the police and social agencies. The tone of the meeting intensified as women shared their personal stories.

On the spot, Eldridge proposed a public hearing in the prison on the relationship between domestic violence and incarceration. On the spot, Superintendent Lord agreed to it.

The twelve women who testified at the hearing were all survivors of domestic violence and most had been convicted of killing their spouses, former spouses, or common-law husbands. Three had maximum life sentences. The others had maximum sentences averaging fifteen years. As a report on the hearing notes: "Nearly all are women who had never been convicted of a crime until they committed the crimes to which they were inexorably led: the killing of men who had brutalized them. The nature of their crimes and the existence of a very low recidivism rate for those who have committed murder and manslaughter provide substantial evidence that these women and others like them are not a danger to society. The wisdom of imprisoning them at all is certainly questionable. The extremely long sentences of the women who testified raise even more serious questions about the fairness of our criminal justice system" (CDVIW, 1987).

At the hearing, the women did not talk about the crime, Lofredo pointed out. They talked about their lives and what led up to the crime.

"The stories of the women were never told," as Lofredo explained it. "What was never told was the abuse. The only part of their lives that was publicly examined was the actual crime that took place as a result of the abuse."

Sponsors of the hearing wanted to provide a supportive atmosphere for the women testifying and make sure that it did not resemble the courtroom. So they invited women's advocates from a variety of organizations, including those working in battered women's shelters. Each woman testifying was allowed to invite ten guests.

"It was very, very emotional," Lord explained, "and we felt the best way to go was to allow *them* to invite, since they were revealing things about themselves."

Close to three hundred people attended the hearing.

4. Annette Johnson from the New York State AIDS Institute assisted Lofredo and MacArthur in pulling the meeting together, giving them names of people working on the women and AIDS issue.

During the discussion at the first meeting, Suki Ports, director of the Minority AIDS Task Force, said that with AIDS we were not just going to lose one generation; we were going to lose two.

At that moment, MacArthur caught her first glimmer that this disease was going to be different for women than it was for men. An infected woman has to choose whether she is even going to *have* children. If she is pregnant, she has to decide whether to abort. If she's HIV-infected and her child is sick, she must make arrangements for the care of her child during her illness, and perhaps after her death.

5. Not all drug experts subscribe to the theory that "setting" is crucial. The theory of the so-called addictive personality is another, and opposing, view.

6. See Worth, 1990a, b.

7. Guinan, 1989.

8. One of these researchers, Dr. Mindy Thompson Fullilove, later supervised a student who conducted a "focus group" of IV drug and crack users. The group discussed whether what went on in the crack houses was intercourse or oral sex:

> Participant: ". . . Basically a mother fucker ain't got time for nothin' else, getting some head and then go on about his business, especially in them crack houses. I've rarely seen any of those female crackheads that wore panties. They come in ready."
> Moderator: "What does that mean?"
> Participant: "That means they come in ready for sex."
> Moderator: "What I'm hearing is that they are doing oral sex."
> Participant: "If she's good and can get them off, cool. But if you don't get off with that, well, baby, I got to go up on in there and get it. Because he don't give up his crack and not get off."

Sources on crack and women: Bowser et al., 1990; Worth, 1990a, b; Weissman, 1991.

9. Source on Helen Cover's early life: O'Hara, 1989.

10. Sources on Boudin and Clark: Frankfort, 1983; Morgan, 1990.

1987

....

1. This was important because in public hospitals physicians did not always order, for example, expensive broncoscopies to diagnose pneumocystis carinii pneumonia (PCP), an opportunistic infection often seen in people with AIDS. They would just say, "Probably that person has PCP because it looks, acts, and responds to treatment like PCP." Before 1987, such cases had not been officially defined as AIDS.

2. ACT UP, 1991.

3. T. D. Verdegem, 1988; Anastos and Marte, 1989.

4. ACT UP, May 1991.

5. Thomas, July 27, 1987.

6. On prostitutes in the U.S. not being vectors of HIV to men: testimony of Anna Forbes before the Joint House Health and Welfare Committee and House Judiciary Committee Hearing on Pennsylvania House Bill 624 and Related Legislative Matters, April 27, 1989; Richardson, 1988; CWPS, 1991. CWPS cites as a paper stating that no AIDS cases in the U.S. had been definitely traced to prostitution: Decker, 1987.

7. On prostitution in Thailand: presentation by Nampet Panichpant at the Women and HIV Conference sponsored by the Public Health Service in Washington, D.C., in December 1990, and follow-up telephone interview. Panichpant described the process to me. I used my own language in writing of it. Where I would write of women and men "used" in prostitution, Panichpant would choose words such as "commercially sexually involved with." Where I use the word "poor," she would choose "economically disadvantaged."

8. A few more details on the sex industry provided by Nampet Panichpant, interim president of the United Thai Council of North America:

The first acknowledged gay bar in Bangkok opened around 1970. Some Asians and Westerners from the former colonialist nations—Britain, France, and the Netherlands—as well as American and Australian men went to this bar, among other places, to search out Thai men for sex. In Thailand on business and pleasure, these "sugar daddies" were never numerically substantial.

The numbers of foreign sugar daddies increased when sex tours from Europe, many of which originated in Amsterdam, Frankfurt, and Paris, and from Japan and the Middle East, accelerated in the mid-1970s.

From a handful of AIDS cases in Thailand in 1986, the numbers exploded to 400,000 in 1992 and are expected to rival the case numbers in Africa by the end of the century.

In the international brothel network, Thai women were also flown in to go-go bars and massage parlors in Germany. People working at the Thai embassy in Germany related to Panichpant horrifying incidents they dealt with involving such Thai women.

For a ground-breaking analysis of and a profoundly disturbing report on the use of women in international sexual slavery, read Kathleen Barry's *Female Sexual Slavery* (1987). Also see the collection of essays *Sexual Liberals and the Attack on Feminism* (Leidholdt and Raymond, eds., 1990).

Large numbers of girls and women from Burma, now ruled by a military dictatorship, are being sold by middlemen to brothel owners in Thailand, according to consistent reports. In 1991, a report by Anti-Slavery

International, submitted to the United Nations Working Group on Contemporary Forms of Slavery, estimated that there were more than 1,500 Burmese girls and women forced to work as prostitutes in one Thai city alone—Ranong, a fishing port on the west coast of Thailand, opposite the southernmost tip of Burma. Many of the women are treated as virtual slaves.

Journalist Teresa Poole reported in 1992: "Such is the demand of Thailand's sex industry for new girls, and the appetite for younger 'AIDS-free' girls, that Ranong is only one of many transit points. . . . If they are found to be HIV-positive they are thrown back over the border where there is little health care" (Poole, 1992).

The problem is apparently more serious than a lack of health care. In April 1992, reports that Burmese girls and women infected with AIDS were being injected with cyanide to stop the spread of the virus in Burma prompted Thai police to stop deporting any women caught working as prostitutes in Thailand.

Thailand's Crime Suppression Division (CSD) Deputy Commander Pol Col Bancha Jarujareet, who leads an antiprostitution center under the police department, stated that in June 1991 the CSD rescued twenty-five Burmese women, age eighteen to thirty-five, from a brothel in Ranong Province following the complaint of one of the women's relatives. All the women were found to be HIV-infected, Bancha said.

After the women were deported to Burma, he learned that they were all missing from their villages and later was told they had been injected with cyanide to prevent them from spreading the virus. He could not say who gave them the injections. Because of this incident, Bancha said no other Burmese women released from brothels would be deported (Veerakul, 1992).

Nitiya Thippayanuruksakul, director of a Bangkok shelter for abused women, said that Thai police at a northern border crossing told her a group of twenty Burmese prostitutes deported in 1991 from the shelter she directs were murdered by troops of Burma's military regime. "The police told us the girls were injected with something and buried," she said (Ostrom, 1992).

This and a similar incident were independently confirmed by the Institute on Women and Technology, according to Dr. Janice Raymond, associate director of the Institute and international coordinator of the Coalition Against Trafficking in Women.

9. HIV infection among women in prostitution in Africa and Asia: Fitzgerald, 1990; Mantell et al., 1988; Mann, 1991; *HAT News,* Aug. 1991.

10. Dr. June Osbourne: presentation at Women and AIDS breakfast at *Vogue* magazine offices, Oct. 19, 1990.

11. Anthony, 1992.

12. We might add as well a word on prurient conference organizing: soliciting and accepting papers on prostitutes-as-vectors for presentations at international AIDS conferences and leaving unaddressed almost all scientific issues concerning women in the AIDS epidemic.

13. On women in Puerto Rico not falling into the "woman with multiple sex partners" risk category, and on woman's ten times greater risk of HIV infection from intercourse: interview with Dr. Helen Rodriquez.

14. Beckman and Amaro, 1984, quoted in NIDA training manual: Rosenshine et. al, 1990.

15. Johnson's conviction was finally overturned by the Supreme Court of Florida July 23, 1992 (Lewin, Tamar, "Drug Verdict over Infants Is Voided," *New York Times,* July 24, 1992). On Florida appeals court upholding a drug-dealing conviction against a pregnant woman: Lewin, April 20, 1991; on Johnson having sought drug treatment and been turned away: Lewin, Feb. 5, 1990. Other sources on construction of reality in "fetal rights" and "fetal abuse" scenarios: Pollitt, 1990; OBN, Feb. 15–28, 1990; Chambers, Nov. 1, 1986; Lewin, Jan. 9, 1989; Roberts, Aug. 11, 1990; Kolder, Gallagher, and Parsons, May 7, 1987.

16. Williams, Oct. 17, 1990.

17. Ibid.

18. Weissman, 1991.

19. Rosenshine et al, 1990.

20. What is our *explicit* policy on ending drug addiction? It is a policy that ignores the demand in the United States for mood-altering drugs and the histories of severe sexual abuse lying beneath much of that demand. Drug suppliers in foreign lands far away are seen as causing the problem. The way to solve it, says the government, is to wage a war on drugs.

The Pentagon, now running out of enemies with the demise of the Cold War, has had its antinarcotics spending increased from $440 million in 1989 to a projected $1.2 billion in 1992. One phase of this war on drugs: The U.S. sends military trainers and equipment, in a $35 million American aid program, to Peru to help the Peruvian military (notorious for its human rights violations) fight cocaine traffickers. Though American officials have accused elements of the Peruvian army of taking payoffs from drug traffickers and of blocking Peruvian police efforts to interrupt the cocaine trade, the United States has decided it is preferable to pour money into this army than to provide drug treatment programs, including child care, for U.S. women who want treatment.

Source on U.S. aid plan to counter drug traffickers in Peru: Krauss, 1991, and Wicker, 1991. Also see Lizarazo, 1992, for U.S. military aid to Colombia in the "drug war."

21. Kinsella, 1989:193–203.

1988

....

1. Guinan and Hardy, Sept./Oct. 1987.

2. Norwood, 1990.

3. Kinsella, 1989:269.

4. Corea, 1985a.

5. Marte banded together with several other medical students and managed to win the dean's acceptance and the ob/gyn department's acquiescence to (though not approval of) the Gynecologic Teaching Associate Program. It involved training women, who often had a background in the women's health movement, to work in teams of two to teach the pelvic exam. With one of the women serving as the model, the team would demonstrate an exam to a group of three or four medical students, and then talk the students through the exam as each practiced it. Some male MDs in the Midwest also pushed for and got the GTA Program introduced in their medical schools. Source on teaching pelvic exams in medical schools: Corea, 1985a.

6. Cervical dysplasia is also called cervical intraepithelia neoplasia, or CIN, since it occurs in the epithelium, the surface layer of cells in the tissue. One grade of cervical dysplasia, CIN III, is severe dysplasia or carcinoma in situ.

7. Why is cervical cancer associated with poverty? It's not fully understood, Rachel Fruchter explains. Cervical cancer has been associated with sexually transmitted diseases, and the assumption has been that poor women were more likely to have intercourse earlier and have more partners. This assumption may no longer be true, but historically it has been the case. Possibly in early adolescence the cervix is more sensitive to trauma associated with infection. There are questions on whether other factors such as nutritional status might be involved but there's been no clear evidence on it. It's not clear how these various factors interact and whether the class phenomenon continues.

More affluent women are more likely to have pap smears and so have cervical abnormalities treated well before they progress to cancer.

8. About half the women with cervical cancer are over fifty.

9. In contrast, it had been easy to establish that men with HIV disease were susceptible to two cancers: Kaposi's sarcoma and B-cell lymphomas. Both cancers had a very low incidence before the HIV epidemic, so when they increased in young men, it showed up fast. With a very high rate in unmarried men in San Francisco, a quick extrapolation to gay men was possible.

But cervical cancer is one of the most common cancers in low-income women in precisely those areas—poor minority communities like Brooklyn—where there is a lot of HIV infection. That rate is going down (perhaps as a result of the preventative work Kings County had been doing), so in order to detect an increase in cervical cancer, there would first have to be a leveling off. In all of Brooklyn, there were about 160 new cases of cervical cancer a year, only half of them in young women. This cancer takes awhile to develop, so a good deal of time would be needed in order to detect an increase in cervical cancer that might be attributable to HIV.

Further complicating the difficulty of finding an association between cervical cancer and HIV is that no registry system for cervical dysplasia exists. So it is impossible to find out if the rate of cervical dysplasia has been increasing.

Before actually doing the study, this was the evidence Fruchter and Maiman could muster in support of their hypothesis that cervical cancer would be more common and more aggressive in women with HIV disease:

Several case histories of women who had died.

The fact that many of their younger women patients had been dying more rapidly in recent years. (But Fruchter and Maiman didn't know why; there could have been causes other than HIV.)

The anonymous survey showing an 11 percent HIV infection rate in the women at the Kings County colposcopy clinic. (But it was a retrospective survey on a limited number of patients.)

10. From the American Cancer Society, Maiman and Fruchter wanted funding for the position of a counselor for women before and after they were tested for HIV. Adequately done, such counseling is time-consuming.

With the grant money from the American Cancer Society, they did hire a counselor part-time.

11. Yet that same difficulty remained: it is precisely the women who are liable to get carcinoma in situ who are at risk for HIV.

Sources on cervical dysplasia/cervical cancer/HIV link: Stillman, 1987; Maiman et al., 1990; Maiman et al., 1991.

12. Sources on Mays and Cochran study: Cochran, 1989; Cochran and Mays, 1989; Cochran and Mays, 1990; Goleman, 1988.

13. The federal government had placed restrictions on AIDS education money through the Helms Amendment to an appropriations bill. That amendment, put forth in 1987 by the conservative Rep. Jesse Helms of North Carolina, barred the CDC from funding AIDS education, information, or prevention materials that could be interpreted as promoting or encouraging homosexuality or drug use.

Another problem with AIDS education was that there was much duplication of effort. No centralized registry existed where health providers and community groups could let others know what they were doing and what yet needed to be done.

14. Once the stories were developed, the script was read by addicted women and professionals working with them.

"Read this for believability," they were told.

Blair Durant, an African-American anthropologist with street smarts, worked with the writer to get the language just right.

After fine-tuning the script, they auditioned actors, shot the script, and edited the video.

The important ingredient in the model, Elkin believed, was in going to the source: the people the video was attempting to reach. The video worked because the community, researchers, and experienced media professionals collaborated.

1989

....

1. See BWHBC, 1992; Cohen and Estner, 1983; Corea, 1985a; Scully, 1980; Seaman and Seaman, 1977.

2. Helen Cover had lived with her boyfriend for many years and he had repeatedly tested negative for HIV, attorney Jack Lynch pointed out. So Cover must have been practicing "safe sex."

3. See Faludi, 1991, xiv. Ample evidence demonstrates the failure to protect the community of women from male violence. For example, see Jones, 1980, pp. 281–95; McNulty, 1980; Dworkin, 1981; Daly, 1978; Walker, 1989.

That evidence also includes testimony of female inmates at the state hearing on domestic violence and incarceration held at Bedford Hills in 1985 (CDVIW, 1987) and mentioned in Chapter 5.

One inmate, never convicted of a crime before killing the husband who had beaten and injured her repeatedly over nine years, testified: ". . . The police would come and he would talk his way out of being the cause of my injuries. If they did take him to the police station, his boss would get the charges dropped."

Another battered imprisoned woman testified: "A couple of times the police entered my home because of a 'domestic squabble.' They would take my husband to the nearest motel to cool off. I asked him that they make him leave his house key and was told, 'We can't do that.' I felt totally unprotected by the police department. I felt that they were giving my husband consent to come back and beat me some more after they left, and he did." He was never arrested (CDVIW, 1987).

The women's stories showed that when they had sought help from police, they had not received it. There was little outrage in police departments, courts, or the media over this threat to the community of women. In a report on the hearings at Bedford Hills, the Committee on Domestic Violence and Incarcerated Women commented that the battered woman must face the consequences of the message behind this police inaction: "that the violence against her is of no importance and will be ignored or trivialized (CDVIW, 1987)."

4. The Contagious Diseases Acts (CDA) of the 1860s in England required the forcible cleansing of women for soldiers' use. Prostitutes in nineteen English garrison towns were required to register, submit to periodic examination, and, if found diseased, be confined up to nine months in a "lock hospital." Only diseased women, not men, were locked up because the aim of the law was to protect male, not female, health. Physician William Acton said so outright in 1869 when he advocated the extension of the CDA to women in civilian towns "so as to protect our adult male population from the effects of syphilis."

In the United States, at the approach of World War I, government and civic officials urged the quarantine and internment of women arrested for prostitution to protect soldiers' health and therefore their "military efficiency." (Allan Brandt has documented this in *No Magic Bullet* [Brandt, 1987]). By March 1918, thirty-two states had passed laws requiring examination of these women for VD. The Department of Justice endorsed the regulations.

Again, the law was directed exclusively against women. The state made no effort to forcibly examine men's genitals and quarantine infected men.

Most courts upheld the laws. With hundreds of women sometimes arrested at a time, local jails filled quickly. In February 1918, President Woodrow Wilson allocated $250,000 from the National Security and Defense Fund to construct and maintain detention buildings for women. A few months later, Congress passed the Chamberlain-Kahn Bill providing $1 million to aid states in establishing "reformatories" for women "for the protection of military and naval forces of the United States against venereal disease." Most detention institutions did not allow visitors. Guards and barbed wire used at many detention centers ensured that the women could not get out.

Dr. W. F. Draper, director of the venereal detention hospital at Newport News, Virginia, argued for lifelong imprisonment of unreformable women who were, he said, "a far greater menace to the happiness and welfare of society than many murderers. . . ."

Dr. C. C. Pierce, director of the U.S. Public Health Service Division of Venereal Disease, also advocated "permanent custodial care" for prostitutes. In a 1919 lecture on VD control, he compared the woman in prostitution to a mosquito spreading yellow fever: Human hosts were more difficult to deal with than insect hosts because you couldn't kill the women. You had to be humane and simply imprison them for life.

The military policy on VD in World War II mirrored that of the First World War. Again, men conceptualized a one-way transmission of VD, from woman to man. In July 1941, the May Act became law. It made prostitution near military installations a federal offense. Again, women arrested for prostitution were subject to mandatory genital examinations and treatment under detention. Some thirty "civilian conservation camps" were created for imprisoning thousands of women, since the jails again overflowed.

When army physicians reported that women in prostitution represented only a minority of the soldiers' sexual contacts, army posters focused on the "promiscuous" girl as the new plague source. One federal committee noted of her: "She is more dangerous to the community than a mad dog. Rabies can be recognized. Gonorrhea and syphilis ordinarily cannot."

More than forty years later, Helen Cover, too, was treated as a plague source "more dangerous to the community than a mad dog." With the AIDS epidemic, it is clear that the view of woman as disease vector has not changed. The strategy of the nineteenth-century Contagious Diseases Act had been to keep prostitution intact as an institution by medicalizing it. Women were medically inspected and medically detained to protect the community of men. There is no more readiness today than there was then to abolish prostitution and the exploitation of women integral to prostitution.

5. Brandt, 1987.

6. Commenting on the nineteenth-century Contagious Diseases Act and

twentieth-century laws mandating pelvic examinations and internment of women arrested for prostitution, Dr. Janice Raymond notes that the system could easily have required that johns be examined. That practice would have stamped out sexually transmitted diseases much faster than examining women because it would have dismantled the institution of prostitution.

The same is true in the Helen Cover case, she observes. Making Cover a scapegoat responsible for the health of the male community keeps the prostitution system intact. It tries to exercise quality control over those women perceived to be contagious and likely to infect men. There's a simple answer to this particular contagion problem, Raymond points out: criminalize prostitution for men. Yet no one suggests that, except feminist groups that have long fought the sexual exploitation of women in prostitution.

7. Sources on Cover story include (in addition to interviews): Decker, 1987; Gigliotti and McQuat, Sept. 11, 1989; O'Brien, March 4, 1989; O'Brien, March 2, 1989; O'Hara, Jan. 29, 1989; O'Hara, Feb. 11, 1989; O'Hara, March 2, 1989; O'Hara, March 4, 1989; O'Hara, March 27, 1989a; O'Hara, March 27, 1989b; Porter, 1989.

8. Brandt, 1987.

9. " . . . As of 1986, there were no documented cases of AIDS transmitted through oral-genital sex," Porter argued. " . . . It has been noted that: 'The theory that prostitutes in the United States are a significant element in the spread of AIDS is likewise not supported by the evidence. . . . By conservative estimate, there are more than 200,000 female prostitutes in the United States, who engage in more than 300 million acts of prostitution annually. Yet, of the thousands of AIDS cases in the United States, not a single one has been definitively traced to prostitution. In short, although caution is in order, there is no justification for alarmist conclusions in light of current scientific evidence.'" (Porter, 1989.)

10. Repeated telephone calls to the district attorney's office for confirmation were unreturned.

11. Many women in cities like Kigali, Rwanda, where, by 1991, there would be a 30 percent HIV infection rate among adults, saw their survival tied to their production of children. As *New York Times* correspondent Jane Perlez reported, there are few sources of revenue for most women in Kigali, the main ones being prostitution and the sale of a few vegetables in front of their shack door:

"To escape these unappealing choices, women often choose to have a child in the belief—most often mistaken—that the man who fathers the baby will then provide support for mother and child."

Eugenie Makabutera, a social worker at the AIDS clinic in Kigali, explained that HIV-positive women, knowing their chances of bearing an infected child, choose to become pregnant. Makabutera told Perlez that most of the women were not legally married and depend on men:

"The women are frightened. If the man wants a child, the woman accepts. The woman thinks the men will continue to give money because of the child." But in most cases, the woman has miscalculated. The man leaves her.

African social workers like E. Maxine Ankrah at Makerere University in Kampala, Uganda, contend that the economic impoverishment of women combined with the sexual demands of men left women vulnerable to AIDS. "An unassailable facet of African culture—the customary and legal right of males to unlimited numbers of partners according to his wishes—would now be questioned," she wrote, adding, "and jettisoned." In a survey among 144 Ugandan women in 1989, Dr. Ankrah found that "because of their lack of decision-making power in matters of sex," as well as others factors, the women believed they faced a greater risk of HIV infection than men.

Clearly, technological solutions, without social justice for women, will never be enough to halt the epidemic. Still, a virucide is urgently needed to slow the spread of the virus. (Perlez, Oct. 28, 1990; Perlez, April 20, 1991.)

JANUARY–JUNE 1990

1. CDC, "Risk for cervical disease in HIV-infected women—New York City," *Morbidity and Mortality Weekly Report* 39(47):846–49.

2. Dooley Worth at congressional hearing, April 17. Legislation and National Security Subcommittee of the Committee on Government Operations.

3. Source, in addition to interviews, ACT UP, May 1991.

4. Sources, in addition to interviews, Ganley, Oct. 5, 1990; Meredith, Nov. 1990; Jennings and Galdwell, 1990.

5. S.P. et al., 1990.

6. These are the study results updated as of December 1990. Zierler et al., 1991, reported results at a slightly earlier stage of the study. These earlier results were:

Approximately half the women in the study reported that they had been raped or forced to have sex in their lifetime. Almost a third of these had been abused for the first time in childhood or teenage years.

Compared with the women who had not been assaulted, sexual assault survivors were more likely to be prescribed tranquilizers and to be heavy consumers of alcohol. They had, respectively, a 70 and an 80 percent excess use of tranquilizers and alcohol.

Childhood sexual abuse survivors were four times more likely to work in prostitution.

Zierler and her colleagues wrote: "We have evidence that early sexual abuse is associated with behavioral outcomes that may be having devastating effects on the public health, particularly in relation to the HIV epidemic. In our study, sexually abused women and men were more likely to engage in sex work, to change sexual partners frequently, and to engage in sexual activities with casual acquaintances than people who were never sexually abused. Women survivors of sexual assault reported more frequent use of large quantities of alcoholic beverages and both genders used tranquilizers more frequently than individuals who had never been assaulted.

"The disturbing prevalence of early sexual abuse and its possible consequences on increasing behaviors that could lead to HIV infection and other poor health outcomes have implications for medical and public health practitioners."

One implication: "Safer sex" messages instructing women to interview potential lovers on their sexual and drug-using past and persuade them to use condoms were not terribly relevant to women being knocked to the ground and sexually assaulted. Nor were "safer sex" messages relevant in the situations (never called "rape") in which women did not feel free to say what they wanted or did not want sexually. The assumption that sex for women was always consensual was ill-founded.

7. The study did not find a difference in intravenous drug use between sexually assaulted women and others. This was surprising. Many studies have found a high association of chemical substance use and sexual assault, Zierler knew. One motivation for substance use was a continuing need to be numbed from the experience of sexual assault. Zierler speculated that more women may report previous sexual assault only after they go into recovery from their addiction and become clearer.

8. Zierler et al., 1991.

JULY–NOVEMBER 1990

·····························

1. On the National Academy of Science book, see: Chavkin et al., Jan. 25, 1991; Miller, Turner, and Moses, 1990.

2. On studies on the endocrine system in HIV disease not focusing on women: interview with Dr. Patricia Warne of the HIV Center; Dobs, Dempsey, Ladenson, and Polk, 1988; Croxson, Chapman, Mill, Levit, Senie, and Zumoff, 1989. The study that excluded the six women from the analysis of sex hormone data: Merenich, McDermott, Asp, Harrison, and Kidd, 1990.

3. The reviewers also questioned whether the study would provide new information because it had no "comparison group." But the Center felt fully justified in limiting the study to inner-city women rather than including a white, middle-class group. More than 70 percent of women with AIDS in the United States were then African-American or Hispanic; in New York City, more than 84 percent.

4. ". . . Knowing one is HIV-positive can be a terrific 'memory aid,' both for recalling specific instances of past promiscuous behavior and for making an overall judgment about it," the reviewers wrote. "Given the stress the subjects will be experiencing, they may be even more prone to 'make sense' of their current situation by selective retrospective recall. . . ."

Researchers would ask the women about their medical and medication histories.

"Again," the reviewers wrote, "it is unlikely that this will be accurately reported by the subjects since the names given to illnesses and the illnesses themselves are culturally bound and often inconsistent with traditional definitions of illness."

5. The reports by Drs. Carpenter, Kloster, Mitchell, and Zorilla were all given at the conference on women and HIV run by the Public Health Service in Washington, D.C., Dec. 1990.

6. Berkelman presentation at Public Health Service conference on women and HIV in Washington, D.C., Dec. 1990.

7. For example, the definition included herpes simplex with an ulcer that lasts more than a month and diarrhea that lasts more than a month. Why couldn't CDC add similar caveats to distinguish the kind of vaginal candidiasis appearing in a woman who is immunosuppressed? A caveat indicating that the candidiasis is recurring and resistant to treatment? Didn't they think physicians

were able to differentiate between a common disorder and that same disorder appearing when something else—immunosuppression—was at play?

Furthermore, since all women are getting these diseases, Maxine Wolfe pointed out, then we know what "normal" is and also know what "abnormal" is—how these same conditions appear in women with an impaired immune system.

"You don't have to be a genius to understand that," Wolfe impatiently told the CDC officials at the meeting. "I don't get it. It's a way of dismissing things. It's just like saying, 'We don't have to take care of this because it's too prevalent.'"

8. For example, oophorectomy (female castration) can be merely good preventive health care, sparing the woman future ovarian cancer by excising the ovaries. Just as prophylactic mastectomies prevent breast cancer by simply cutting off healthy breasts. See Corea, 1985a; Hynes, 1990; Scully, 1980; BWHBC, 1992; Seaman and Seaman, 1977.

9. Nor need they fear that if they added severe, recurring vaginal candidiasis unresponsive to treatment to the CDC AIDS definition, physicians would suddenly rush to report ordinary cases of candidiasis as AIDS, the activists said.

As it was, physicians were reluctant to make an AIDS diagnosis in their patients, one condition that led to an undercount of women with AIDS. CDC trusted the clinical judgment of physicians in other instances, for example, judging whether a condition was "*with* an AIDS-like disease" or "*due to* an AIDS-like disease."

". . . But somehow, when we get to women, no one is willing to trust that clinical decision. Somehow we can't come up with a way to phrase it that would be acceptable . . . ," Wolfe said. "I can't believe it's impossible to do. Medicine is not an exact science and yet we've learned to live with it, in its inexactness, for men, but we can't figure out how to do it under this circumstance [i.e., with women]. . . . "

10. It was fascinating to Maxine Wolfe that the issue of vaginal candidiasis made the CDC people so crazy. Many HIV-infected women ACT UP had worked with had told them how frustrating it was to try to explain to a medical or social service professional, even another woman, that they had a vaginal yeast infection that would not go away and that was so severe they could not work. Professionals would laugh at the women.

They dismissed it as "just a little thing." Yet thrush in men was serious, worthy of inclusion in the AIDS definition, even though it was, in most cases, easier to deal with than vaginal candidiasis. Again, male suffering was serious suffering. Female suffering provided comic relief.

11. Source, in addition to interviews: Sprecher, Dec. 1990.

12. On plans for federal conference on women and HIV infection: Meredith, 1990; Ryan, 1990. Correspondence between NIAID and ACT UP, Aug. 13 and 21, 1990; Sept. 13, 1990; Nov. 5, 25, and 26, 1990.

DECEMBER 1990

1. The lack of a study for women comparable to the MACS for men would slow up medical and government actions to benefit HIV-infected women because results coming in from a study in one geographic location would have to be repeated and confirmed at other sites (a time-consuming process) before they would affect policy. For men, with the MACS studies going on simultaneously in several different sites, results could be rapidly confirmed and acted upon.

By 1991, $80 million had been spent on studying the natural history of HIV disease in men. That same year, CDC reported that it had allocated approximately $4.5 million in fiscal year 1991 to conduct studies in women and a similar amount for the following year (HRIRS, 1992:117).

In 1993, NIAID plans to begin recruiting women into a fund-starved women's natural history study of HIV. At congressional hearings on women and HIV disease in June 1991, Dr. Fauci gave no exact figures on how much would be spent on the women's "MACS" study. In questioning him, Rep. Ted Weiss of New York observed: "NIAID staff stated at a recent meeting that one of the problems with current epidemiology research on women is difficulties in resource allocation. I guess this means you don't have the funds to do an adequate study. Is that true?"

Fauci replied: "That is a rather convoluted way of saying that, yes, sir." (HRIRS, 1992:116–17.)

2. The legislation supported by the Center for Women Policy Studies, updated as of 1991, includes the following bills:

a. Women and AIDS Research Initiative (H.R. 1078). Rep. Constance Morella (R-MD).
—Authorizes additional, targeted funds for the NIH and the Alcohol, Drug Abuse and Mental Health Administration (ADAMHA) to conduct woman-focused AIDS research.
—Creates a new program under the community-based Clinical Research Initiative to expand clinical trials of AIDS treatments for

women. Funds for expenses such as child care and transportation are included so that low-income women can participate.

b. Women and AIDS Outreach and Prevention Act (H.R. 1072). Rep. Constance Morella (R-MD).
—Authorizes additional funds for HIV prevention and education efforts to health-care providers that already serve low-income women—including family planning clinics, community health centers, and other women's health providers, in areas with high HIV infection rates.
—Funds will improve outreach to women and women's access to HIV testing and woman-focused counseling, increase access to other preventive health services, and cover funding for referrals for treatment for HIV disease, substance abuse, pregnancy, and housing.

c. Social Security and SSI AIDS Disability Act of 1991 (H.R. 2299) Rep. Robert Matsui (D-CA).
—Requires the Social Security Administration to adopt an interim definition of HIV disability that includes symptomatology of women, IV drug users, and children rather than using the CDC AIDS definition for determining who is disabled and eligible for Social Security benefits.
—Provides that women will no longer be denied immediate Supplemental Security Income (SSI) because they do not exhibit CDC-defined conditions.
—Mandates that a panel of experts study and recommend to Congress changes in the current evaluation of disability in all HIV-positive individuals so that all these individuals who develop serious AIDS-related conditions are eligibile for benefits.

3. See Corea, 1985b, for information on male research challenging the current reality that new life cannot be created without live women.

AFTERWORD

....

1. Navarro, Aug. 8, 1991; Navarro, July 8, 1991; Navarro, Feb. 10, 1992.

2. An international meeting of experts held by the Coalition Against Trafficking in Women with UNESCO in 1991 at the State College of Pennsylvania explains in *The Penn State Report:* "Sexual exploitation involves the use of sex to dehumanize another by objectifying human beings, reducing and

equating them to sex and nothing more, thereby violating their human dignity. Sexual exploitation threatens the integrity of women's identity and promotes devaluation of women's self-worth. . . ."

Introducing a new concept of prostitution under the umbrella of sexual exploitation, the *Report* further states: "The sexual exploitation of women through prostitution victimizes women both within and outside prostitution. When prostitution is accepted and normalized, what is legitimized is the sale of body and sex of the individual prostitute and it is the sale of any woman. By reducing women to a commodity to be bought, sold, appropriated, exchanged, or acquired, prostitution affects women as a group. It reinforces the societal equation of women to sex which reduces women to being less than human, and contributes to sustaining women's second class status throughout the world."

The Penn State Report calls on states to protect against sexual exploitation of women from production or dissemination of pornography by recognizing that according to Article 30 of the International Declaration of Human Rights, one right (freedom of speech) cannot be used to usurp the right to human dignity and equality (UNESCO and the Coalition Against Trafficking in Women, 1992:7–8).

Pornography, using images of women in subordination to trigger orgasms, makes inequality sexy. It teaches men not just in their minds, but *in their very bodies* that women are subordinate, law professor Catharine MacKinnon and writer Andrea Dworkin explain.

They write: "Each time men are sexually aroused to pornography—the sexually explicit subordination of women—they learn to connect women's sexual pleasure to abuse and women's sexual nature to inferiority. They learn this in their bodies, not just their minds, so that it becomes a physical, seemingly natural response. When real women claim not to want inequality or force, they are not credible compared with the continually sexually available 'real women' in pornography."

As MacKinnon further explained in an interview: " . . . Pornography makes inequality sexy. It makes it sex. Every time men masturbate and come to the subordination of women, their body learns: this is sex, this is a real woman."

See: Dworkin and MacKinnon, 1988; Dworkin, 1979; Leidholdt and Raymond, 1990.

3. In the United States, the CDC estimated in 1991 that 80,000 to 100,000 women are HIV infected. During the 1980s, 25 percent of AIDS cases in adults worldwide were women, but in 1990 to 1991 alone, that figure jumped to 40 percent. By the year 2000, the ratio will be reversed, with 60 percent of HIV infections among women and children and 40 percent among adult men. Globally, the spread of HIV by heterosexuals will likely

represent 75 to 80 percent of HIV transmission in the 1990s, predicts Dr. Jonathan Mann, director of the International AIDS Center of Harvard AIDS Institute in Boston and from 1986 to 1990 director of the World Health Organization's Global Program on AIDS.

Mann also warns: "Regardless of which people, with whatever behaviors, were first affected in a community, HIV has demonstrated its ability to cross all social, cultural, economic and political borders. The HIV pandemic is in the process of reaching all human communities. . . . The decade of the 1990s will be much more difficult [in the HIV pandemic] than the very hard 1980s have been. HIV and all the problems it entails is an accelerating problem, gaining momentum worldwide."

BIBLIOGRAPHY

ACT UP/New York Women and AIDS Book Group. 1990. *Women, AIDS and Activism.* South End Press, Boston.

ACT UP DC. 1990, September. Denial of Social Security Benefits to Women with HIV/AIDS Due to the Use of the Centers for Disease Control's Definition of AIDS: A Briefing Paper. Unpublished.

ACT UP. 1991, May. Treatment and Research Agenda for Women with HIV Infection. (For copy, contact: ACT UP/NY, 135 W. 29th Street, #10, New York, NY 10001.)

AIDS hooker is back in jail. 1984, March 13. *New Haven Register.*

Altman, Lawrence K. 1991, July 29. U.S. plans aspirin study of women. *New York Times.*

Amaro, Hortensia. 1990. Women's reproductive rights in the age of AIDS: new threats to informed consent. In *From Abortion to Reproductive Freedom: Transforming a Movement.* M. Gerber Fried, editor. South End Press, Boston.

Anastos, Kathryn, and Carola Marte. 1989, Winter. Women—the missing persons in the AIDS epidemic. *Health/PAC Bulletin:* 6–13.

Anthony, Jane. 1992, January/February. Prostitution as "choice." *Ms.*

Barbuto, Joan. 1984, January 23. AIDS risk: prostitute suspected as carrier. *New Haven Register:*1.

Barry, Kathleen. 1987. *Female Sexual Slavery.* New York University Press, New York.

Becker, M. H., and J. G. Joseph. 1988. AIDS and behavioral change to reduce risk: a review. *American Journal of Public Health.* 78:394–410.

Beckman, L. J., and H. Amaro. 1984. Patterns of women's use of alcohol treatment agencies. In: Wilsnack, S. C., and L. J. Beckman, eds. *Alcohol Problems in Women: Antecedents, Consequences and Intervention.* The Guilford Press, New York.

Berkelman, Ruth L., William L. Heyward, Jeanette K. Stehr-Green, and James W. Curran. 1989, June. Epidemiology of human immunodeficiency virus infection and acquired immunodeficiency syndrome. *The American Journal of Medicine.* 86:761–70.

Bolling, D. R., and B. Voller. 1987. AIDS and heterosexual anal intercourse. *Journal of the American Medical Association.* 258:474.

Boston Women's Health Book Collective (BWHBC). 1992. *The New Our Bodies, Ourselves: Updated and Expanded for the Nineties.* Simon & Schuster, New York.

Bowser, Benjamin P., Mindy Thompson Fullilove, and Robert E. Fullilove. 1990. African-American youth and AIDS high-risk behavior. *Youth & Society.* 22(1):54–66.

Brandt, Allan M. 1987. *No Magic Bullet: A Social History of Venereal Disease in the United States Since 1880.* Oxford University Press, New York, Oxford.

Brody, Jane E. 1989, February 26. Who's having sex? Data are obsolete, experts say. *The New York Times.*

Byron, Peg. 1991, January/February. HIV: The national scandal. *Ms.:* 24–29.

Cauley, Kate, Linda Demkovich, and Caitlin C. Ryan, eds. 1990, October. AIDS and HIV in women: state legislative initiatives. *Intergovernmental AIDS Reports.* 3(7):1–5.

CDVIW (Committee on Domestic Violence and Incarcerated Women). 1987, June. *A Report of the Committee on Domestic Violence and Incarcerated Women: Battered Women and Criminal Justice.* Copies of the report may be obtained from Ruth Cassell and David Leven, Prisoners' Legal Services of New York, 105 Chambers Street, New York, NY 10007; Sister Mary Nerney, STEPS to End Family Violence, 104 East 107th Street, New York, New York 10029.

Chambers, Marcia. 1986, November 1. Are fetal rights equal to infants'? *The New York Times*.

Chavkin, Wendy, Judith Cohen, Anke A. Ehrhardt, Mindy Thompson Fullilove, and Dooley Worth. 1991, January 25. Women and AIDS. *Science* (251):359–60.

Chu, Susan Y., James W. Buehler, Patricia L. Fleming, and Ruth L. Berkelman. 1990, November. Epidemiology of reported cases of AIDS in lesbians, United States 1980–89. *American Journal of Public Health*. 80(11):1380–81.

Chu, Susan Y., James W. Buehler, and Ruth L. Berkelman. 1990. July 11. Impact of the human immunodeficiency virus epidemic on mortality in women of reproductive age, United States. *Journal of the American Medical Association*. 264(2):225–29.

Clark, Judy, and Kathy Boudin. 1990. Community of women organize themselves to cope with the AIDS crisis: a case study from Bedford Hills Correctional Facility. *Social Justice:* 17(2):90–109.

Cochran, Susan D. 1989. Women and HIV infection: issues in prevention and behavior change. In: *Primary Prevention of AIDS*. Vickie M. Mays, George W. Albee, and Stanley F. Schneider, eds. Sage Publications, Newbury Park.

———, and Vickie M. Mays. 1989, March. Women and AIDS-related concerns. *American Psychologist:* 44(3):529–35.

———. 1990, March 15. Sex, lies and HIV. *The New England Journal of Medicine*. Vol. 322(11):774–75.

Cohen, Nancy Wainer, and Lois J. Estner. 1983. *Silent Knife: Cesarean Prevention and Vaginal Birth after Cesarean*. Bergin & Garvey Publishers, Inc., South Hadley, Mass.

Corea, Gena. 1985a. *The Hidden Malpractice: How American Medicine Mistreats Women as Patients and Professionals*. Harper & Row, New York.

———. 1985b. *The Mother Machine: Reproductive Technologies from Artificial Insemination to the Artificial Womb*. Harper & Row, New York.

Croxson, Thomas S., William F. Chapman, Lorraine K. Miller, Charles D. Levit, Ruby Senie, and Barnett Zumoff. 1989. Changes in the hypothalamic-pituitary-gonadal axis in human immunodeficiency virus–infected homosexual men. *Journal of Clinical Endocrine Metabolism*. 68:317–21.

CWPS. 1991, February 27. Proposal for renewal grant to support the Center for Women Policy Studies' National Resource Center on Women and AIDS. Unpublished.

Daly, Mary. 1978. *Gyn/Ecology.* Beacon Press, Boston.

Decker, J. 1987. Prostitution as a public health issue. In H. L. Dalton, ed., *AIDS and the Law:* 81–84. Yale University Press, New Haven.

Dobs, Adrian S., Michael Dempsey, Paul W. Ladenson, and B. Frank Polk. 1988. Endocrine disorders in men infected with human immunodeficiency virus. *American Journal of Medicine.* 84:611–16.

Dworkin, Andrea. 1981. *Our Blood.* Perigee Books, New York.

———. 1979. *Pornography: Men Possessing Women.* G.P. Putnam's Sons, New York.

———. 1991. *Mercy.* Four Walls Eight Windows, New York.

Dworkin, Andrea, and Catharine A. MacKinnon. 1988. *Pornography and Civil Rights: A New Day for Women's Equality.* Organizing Against Pornography: A Resource Center for Education and Action, Minneapolis.

Ehrhardt, Anke A. 1988, July–August. Preventing and treating AIDS: The expertise of the behavioral sciences. *Bulletin of the New York Academy of Medicine.* (64)6:513–19.

Eisenberg, Carola. 1989, November 30. Sounding board: Medicine is no longer a man's profession. *New England Journal of Medicine* (321)22:1542–44.

Ellerock, Tedd V., and Martha F. Rogers. 1990, September. Epidemiology of human immunodeficiency virus infection in women in the United States. *Obstetrics and Gynecology Clinics of North America.* 17(3):523–43.

Faludi, Susan. 1991. *Backlash: The Undeclared War Against American Women.* Crown Publishers, New York.

Feingold, Anat R., Sten H. Vermund, Robert D. Burk, Karen F. Kelley, Lewis K. Schrager, Klaus Schreiber, Gary Munk, Gerald H. Friedland, and Robert S. Klein. 1990. Cervical cytologic abnormalities and papillomavirus in women infected with human immunodeficiency virus. *Journal of Acquired Immune Deficiency Syndromes.* 3:896–903.

Fitzgerald, Mary Anne. 1990, October 27. A red light against AIDS. *New Scientist:* 51.

Flam, Robin, and Zena Stein. 1986. Behavior, infection, and immune response: an epidemiological approach. In: Feldman, D. A., and T. M. Johnson, eds. *The Social Dimension of AIDS: Methods and Theory.* Praeger Press, New York.

Frankfort, Ellen. 1983. *Kathy Boudin and the Dance of Death.* Stein and Day, Briarcliff Manor, New York.

Fullilove, Mindy Thompson. 1990, June 22. Epidemiology and primary prevention of AIDS among adolescents. Paper presented at the Sixth International Conference on AIDS.

Fullilove, Mindy Thompson, Robert E. Fullilove II, Katherine Haynes, and Shirley Gross. 1990, February. Black women and AIDS prevention: a view towards understanding the gender rules. *The Journal of Sex Research.* 27(1):47–64.

Fullilove, Robert E., Mindy Thompson Fullilove, Benjamin P. Bowser, and Shirley A. Gross. 1990, February 9. Risk of sexually transmitted disease among black adolescent crack users in Oakland and San Francisco, Calif. *Journal of the American Medical Association.* 263(6):851–55.

Ganley, Susan. 1990, October 5. Protesters say policies are killing women with AIDS. *The Washington Blade.*

Gardiner-Caldwell SynerMed. 1991, August. U.S. Public Health Service National Conference, Women and HIV Infection. *Clinical Courier,* 9(6).

Garnett, Lynne. 1984, January 23. Debate now centers on quarantine issue. *New Haven Register.*

Gigliotti, Anthony J., and Howard J. McQuat. 1989, September 11. State of New York, Supreme Court, Appellate Division. *The People of the State of New York, respondent,* v. *Helen Cover, appellant.* Indictment No. 87-680-1. Index No. 87-577 (criminal). The People's Brief.

Gillespie, Marcia Ann. 1991, January/February. HIV: The Global Crisis. *Ms.:*16–22.

Gross, Jane. 1991, July 14. Female surgeon's quitting touches nerve at medical schools. *New York Times.*

Guilfoy, Christine. 1984, March 24. Media indicts woman rumored to have AIDS. *Gay Community News* (Boston).

Guinan, Mary E. 1989, July/August. Women and crack addiction. *Journal of the American Medical Women's Association.*

————. 1987, November/December. Women, children and AIDS. *Journal of the American Medical Women's Association.*

Guinan, Mary E., and Ann Hardy. 1987, September/October. Women and AIDS: The future is grim. *Journal of the American Medical Women's Association.*

————. 1987. Epidemiology of AIDS in women in the United States. *Journal of the American Medical Women's Association.* 257(15):2039–42.

Gunn, A. E. 1988. The CDC and abortion in HIV-positive women. Letter to the Editor. *Journal of the American Medical Association.* 259(27):217–218.

Hager, George. 1989, August 19. Every voter's a critic on arts funding. *Congressional Quarterly Weekly Report.* Vol. 47:2174–76.

HAI News. 1991, August. AIDS and the sex industry. 60:7.

Hamm, Steve. 1984, February 15. Prostitute fears for safety. *New Haven Register.*

————. 1984, March 21. Deal alleged in AIDS case. *New Haven Register.*

Hearst, N., and S. B. Hulley. 1988. Preventing the heterosexual spread of AIDS. Are we giving our patients the best advice? *Journal of the American Medical Association.* 259:2428–32.

Hilts, Philip J. 1990, September 11. N.I.H. starts women's health office. *New York Times.*

————. 1991, May 7. Lab mix-ups fueled dispute on discovery of AIDS virus. *The New York Times.*

————. 1991, September 10. Women still behind in medicine. *New York Times.*

————. 1991, September 15. Censure is urged for AIDS scientist. *New York Times.*

Hladky, Gregory B. 1984, February 18. Prostitute warned to stay in hospital. *New Haven Register.*

HRIRS. Human Resources and Intergovernmental Relations Subcommittee of the Committee on Government Operations, House of Representatives, 102nd Congress. 1992. *Women and HIV Disease: Falling Through the Cracks.* U.S. Government Printing Office, Washington, D.C.

Hynes, H. Patricia. 1989. *The Recurring Silent Spring*. The Athene Series. Pergamon Press, Elmsford, N.Y.

―――. 1991. *Reconstructing Babylon: Essays on Women and Technology*. Indiana University Press, Bloomington, Indianapolis.

Jones, Ann. 1980. *Women Who Kill*. Holt, Rinehart, and Winston. New York.

Kasl, Charlotte Davis. 1989. *Women, Sex and Addiction*. Harper & Row. New York.

Kinsella, James. 1989. *Covering the Plague: AIDS and the American Media*. Rutgers University Press, New Brunswick and London.

Kolata, Gina. 1991, August 25. U.S. rule on fetal studies hampers research on AZT. *New York Times*.

Kolberg, Rebecca. 1990, October. AIDS activists target Social Security. UPI.

Kolder, Veronika E. B., Janet Gallagher, and Michael T. Parsons. 1987, May 7. Court-ordered obstetrical interventions. *New England Journal of Medicine*. 316(19):1192–96.

Krauss, Clifford. 1991, August 7. U.S. military team to advise Peru in war against drugs and rebels. *New York Times*.

―――. 1992, January 25. In shift, U.S. will aid Peru's army against drugs and rebels. *New York Times*.

Leidholdt, Dorcheen, and Janice G. Raymond, eds. 1990. *Sexual Liberals and the Attack on Feminism*. Pergamon Press, New York.

Lewin, Tamar. 1989, January 9. When courts take charge of the unborn. *New York Times*.

―――. 1990, February 5. Drug use in pregnancy new issue for the courts. *New York Times*.

―――. 1991, April 20. Appeals court in Florida backs guilt for drug delivery by umbilical cord. *New York Times*.

Lizarazo, Jorge Gomez. 1992, January 28. Colombian blood, U.S. guns. *New York Times*.

MacKinnon, Catharine A. 1987. *Feminism Unmodified*. Harvard University Press, Cambridge Mass.

Maiman, Mitchell, Rachel G. Fruchter, Eli Serur, and John G. Boyce. Prevalence of human immunodeficiency virus in a colposcopy clinic. *Journal of the American Medical Association.* 1988.

Maiman, Mitchell, Rachel G. Fruchter, Eli Serur, Jean Claude Remy, Ferald Feuer, and John Boyce. Human immunodeficiency virus infection and cervical neoplasia. *Gynecologic Oncology.* 1990. 38:377–82.

Maiman, Mitchell, Nicholas Tarricone, Jeffrey Vieira, Jorge Suarez, Eli Serur, and John G. Boyce. 1991, July. Colposcopic evaluation of human immunodeficiency virus–seropositive women. *Obstetrics and Gynecology.* 78(1):84–88.

Mann, Jonathan M. 1991, April 20. AIDS and women: A global perspective. Unpublished typescript.

Mantell, J. E., S. P. Schinke, and S. H. Akabas. 1988. Women and AIDS prevention. *Journal of Primary Prevention,* 9(1&2):18–40.

Marte, Carola, and Kathryn Anastos. 1990, Spring. Women—the missing persons in the AIDS epidemic. Part II. *Health/PAC Bulletin:* 11–18.

Mays, Vickie M., and Susan D. Cochran. March–April 1987. Acquired immunodeficiency syndrome and black Americans: special psychosocial issues. *Public Health Reports.* 102(2):224–31.

———. 1988, November. Issues in the perception of AIDS risk and risk reduction activities by black and Hispanic/Latina women. *American Psychologist.* Vol. 43(11):949–57.

McNulty, Faith. 1980. *The Burning Bed.* Bantam Books, New York.

Meredith, Linda. 1990, November. Actions targeting NIAID result in conference on women. *ACT UP/DC FRONTLINES:* 4.

Merenich, John A., and Michael T. McDermott, Arnold A. Asp, Shannon M. Harrison, and Gerald S. Kidd. 1990. Evidence of endocrine involvement early in the course of human immunodeficiency virus infection. *Journal of Clinical Endocrine Metabolism.* 70:566–71.

Mesce, Deborah. 1990, October. Eighteen arrested for protesting lack of benefits for women AIDS victims. Associated Press.

Meyer-Bahlburg, Heino F. L., Theresa M. Exner, Gerda Lorenz, Rhoda S. Gruen, Jack M. Gorman, and Anke A. Ehrhardt. 1991, February. Sexual risk behavior, sexual functioning, and HIV disease progression in gay men. *The Journal of Sex Research.* 28(1):3–27.

Miller, H. G., C. F. Turner, and L. E. Moses. 1990. *AIDS: The Second Decade*. National Academy Press, Washington, D.C.

Minkoff, H. L. 1987. Care of pregnant women infected with human immunodeficiency virus. *Journal of the American Medical Association*. 258(19):2712–17.

———, and Jack A. DeHovitz. 1991, October 23/30. Care of women infected with the human immunodeficiency virus. *Journal of the American Medical Association*. 266(16):2253–58.

Mitchell, Janet L. 1988. Women, AIDS, and public policy. *AIDS and Public Policy Journal* (3)2:50–52.

Morgan, Robin. 1989. *The Demon Lover: On the Sexuality of Terrorism*. W.W. Norton & Co., New York.

National Commission on AIDS. 1991, March. Report: *HIV Disease in Correctional Facilities*.

Navarro, Mireya. 1991, July 8. Dated AIDS definition keeps benefits from many patients. *New York Times*.

———. 1991, August 8. U.S. widens rules on who has AIDS. *New York Times*.

———. 1992, February 10. Agencies slowed in effort to widen definitions of AIDS. *New York Times*.

Nelson, Chris. 1990, October 7–October 13. Actions focus on women with AIDS/HIV. *Gay Community News*. 18 (13):1.

Newman, A. 1987. Patterns in AIDS spread elicit proposal to tighten precautions for involuntary sterilizations. *Obstetrics and Gynecology*. 22 (12):1. 36–37.

New York City Commission on Human Rights (NYCCHR). November 1983–April 1986. *Report on Discrimination Against People with AIDS*. Typescript.

New York City Commission on Human Rights (NYCCHR), the AIDS Discrimination Unit. January 1986–August 1987. *Report on Discrimination Against People with AIDS and People Perceived to Have AIDS*. Typescript.

New York City Commission on Human Rights (NYCCHR), the AIDS Discrimination Unit. August 1987. *AIDS and People of Color: The Discriminatory Impact*. Typescript.

New York Times. 1991, July 26. Take women's health to heart (editorial). *New York Times.*

New York Times. 1991, June 4. Citing sexism, Stanford doctor quits. *New York Times.*

New York Times. 1991, September 9. Toward healthy women (editorial). *New York Times.*

Norwood, Chris. 1987. *Advice for Life: A Woman's Guide to AIDS.* Pantheon Books, New York.

———. 1988, November/December. Women and the "hidden" AIDS epidemic. *The Network News.*

———. 1990, May. Media coverage of women and AIDS. In *The Guide to Resources on Women and AIDS.* Center for Women Policy Studies, Washington, D.C.

Nova Research. 1990. Preventing AIDS among female sexual partners of injection drug users. NOVA Research Co., Bethesda, Maryland. (The training manual is based on an AIDS prevention model developed by Nancy Rosenshine, Barbara Sowder, and Peggy L. Young, principal investigators.)

O'Brien, John. 1989, March 2. Lawyer says prison term can worsen client's AIDS. *Syracuse Post-Standard.*

———. 1989, March 4. Judge sends victim of AIDS to prison. *Syracuse Post-Standard.*

OGN. 1990, February 15–28. Laws on fetal abuse expected to erode trust in MDs and deter prenatal care. *Ob/Gyn News.*

O'Hara, Jim. 1989, January 29. Prostitution suspect has AIDS; officials try to keep her jailed. *Syracuse Herald American.*

———. 1989, February 11. Wildridge wants stiff penalties for those who spread AIDS. *Syracuse Herald-Journal.*

———. 1989, March 2. AIDS victim faces up to 7 years in prison. *Syracuse Herald-Journal.*

———. 1989, March 4. Woman with AIDS sentenced to prison. *Syracuse Herald-Journal.*

———. 1989, March 27. Dreams shattered, Helen Cover lives to show kids her mistakes. *Syracuse Herald-Journal.*

———. 1989, March 27. State group is monitoring Cover's case. *Syracuse Herald-Journal.*

Ostrom, Neenyah. 1992, April 27. Prostitutes injected with cyanide in Burma. *New York Native.*

Perlez, Jane. 1990, October 28. Toll of AIDS on Uganda's women puts their roles and rights in question. *New York Times.*

———. 1991, April 21. AIDS outweighed by the desire to have a child. *New York Times.*

Pollitt, Katha. 1990, March 26. "Fetal Rights": A new assault on feminism. *The Nation:* 409–17.

Poole, Teresa. 1992, March 9. Burmese girls sold into sex slavery. *The Independent.*

Porter, Scott J. 1989. State of New York Supreme Court, Appellate Division, Fourth Department, *The People of the State of New York, respondent,* v *Helen S. Cover, appellant.* Brief for appellant. Indictment No. 87-680-1. Index No. 87-577. Syracuse.

Reid, Elizabeth. In press. The development implications of the AIDS epidemic in Africa. In *AIDS in Africa and the Caribbean: The Documentation of an Epidemic.* George C. Bond, John Kreniske, Ida S. Susser, and Joan Vincent, eds. Institute of African Studies and the HIV Center, New York.

Richardson, Diane. 1988. *Women and AIDS.* Methuen Press, New York.

Rieder, Ines, and Patricia Ruppelt, eds. 1988. *AIDS: The Women.* Cleis Press, San Francisco.

Roberts, Dorothy. 1990, August 11. The bias in drug arrests of pregnant women. *New York Times.*

Scully, Diana. 1980. *Men Who Control Women's Health: The Miseducation of Obstetricians-Gynecologists.* Houghton Mifflin Company, Boston.

Seaman, Barbara, and Gideon Seaman. 1977. *Women and the Crisis in Sex Hormones.* Rawson Associates Publishers, Inc., New York.

Selik, Richard M., Ann M. Hardy, and James W. Curran. 1989. Epidemiology of AIDS and HIV infection in women in the United States. *Clinical Practice of Gynecology.* 1:33–42.

Selwyn, P. A., E. E. Schoenbaum, K. Davenyy, V. J. Robertson, A. R. Feingold, J. F. Shulman, M. M. Mayers, R. Klein, G. H. Friedland, and M. F. Rogers. 1989. Prospective study of human immunodeficiency virus infection and pregnancy outcomes in intravenous drug users. *Journal of the American Medical Association.* 261(9):1289–94.

Shilts, Randy. 1987. *And the Band Played On.* Penguin Books, New York.

S.P., M.C., K.P., R.G., G.S., M.X.C., C.M., R.C., D.C., L.K., and P.S. On behalf of themselves and all others similarly situated, plaintiffs, against Louis W. Sullivan, M.D., Secretary of the United States Department of Health and Human Services, defendant. 1990. 90 Civ. 6294 (MGC). Second amended class action complaint. United States District Court, Southern District of New York.

Spender, Dale. 1980. *Man-Made Language.* Routledge & Kegan Paul, London.

Sprecher, Lorrie. 1990, December. Women with AIDS: dead but not disabled. *The Positive Woman: A Newsletter by, for and About the HIV-Positive Woman* 1(2):4. (Available from P.O. Box 33061, Washington, D.C. 20033-0061.]

Stein, Zena A. 1990. HIV prevention: the need for methods women can use. *American Journal of Public Health.* 80:460–462.

Stemerding, Beatrijs, and Conchita de Roba. 1991, April-June. Women and AIDS: The Seventh International Conference on AIDS. *Women's Global Network of Reproductive Rights Newsletter.* 35:33.

Stephens, P. Clay. 1988. Women and AIDS in the U.S. *New England Journal of Public Policy.* 4(1):381–401.

Stillman, Frederick H., and Alexander Sedlis. 1987, June. Anogenital papillomavirus infection and neoplasia in immunodeficient women. *Obstetrics and Gynecology Clinics of North America.* 14(2):537–58.

Thomas, Patricia. 1987, July 27. AIDS agenda slights women. *Medical World News:* 12–13.

Thompson, Larry. 1990, December 11. The alarming spread of AIDS among women. *Washington Post.*

Tilleraas, Perry. 1988. *The Color of Light: Daily Meditations for All of Us Living with AIDS.* Hazelton, Center City, Minn.

UNESCO and Coalition Against Trafficking in Women. 1992. *The Penn State Report.* Coalition Against Trafficking in Women. P.O. Box 10077, Calder Square, State College, PA 16805.

Veerakul, Suevit. 1992, April 3. Cyanide jab reports halt deporting of Burma girls. *The Nation*.

Verdegem, T. D., et al., 1988. Increased fatality from pneumocystis carinii pneumonia in women with AIDS. Fourth International Conference on AIDS, Stockholm, Sweden. Abstract:445.

Vermund, Sten H., and Karen F. Kelley. 1990. Human papillomavirus in women: methodologic issues and role of immunosuppression. *Reproductive and Perinatal Epidemiology*. Editor, Michele Kiely. CRC Press, Boca Raton.

Vermund, Sten H., Karen Hein, Helene D. Gayle, Joan M. Cary, Pauline A. Thomas, and Ernest Drucker. 1989, October. Acquired Immunodeficiency Syndrome among adolescents. *American Journal of Diseases of Children*. 143:1220–25.

Vermund, Sten H., Terry Alexander-Rodriquez, Sheila MacLeod, and Karen F. Kelley. 1990. History of sexual abuse in incarcerated adolescents with gonorrhea or syphilis. *Journal of Adolescent Health Care*. 11:449–52.

Vermund, Sten H., and Daniel F. Hoth. December 1990. How can epidemiology assist in guiding interventions for the Acquired Immunodeficiency Syndrome/Human Immunodeficiency Virus? *Epidemiology and HIV/AIDS:* 141–55.

Walker, Lenore E., 1989. *Terrifying Love: Why Battered Women Kill and How Society Responds*. Harper & Row, New York.

Wallace, Joyce, and Felice S. Coral, Ilonna J. Rimm, Heather Lane, Herbert Levine, Ellis L. Reinherz, Stuart F. Schlossman, and Joseph Sonnabend. 1982, April 17. T-cell ratios in homosexuals. *The Lancet:* 908.

Wallace, Joyce, Joanne Downes, Albert Ott, Rebecca Reise, James Monroe, Denise Jordan, Yolene Thomas, Eva Glickman, Linda Rogozinski, and Leonard Chess. 1983, January 1/8. T-cell ratios in New York City prostitutes. *The Lancet:* Appendix B.

Wallace, Joyce I. 1988. Human immunodeficiency virus infection in women. *The New York Medical Quarterly:* 140–43.

Wallace, Roderick. 1989. Minority AIDS and "planned shrinkage" in New York City. *MIRA: Multicultural Inquiry and Research on AIDS*. 3(1):1–2.

———. 1990b. Urban desertification, public health and public order: 'Planned shrinkage,' violent death, substance abuse and AIDS in the Bronx. *Social Science Medicine* 31 (7):801–13.

————, and Deborah Wallace. 1990, Sept.–Oct. Origins of public health collapse in New York City: the dynamics of planned shrinkage, contagious urban decay and social disintegration. *Bulletin of the New York Academy of Medicine.* 66(5):391–34.

Waring, Marilyn. 1988. *If Women Counted: A New Feminist Economics.* Harper & Row, New York.

Weissman, Gloria. 1991, March 27. Breaking the barriers to effective drug treatment for women: challenges for the 90s. Speech delivered at the conference "Breaking the Barriers: Women Finding Solutions to the Problems of Addiction," at the Josette Mondanaro Women's Resource Center/Prototypes, Los Angeles, California.

Wicker, Tom. 1991, August 8. The Peru syndrome. *The New York Times.*

Williams, Monte. 1990, October 17. Mother-child controversy: fetal-rights opponents worry the movement will go too far. *Daily News.*

Wofsy, Constance B. 1987, April 17. Human immunodeficiency virus infection in women. *Journal of the American Medical Association.* 257(15):2074–76.

Working Group on HIV Testing of Pregnant Women and Newborns. 1990, November 14. HIV infection, pregnant women, and newborns: a policy proposal for information and testing. *Journal of the American Medical Association.* 264(18):2416–20.

Worth, Dooley. 1990. Women at high risk of HIV infection: behavioral, prevention, and intervention aspects. In *Behavioral Aspects of AIDS and Other Sexually Transmitted Diseases.* David Ostrow, ed. Plenum Press, New York.

————. 1990. "Minority Women and AIDS: Culture, Race and Gender." In *Cultural Aspects of AIDS.* Douglas Feldman, ed. Praeger, New York.

Zierler, Sally, Deborah Laufer, Lisa Feingold, Ira Kantrowitz-Gordon, Charles Carpenter, and Kenneth Mayer. 1990, July. Heterosexual behavior and HIV infection: the New England Behavioral Health Study. *Rhode Island Medical Journal:* 285–92.

Zierler, Sally, Lisa Feingold, Deborah Laufer, Priscilla Velentgas, Ira Kantrowitz-Gordon, and Kenneth Mayer. 1991, April. Adult survivors of childhood sexual abuse and subsequent risk of HIV infection. *American Journal of Public Health* 88(4):1–4.

INDEX